REVIEW QUESTIONS IN

Ophthalmology

A Question and Answer Book

Second Edition

REVIEW QUESTIONS IN

Ophthalmology

A Question and Answer Book

Second Edition

Kenneth C. Chern, MD
Ophthalmic Consultants of Boston
Tufts/New England Medical Center
Boston, Massachusetts

Kenneth W. Wright, MD
Director of Pediatric Ophthalmology
Cedars-Sinai Medical Center
Clinical Professor of Ophthalmology
Keck School of Medicine
University of Southern California
Los Angeles, California

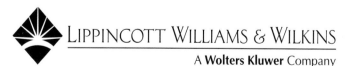
LIPPINCOTT WILLIAMS & WILKINS
A **Wolters Kluwer** Company

Philadelphia · Baltimore · New York · London
Buenos Aires · Hong Kong · Sydney · Tokyo

Acquisition Editor: Jonathan Pine
Development Editor: Jenny Kim
Marketing Manager: Scott Lavine
Production Services: Maryland Composition, Inc.
Project Manager: Fran Gunning
Compositor: Maryland Composition, Inc.
Printer: Quebecor World Bogotá S.A.

Library of Congress Cataloging-in-Publication Data

Review questions in ophthalmology : a question and answer book / editors,
  Kenneth C. Chern, Kenneth W. Wright—2nd ed.
    p. ; cm.
  Includes bibliographical references and index.
  ISBN-13: 0-7817-5203-5
  ISBN-10: 978-0-7817-5203-09
  1. Ophthalmology—Examinations, questions, etc. 2. Ophthalmology—Miscellanea.
  I. Chern, Kenneth C. II. Wright, Kenneth W. (Kenneth Weston), 1950–
  [DNLM: 1. Eye Diseases—Examination Questions. WW 18.2 R453 2004]
  RE49.R48 2004
  617.790076—dc22
                                2004015187

07 08 09
4 5 6 7 8 9 10

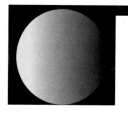

Preface

Ophthalmology is a vast and expanding specialty. Day by day, more is being discovered and elucidated. There is such an overwhelming body of knowledge that it is difficult to discern what is critical to know. We assembled this book as a means of self-assessment of learned material. By answering questions, you apply and assimilate a wide variety of information. This may help to identify areas of weakness and need for further study. We hope that you find this format useful and educational. We have tried to shy away from the esoteric and trivial, and to emphasize the diseases that are important to recognize and commonly encountered. This is not meant to be a definitive text, but a supplement to the textbooks and journals as part of a structured study program. As a result, the explanations have been kept brief and concise.

We have endeavored to include in each section a series of clinical case presentations. These describe actual patients and scenarios that you might see in your clinic. We hope that they stimulate your thought processes and expand the differential that you might consider.

We are aware of and respect the position of the American Board of Ophthalmology (ABO) in continuing to ensure the qualification and certification of ophthalmologists and the role that the written and the oral examinations play in this regard. Every effort has been made to ensure that no material from the written or the oral examinations has been duplicated in this book. It is inevitable that some of the same topics in this book may also be covered on the Ophthalmology Knowledge Assessment Program examination administered by the ABO, but this is merely because these subjects are of sufficient relevance to warrant their inclusion in any comprehensive ophthalmology text.

We hope that the many hours expended in assembling this book will provide you with an equally great basis for enriching and expanding your knowledge of ophthalmology.

Kenneth C. Chern
Kenneth W. Wright

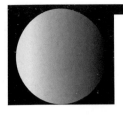

Acknowledgment

Any book such as this encompasses the work and effort of many people, and to each of them we are extremely thankful. In particular, we would like to acknowledge the assistance of the photographers of the Cleveland Clinic Foundation Department of Ophthalmology, Tami Fecko, Michael Kelly, Deborah Ross, and Pam Vargo, who have taken the majority of the clinical photographs displayed in this book.

This book would not be possible without the time and contributions of the many authors. In this second edition, we would like to acknowledge the ophthalmologists who were instrumental in making the first edition possible.

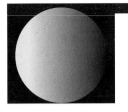

Dedication

To the residents and fellows which we have trained over the years. May the knowledge and skills you acquire serve you well in helping the thousands of patients who you will treat and aid.

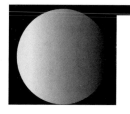

Section Contributors

Kenneth C. Chern, MD
Department of Ophthalmology
Tufts/New England Medical Center
Boston, Massachusetts;
Ophthalmic Consultants of Boston
Beverly, Massachusetts

Monica Evans, MD
Ocular Pathology Fellow
University of Southern California;
Ophthalmologist
Doheny Eye Institute
Los Angeles, California

Laura Fine, MD
Ophthalmic Consultants of Boston
Boston, Massachusetts

Nicoletta Fynn-Thompson, M.D.
Fellow, Cornea and Anterior Segment
Department of Ophthalmology
New England Eye Center, Tufts University
Boston, Massachusetts

Supriya Goyal, MD
Fellow, Glaucoma
Department of Ophthalmology
New England Eye Center, Tufts University
Boston, Massachusetts

Wendy Lee, MD
Assistant Professor
Department of Ophthalmology
Bascom Palmer Eye Institute
University of Miami School of Medicine
Miami, Florida

Jason Rothman, MD
Fellow, Cornea and Anterior Segment
Department of Ophthalmology
New England Eye Center, Tufts University
Boston, Massachusetts

Kenneth W. Wright, MD
Director, Wright Foundation for Pediatric
    Ophthalmology
Clinical Professor of Ophthalmology
Keck School of Medicine
University of Southern California;
Director, Pediatric Ophthalmology
Cedars-Sinai Medical Center
Los Angeles, California

Contents

1

Fundamentals

QUESTIONS

1. In a Gaussian distribution, what percentage of data is encompassed within two standard deviations of the mean?

   A) 50%
   B) 68.3%
   C) 95.5%
   D) 99.7%

2. A diurnal curve of IOP taken in a patient revealed the following measurements:16, 17, 18, 18, 19, 20, 21, 23. What is the mean/mode/median IOP?

	Mean	Mode	Median
A)	18.5,	18.5,	18.5
B)	18.0,	18.5,	19.0
C)	19.0,	18.0,	18.5
D)	19.0,	18.5,	18.0

3. Life table analysis of a particular disease comparing treatment A to treatment B is graphed in Figure 1-1. Which of the following conclusions is valid?

   A) Treatment A will continue to be better than treatment B.
   B) The 4-year outcome of the two treatments is comparable.
   C) Treatment B results in an initial greater loss of visual acuity but with stabilization at this level.
   D) The natural course of the disease is loss of vision.

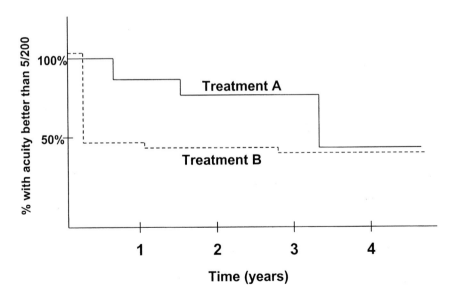

FIGURE 1-1.

Questions 4–5

You are testing the vision of a patient with a blind eye. Five out of 15 times he says he sees the light when the light is actually off. Two out of 10 times he says the light is off when it is actually on.

4. What is the number of true-positive responses for this patient?

    A) 2
    B) 10
    C) 8
    D) 5

5. What are the sensitivity and specificity of this test?

    A) 80%, 66.7%
    B) 61.5%, 20%
    C) 83.3%, 56%
    D) 33.3%, 20%

6. The null hypothesis for the Diabetic Retinopathy Study is that no difference exists between photocoagulation and no photocoagulation for proliferative diabetic retinopathy. In fact, there is a significant difference. If we accept the null hypothesis and conclude that photocoagulation does not make a difference in PDR, this is an example of:

    A) type I error
    B) type II error
    C) sampling error
    D) power

7. To properly analyze data to ensure that the conclusions are NOT a result of confounding variables, which test would be the most appropriate?

    A) ANOVA test
    B) Student's t-test
    C) Chi-square test
    D) Multivariate analysis

8. A prospective study is designed so that neither the patient nor the physician knows whether the patient is receiving treatment or placebo. What type of study is this?

    A) Longitudinal study
    B) Single masked study
    C) Case-controlled study
    D) Double-blind study

9. A study was performed that examined whether patients with ARMD and CNVM had evidence of prior laser photocoagulation. Records of all patients with the diagnosis of ARMD and CNVM over the past 5 years were compiled. What type of study is this?

    A) Prospective study
    B) Retrospective study
    C) Longitudinal study
    D) Cohort study

10. The p value of a study is calculated to be $p<0.03$. What does this indicate?

    A) The incidence of the disease is 3%.
    B) The likelihood of results occurring as a matter of chance is 3%.
    C) There is a 3% confidence interval.
    D) Three percent of the data was biased.

11. At a conference, a speaker reports that the visual acuity of five of five patients using a new eye drop improved from 20/50 to 20/20. These results may be due to all of the following study weaknesses EXCEPT:

    A) selection bias
    B) no control group
    C) lack of significance
    D) unblinded researchers

12. All of the following options are ways to increase the amount of drug absorption from an eye drop EXCEPT:

    A) prior administration of a topical anesthetic
    B) nasolacrimal duct occlusion
    C) eye closure after drop administration
    D) increased hydrophilicity of the drug

13. All of the following drugs would have a higher uptake in the eye as an ointment rather than as a topical drop EXCEPT:

    A) tetracycline
    B) chloramphenicol
    C) fluorometholone
    D) penicillin

14. Mitomycin C has been used in all of the following situations EXCEPT:

    A) proliferative vitreoretinopathy after vitrectomy
    B) conjunctival fibrosis following trabeculectomy
    C) pterygium recurrence
    D) stromal haze formation after PRK

15. All of the following effects are seen when a direct-acting cholinergic agonist is used EXCEPT:

    A) miosis
    B) increase in zonular tension
    C) increased outflow facility
    D) traction on peripheral retina

16. A patient's medication list includes drug X. He is going to undergo a combined trabeculectomy and cataract extraction under general anesthesia. The anesthesiologist is hesitant to use succinylcholine. What could drug X be?

    A) Levobunolol
    B) Pilocarpine
    C) Echothiophate iodide (Phospholine Iodide)
    D) Dorzolamide (Trusopt)

17. Which series is in correct order of decreasing mydriatic duration?

    A) Homatropine, scopolamine, cyclopentolate, tropicamide
    B) Atropine, homatropine, tropicamide, cyclopentolate
    C) Tropicamide, homatropine, cyclopentolate, scopolamine
    D) Atropine, scopolamine, homatropine, tropicamide

18. The production of which inflammatory mediator is NOT affected by the use of NSAIDs like diclofenac and ketorolac?

    A) leukotriene
    B) thromboxane
    C) prostaglandin
    D) prostacyclin

19. The mechanism of action of topical cyclosporine (Restasis) is via:

    A) prevention of the degranulation of mast cells
    B) suppression of T cells
    C) inhibition of vascular endothelial growth factor
    D) disruption of the bacterial cell wall

20. All of the following side effects may be seen when using apraclonidine EXCEPT:

    A) dry mouth
    B) lid drooping
    C) conjunctival blanching
    D) lethargy

21. Which of the following agents may be implicated in causing black deposits in the conjunctiva?

    A) Pilocarpine
    B) Epinephrine
    C) Dipivefrin (Propine)
    D) Echothiophate

22. All of the following side effects may be seen with the use of a prostaglandin analogue EXCEPT:

    A) anterior uveitis
    B) cystoid macular edema
    C) necrotizing scleritis
    D) eyelash growth

23. Which of the following topical beta-blockers would be best suited for someone with mild bronchoconstrictive disease?

    A) Timolol
    B) Betaxolol
    C) Metipranolol
    D) Levobunolol

24. All of the following effects may be associated with the use of dorzolamide EXCEPT:

    A) metallic taste
    B) tingling in the hands and feet
    C) skin rash
    D) optic neuritis

25. In a susceptible patient, which of the following topical agents would increase IOP the most?

    A) Dexamethasone
    B) Fluorometholone
    C) Prednisolone
    D) Loteprednol etabonate (Lotemax)

26. What percentage of patients on medium to high dosages of topical dexamethasone for 6 weeks develops elevated IOP?

    A) 20%
    B) 42%
    C) 66%
    D) 83%

27. Ciprofloxacin has good antibacterial properties against all of the following organisms EXCEPT:

    A) Haemophilus
    B) Pseudomonas
    C) Staphylococcus
    D) Streptococcus

28. What percentage of patients that have sensitivity to penicillin will have cross-reactivity to cephalosporins?

    A) 10%
    B) 20%
    C) 30%
    D) 40%

29. Allergy to which one of the following medications is a relative contraindication to the use of a carbonic anhydrase inhibitor?

A) Sulfonamides
B) Penicillin
C) Iodine dye
D) Codeine

30. A patient allergic to latanoprost (Xalatan) would be least likely to have a cross-allergy to

A) isopropyl unoprostone (Rescula)
B) travoprost (Travatan)
C) bimatoprost (Lumigan)
D) brimonidine tartrate (Alphagan)

31. Which drug and side effect are mismatched?

A) Ciprofloxacin—epithelial plaques
B) Pilocarpine—brow ache
C) Ketorolac tromethamine (Acular)—stinging sensation
D) Methazolamide—fever

32. Natamycin may be effective in the treatment of all of the following infectious agents EXCEPT:

A) Aspergillus
B) Candida albicans
C) Fusarium
D) Mucor

33. Agents reported to be effective in the treatment of Acanthamoeba include all of the following EXCEPT:

A) neomycin
B) polyhexamethylene biguanide
C) propamidine
D) trifluridine

34. Which of the following characteristics is undesirable in the design of a viscoelastic?

A) Isosmotic
B) Hydrophilic
C) Inert
D) Clear

35. What is the anesthetic duration of topical proparacaine?

A) 5 minutes
B) 10 minutes
C) 15 minutes
D) 20 minutes

36. Which drug and mechanism of action is paired correctly?

    A) Cromolyn sodium (Crolom)—NSAID
    B) Levocabastine (Livostin)—prostaglandin inhibitor
    C) Lodoxamide tromethamine (Alomide)—mast cell stabilizer
    D) Diclofenac sodium (Voltaren)—antihistamine

37. Which statement concerning the cornea is FALSE?

    A) Oxygen for the nourishment of epithelial cells is provided by the tear film.
    B) Endothelial cells actively pump water into the aqueous to deturgesce the cornea.
    C) Descemet's membrane consists of two layers: a fetal banded layer and an adult unbanded layer.
    D) Bowman's membrane is a true basement membrane secreted by the basal epithelial cells.

38. Which component of the tear film is the thickest?

    A) Marginal strip
    B) Lipid layer
    C) Aqueous layer
    D) Glycoprotein layer

39. Which one of the following is the main reflex tear secretor?

    A) Gland of Wolfring
    B) Gland of Krause
    C) Lacrimal gland
    D) Meibomian gland

40. What are the main contributors to the innervation of the cornea?

    A) Short anterior ciliary nerves
    B) Long anterior ciliary nerves
    C) Short posterior ciliary nerves
    D) Long posterior ciliary nerves

41. Which one of the following associations is FALSE?

    A) Stromal wound healing—type I collagen
    B) Descemet's membrane—type IV collagen
    C) Vitreous—type II collagen
    D) Lens capsule—type IV collagen

42. Which one of the following most closely approximates normal aqueous humor production?

    A) 2 μl/min
    B) 4 μl/min
    C) 6 μl/min
    D) 8 μl/min

43. Which of the following electrolytes are found in the aqueous humor at half the level of the plasma?

    A) Na^+, K^+
    B) Ca^{2+}, PO_4^{2-}
    C) Cl^-, HCO_3^-
    D) Cu^{2+}, Zn^{2+}

44. All of the following substances found in the anterior chamber are indicative of a disruption of the blood–aqueous barrier EXCEPT:

    A) pigment
    B) fibrin
    C) white blood cells
    D) protein

45. The accumulation in the lens of which one of the following leads to brunescent cataracts?

    A) High molecular weight crystallin
    B) Alpha crystallin
    C) Gamma crystallin
    D) Water-insoluble protein

46. Which one of the following is NOT a protective mechanism against oxidation in the lens?

    A) Glutathione peroxidase
    B) Vitamin A
    C) Superoxide dismutase
    D) Catalase

47. Which one of the following is NOT associated with a decrease in hyaluronate concentration in the vitreous?

    A) Vitreous hemorrhage
    B) Hyperopia
    C) Diabetes
    D) Aphakia

48. How long does it take for a photoreceptor to renew its outer segment?

    A) 1 hour
    B) 1 day
    C) 10 days
    D) 100 days

49. Which one of the following characteristics of the retinal pigment epithelium is NOT correct?

    A) Active Na^+-K^+ pump on the basal surface to maintain the ion gradient in the interphotoreceptor matrix
    B) Contributes to blood–retinal barrier
    C) Contributes to adhesion of sensory retina
    D) Involved in isomerization of vitamin A

50. What is the difference in light sensitivity of the rods compared with the cones?

    A) Equal in sensitivity
    B) 10 times more sensitive
    C) 1000 times more sensitive
    D) 10,000 times more sensitive

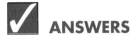 **ANSWERS**

1. C)   95.5%

    A Gaussian distribution describes a normal curve. When plotted on a graph, it assumes the shape of a bell curve. The mean lies at the center of the distribution. The mean ± one S.D. will encompass 68.3% of all items, ±2 S.D. = 95.5%, and ± 3 S.D. = 99.7% (Fig. 1-2).

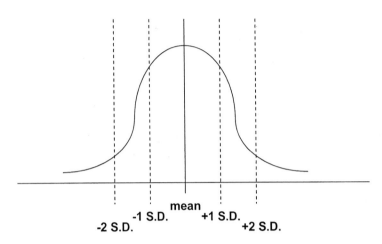

FIGURE 1-2.

2. C)   19.0, 18.0, 18.5

    To calculate the *mean,* or average, the sum of the data values is divided by the total number of values, i.e., 152/8 = 19. The *mode* is the value that occurs most frequently within the data, i.e., 18. If more than one number appears most frequently, the data can be termed *bimodal, trimodal,* and so on. The *median* is the middlemost number when the values are arranged from low to high. In this case, there are eight values; the median is the average of the fourth and fifth data points, i.e., (18 + 19)/2 = 18.5.

3. B)   The 4-year outcome of the two treatments is comparable.

    Life table analysis plots the percentage of patients reaching a particular endpoint (in this case, maintaining visual acuity of 5/200 or better) against time. As time progresses to the right, more and more patients have visual acuity less than 5/200 and thus drop out of the analysis. At a particular point in time, the two treatments can be compared by looking at the difference in position of the lines. The outcome of both treatments is approximately the same at 4 years. The data cannot be extrapolated for long-term results. The natural course of the disease is not evaluated in this study because both arms received treatment.

4. C) 8

The chart below divides the patient's responses according to whether the light is on or off and whether the patient "sees" the light or not.

		Light	
		ON	OFF
Patient's response	ON	8 (TP)	5 (FP)
	OFF	2 (FN)	10 (TN)

TP=true-positive, FP=false-positive, FN=false-negative, TN=true-negative

The number of true-positive responses is the number of times he saw the light when it was actually on. This occurred eight times.

5. A) 80%, 66.7%

The sensitivity and specificity are indices of the reliability of the patient for a particular test. Higher sensitivity and specificity rates indicate a very reliable patient. They are calculated as follows:

Sensitivity = TP/(TP + FN) = 8/(8 + 2) = 80%
Specificity = TN/(TN + FP) = 5/(5 + 10) = 66.7%
Positive predictive value = TP/(TP + FP)
Negative predictive value = TN/(TN + FN)

6. B) type II error

Errors may be made regarding the null hypothesis (H_o), which states that no difference exists between the control group and the intervention group. If one rejects the null hypothesis when in fact the results occurred by chance, this is called a *type I error* or *alpha error*. If one accepts the null hypothesis when in fact there really was a difference, this is called a *type II error* or *beta error*. The power of the study is −beta, or the ability of the study to detect a difference when a difference is present. Sampling error is bias of the data secondary to the use of a nonrepresentative population.

7. D) Multivariate analysis

When many factors can affect an outcome variable, all of them must be examined. Therefore, one may use many types of multivariate analyses such as a multiple regression analysis, logistic regression, or Cox hazard function. An ANOVA (analysis of variance) determines whether the means of the normal distributions are identical. A student's t-test determines whether the means of two normal populations are far enough apart to conclude that the distributions are different. A Chi-square test determines whether more than two sampled populations can be considered equal.

8. D) Double-blind study

9. B) Retrospective study

Two types of studies exist: retrospective (observational) and prospective (experimental). Within the *retrospective*, or *case-control* variety, either a case report or a case series may be employed. In a retrospective study, patients are taken at a single point in time and examined for a variable that occurred antecedent to the date of examination. In a *prospective, longitudinal,* or *cohort study,* patients are enrolled and then followed for the development of an outcome variable. Prospective studies in which neither the investigator nor the patient knows whether the patient is receiving intervention or placebo is the best type of study to eliminate bias. This is referred to as a *double-blind, placebo-controlled trial.*

10.   B)   The likelihood of results occurring as a matter of chance is 3%.

The *p* value, also called the *significance level,* is a measure of the probability that the results occurred by chance alone. For example, $p < 0.03$ means that if an experiment were done 100 times, you would get the same result 97 times and you would get a different result 3 times because of chance.

11.   C)   lack of significance

With small case series and studies, the results must be evaluated carefully because errors can be introduced due to the small number of cases involved. Selection bias means setting criteria that eliminate cases that do not conform to the desired results. A control group helps determine whether results are due to random chance or selection bias. Researchers should be blinded as to which eye received the eye drop to avoid giving extra encouragement when testing the eye that received the drop. If all five patients improved, this could be viewed as a significant result. *p* values can be calculated, but they are not as meaningful when the number of cases is small.

12.   D)   increased hydrophilicity of the drug

Ways to increase absorption include decreasing the nasolacrimal pumping, decreasing the washout by another drop by increasing the interval between administrations of drops, and increasing the lipid solubility to facilitate corneal penetration. A topical anesthetic disrupts epithelial integrity, allowing greater drug absorption.

13.   D)   penicillin

Drugs administered in ointment form require high lipid solubility and some water solubility. Higher aqueous humor levels are achieved with all of the listed medications except penicillin. Penicillin penetrates the blood–ocular barrier poorly and also is actively transported out of the eye.

14.   A)   proliferative vitreoretinopathy after vitrectomy

Mitomycin C is a potent antifibrotic and chemotherapeutic agent. In small doses, it is toxic to the corneal endothelium and other intraocular structures. Mitomycin C has only been used on the external ocular surface.

15.   B)   increase in zonular tension

Direct-acting cholinergics (acetylcholine, carbachol, pilocarpine) excite the postsynaptic receptor. This causes contraction of the iris sphincter; contraction of the circular fibers of the ciliary muscle causing relaxation of the zonular tension; contraction of the longitudinal fibers of the ciliary muscles, which pull on the scleral spur and open the meshwork, and contraction of the ciliary muscles, which may cause a retinal tear.

16. C) echothiophate iodide (Phospholine Iodide)

All of the listed agents are antiglaucoma medications. Succinylcholine is a depolarizing agent used in induction of anesthesia. Any medication that would retard cholinesterase activity would prolong respiratory paralysis and become hazardous. Echothiophate iodide is an irreversible cholinesterase inhibitor whose effects may persist for days after discontinuation of the drug. Levobunolol is a non-selective beta-blocker; pilocarpine functions as a direct-acting cholinergic; and dorzolamide is a carbonic anhydrase inhibitor.

17. D) Atropine, scopolamine, homatropine, tropicamide

Mydriatic recovery in normal eyes is as follows: atropine (7–10 days), scopolamine (3–7 days), homatropine (1–3 days), cyclopentolate (1 day), and tropicamide (6 hours).

18. A) leukotriene receptor inhibitor

Phospholipids are metabolized into a number of pro-inflammatory mediators as indicated in Figure 1-3. Corticosteroids block the metabolic pathway at the highest level, preventing the formation of all of the mediators. NSAIDs block the cyclo-oxygenase pathway, eliminating production of prostaglandins, prostacyclin, and thromboxane. The lipoxygenase pathway is still functional and results in the formation of leukotrienes.

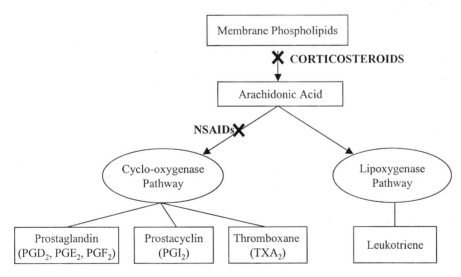

FIGURE 1-3

19.   B)   suppression of T cells

Cyclosporine is a potent immunosuppressive agent that acts by suppressing T cells. This is helpful in many ocular surface conditions from atopic keratoconjunctivitis to dry eyes to graft rejection.

20.   B)   lid drooping

Side effects of apraclonidine (an α_2-adrenergic agonist) include conjunctival blanching, lid retraction, dry mouth, lethargy, and local allergy. Cardiovascular or respiratory effects are extremely rare.

21.   B)   Epinephrine

Oxidative products of epinephrine can produce black deposits on the conjunctiva known as *adrenochrome* deposits. Although they may be mistaken for foreign bodies or melanoma, they are harmless. Dipivefrin is a conjugated epinephrine compound broken down by corneal esterases to active forms. Adrenochrome deposits are infrequently formed with this preparation.

22.   C)   necrotizing scleritis

The prostaglandin analogues have pro-inflammatory properties in susceptible patients. Conjunctival hyperemia is commonly seen; however, more severe inflammation such as necrotizing scleritis is not a result of the prostaglandin and a systemic etiology should be considered. Eyelash growth is seen to varying degrees with the prostaglandin analogues.

23.   B)   Betaxolol

All of the agents listed are β-adrenergic receptor antagonists. However, betaxolol is B_1-selective, making it a better choice in patients with pulmonary disorders. All of the other listed agents are β_1 β_2-nonselective. All of these drugs are contraindicated in patients with severe asthma or COPD.

24.   D)   optic neuritis

Side effects associated with dorzolamide include many of the same systemic side effects as acetazolamide, such as numbness in the hands, feet, or lips; a metallic taste of carbonated beverages; malaise; anorexia; weight loss; nausea; somnolence, and depression. Additionally, a local skin allergy may be noted. The incidence of side effects with topical therapy is less than that with systemic administration.

25.   A)   Dexamethasone

The IOP-elevating potential, in decreasing order, is dexamethasone > prednisolone > loteprednol etabonate > fluorometholone > hydrocortisone > tetrahydrotriamcinolone.

26.   B)   42%

Steroid-induced elevation of IOP can occur with topical, systemic, or periocular administration. After 6 weeks of therapy, 42% of patients develop pressures above 20 mmHg, and 6% develop pressures greater than 31 mmHg.

27. D)   Streptococcus

Ciprofloxacin has broad gram-positive and gram-negative bacterial activity by interfering with DNA gyrase; however, recent reports have described the growing resistance of streptococci to ciprofloxacin.

28. A)   10%

Allergic reactions include local allergy, rash, itching, hives, bronchoconstrictive disease, and anaphylactic reactions that can be fatal. A strong history of serious allergy to penicillins is a contraindication to cephalosporin administration. Approximately 10% of patients with penicillin allergy will cross-react, making the use of cephalosporins dangerous in some cases.

29. A)   Sulfonamides

Carbonic anhydrase inhibitors are similar to sulfonamides in chemical structure, and allergic cross-reactions may occur.

30. D)   brimonidine tartrate (Alphagan)

Isopropyl unoprostone, travoprost, and bimatoprost are all prostaglandin analogues like latanoprost. There is increased cross-sensitivity between these drugs. Brimonidine is in a different class, and an allergy to latanoprost would not be indicative of an allergy to brimonidine.

31. D)   Methazolamide—fever

All of the drugs and side effects are paired correctly except for methazolamide and fever. The side effects of the carbonic anhydrase inhibitors principally include tingling of the fingers and toes, lethargy, anorexia, depression, and weight loss. Fever, tachycardia, delirium, and dry mouth are signs of anticholinergic toxicity from drugs such as atropine.

32. D)   Mucor

Natamycin is available as a 5% topical ophthalmic solution. It is active against filamentous fungi including *Aspergillus, Cephalosporium, Curvularia, Fusarium, Penicillium,* and *Candida albicans.* Mucor is better treated with amphotericin B.

33. D)   trifluridine

Acanthamoeba is a parasite that inhabits soil, water, and air. It can be associated with homemade contact lens solutions, improperly disinfected swimming pools, and trauma. No single drug is effective in treatment. Agents that have been used include neomycin, natamycin, miconazole, propamidine, dibromopropamidine, polyhexamethylene biguanide, and chlorhexidine. Trifluridine is a nucleoside analog used for viral infections.

34. B)   Hydrophilic

Viscoelastics resist flow and deformation. They facilitate tissue manipulation and maintain intraocular space. For use within the eye, they must be inert, isosmotic, sterile, nonpyogenic, nonantigenic, and optically clear. Many viscoelastics today are preparations of methylcellulose or sodium hyaluronate.

35.   D)   20 minutes

Proparacaine is a topical ester anesthetic. Its duration of action is about 20 minutes. In injectable form, lidocaine lasts 1 to 2 hours, mepivacaine lasts 2 to 3 hours, and bupivacaine (Marcaine) lasts up to 8 hours.

36.   C)   Lodoxamide tromethamine (Alomide)—mast cell stabilizer

The correct pair is lodoxamide and mast cell stabilizer. Cromolyn is also a mast cell stabilizer. Levocabastine is the anti-histamine agent. Diclofenac is an NSAID (along with ketorolac and ibuprofen). Prostaglandin inhibitors for lowering IOP have recently been released.

37.   D)   Bowman's membrane is a true basement membrane secreted by the basal epithelial cells.

Bowman's membrane is NOT actually a basement membrane; it is an organized, compressed collection of collagen fibers of the anterior stroma. It is not secreted by the epithelium nor does it have the typical cell–basement membrane attachments. The oxygen for the cornea is derived from diffusion from the tear film or the aqueous humor. The aqueous provides oxygen for the endothelium while the epithelium is nourished by the tear film. The clarity and dehydration of the cornea is maintained by active water pumping by the endothelium and by evaporation of the tear film. The epithelium and lipid layer of the tear film provide barriers to loss of corneal water. Descemet's membrane is constantly laid down by the endothelial cells. A fetal layer can be distinguished from the material added after birth by its striated pattern.

38.   C)   Aqueous layer

The tear film consists of an anterior lipid layer, a middle aqueous phase, and a posterior mucin layer (Fig. 1-4). The tear film is 7 µl thick, and the aqueous phase is the thickest. The lipid layer is secreted by the meibomian glands and the glands of Zeis. The aqueous layer is produced by the glands of Krause and Wolfring. The mucin layer is secreted by the goblet cells.

39.   C)   Lacrimal gland

The accessory lacrimal glands are the basic secretors. These include the glands of Krause and Wolfring. The reflex secretor is the main lacrimal gland. Stimulation of the first branch of the trigeminal nerve can induce tearing through a reflex arc. Meibomian glands secrete oily fluid for the lipid layer.

40.   D)   Long posterior ciliary nerves

Innervation to the cornea is via the first branch of the trigeminal nerve. Approximately 70 to 80 branches of the long posterior ciliary nerves enter the cornea peripherally after losing their myelin sheath 1 to 2 mm before the limbus.

41.   A)   Stromal wound healing—type I collagen

Although type I collagen exists in the stroma, it is associated with normal stroma. Type III collagen is associated with stromal wound healing. Type IV collagen is

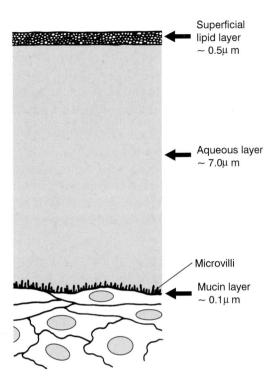

Superficial
lipid layer
~ 0.5μ m

Aqueous layer
~ 7.0μ m

Microvilli

Mucin layer
~ 0.1μ m

FIGURE 1-4. From Wright K. Textbook of ophthalmology. Baltimore: Williams & Wilkins, 1997.

secreted by the endothelial cells in burst fashion, accounting for thickening of Descemet's membrane. The lens capsule is noncellular and associated with type IV glycoprotein-associated collagen. The origin of vitreous collagen has not been fully established, but it is thought to arise from type II collagen.

42. A)   2 μl/min

Aqueous humor enters the posterior chamber through diffusion, ultrafiltration, and active secretion by the nonpigmented epithelium of the ciliary body. The rate of formation in people is 2 μl/min.

43. B) Ca^{2+}, PO_4^{2-}

Only calcium and phosphorus are in concentrations of about one-half that in plasma. Sodium, potassium, magnesium, iron, zinc, and copper all approximate levels found in plasma. Chloride and bicarbonate vary from 20% to 30% above or below plasma levels.

44. A)   Pigment

The blood–aqueous barrier maintains the aqueous as a cell-free, protein-free ultrafiltrate. Red and white blood cells and fibrin are not normally present in the aqueous. Protein may be visible as flare within the aqueous humor. Pigment can be released from the posterior iris in a condition such as pigment dispersion syndrome and does not necessarily indicate disruption of the blood–aqueous barrier.

45.   D)   Water-insoluble protein

Lens proteins can be divided into two sets: the water-soluble proteins and the water-insoluble proteins. The water-soluble proteins are comprised largely of the crystallins. The HM-crystallin is made of both alpha and beta constituents. With accumulation of the water-insoluble fraction, a marked browning of the lens nucleus may occur. The amount of accumulation correlates with the degree of opacification.

46.   B)   Vitamin A

Free radicals are highly reactive species that can lead to damage of lens fibers and subsequent opacification. In addition to superoxide dismutase, glutathione, and catalase, vitamins C and E may be protective against oxidative damage. Vitamin A is essential in the retina and is involved in photoreceptor light transduction.

47.   B)   Hyperopia

Various biochemical changes occur in the vitreous with age and disease. Among the causes of decreased concentration of hyaluronate are syneresis, myopia, aphakia, diabetes mellitus, and injury with hemorrhage, inflammation, or surgery.

48.   C)   10 days

One of the most important functions of the RPE is phagocytosis of the outer segments of the photoreceptor. Each photoreceptor renews its outer segment every 10 days.

49.   A)   Active Na^+-K^+ pump on the basal surface to maintain the ion gradient in the interphotoreceptor matrix

The RPE serves many functions, including development of photoreceptors during embryogenesis; maintenance of the outer blood–retinal barrier; maintenance of the environment of the subretinal space; adhesion of the underlying sensory retina; selective transport of metabolites to and from the retina; uptake, transport, storage, metabolism, and isomerization of vitamin A; phagocytosis of photoreceptor outer segment tips; and stray light absorption by melanin granules. The ATP-dependent Na^+-K^+ pump can be found on the apical surface of the cell.

50.   C)   1000 times more sensitive

The rods are 100 to 1000 times more sensitive to light than the cones, allowing better vision in dim light. At this luminance level, the cones are not triggered; therefore, the world appears as shades of grey. Fine resolution of detail is hampered in this lighting condition because the rods are not concentrated in the fovea like the cones. The highest concentration of rods is actually 20° from the fovea.

Notes

Notes

2

Embryology and Anatomy

QUESTIONS

1. On which day do the optic pits appear on the developing embryo?

    A) Day 17
    B) Day 23
    C) Day 27
    D) Day 33

2. On which day does the embryonic fissure close?

    A) Day 17
    B) Day 23
    C) Day 27
    D) Day 33

3. Which one of the following does NOT result from a failure of the optic fissure to close?

    A) Optic nerve coloboma
    B) Lid coloboma
    C) Iris coloboma
    D) Choroidal coloboma

Questions 4–14   Match the structure with the embryonic tissue from which it is derived.

    A) Mesoderm
    B) Neural crest
    C) Neural ectoderm
    D) Surface ectoderm

4. Lens

5. Corneal endothelium

6. Extraocular muscles

7. Retinal pigment epithelium

8. Corneal epithelium

9. Lacrimal gland

10. Schlemm's canal

11. Choroid

12. Sphincter pupillae

13. Nonpigmented layer of ciliary body

14. Nasolacrimal system

Questions 15–17   Match the following embryonic vitreous structures to their adult counterparts.

A) Zonules
B) Hyaloid canal remnants
C) Vitreous body
D) None of the above

15. Primary vitreous

16. Secondary vitreous

17. Tertiary vitreous

18. The following are all remnants of the hyaloidal vascular system EXCEPT:

A) Mittendorf dot
B) corneal leukoma
C) persistent pupillary membrane
D) Bergmeister's papilla

19. Which is true about the vitreous?

A) Collagen is the major structural component.
B) Its strongest attachments are at the vitreous base, optic nerve, and retinal vessels.
C) Posterior vitreous detachment results from the collapse and contraction of collagen fibers, which occurs with age.
D) All of the above

20. Which one of the following statements about the myelination of the optic nerve is FALSE?

A) Myelination begins during the seventh month of gestation.
B) Myelination is completed after birth.
C) Myelination progresses posteriorly from the lamina cribrosa.
D) Myelination allows more rapid transmission of nerve impulses.

21. Which of the following is true of the optic canal?

A) It is between 8 and 10 mm in length.
B) It is located within the lesser wing of the sphenoid.
C) Sympathetic nerves pass through this canal.
D) All of the above

22. Which bone does NOT form part of the orbital floor?

    A) Maxillary
    B) Lacrimal
    C) Zygomatic
    D) Palatine

23. The medial wall of the orbit includes:

    A) the ethmoid bone, the anterior ethmoidal foramen, the infraorbital foramen
    B) the lacrimal bone, the superior orbital fissure, the zygomaticotemporal foramen
    C) the frontoethmoidal suture line, the posterior ethmoidal foramen, the posterior lacrimal crest
    D) the lacrimal bone, the anterior lacrimal crest, the supraorbital foramen

24. Which one of the following statements concerning the lateral orbital tubercle is TRUE?

    A) The tubercle is positioned at the junction of the frontal and maxillary bones.
    B) The tubercle lies entirely on the maxillary bone.
    C) The tubercle is the primary attachment site of the lateral canthal tendon, Whitnall's ligament, and Lockwood's ligament.
    D) Attachments between the lateral rectus and the tubercle serve as a check ligament of the lateral rectus.

Questions 25–29   Through which foramen does each structure pass?

    A) Superior orbital fissure
    B) Inferior orbital fissure
    C) Optic canal
    D) None of the above

25. Posterior ethmoidal artery

26. Trochlear nerve

27. Maxillary nerve

28. Ophthalmic artery

29. Superior orbital vein

30. All of the extraocular muscles receive blood supply from the ophthalmic artery EXCEPT:

    A) Lateral rectus
    B) Superior oblique
    C) Inferior oblique
    D) Medial rectus

31. All are true of the lacrimal pump and mechanism of lacrimal drainage EXCEPT:

    A) evaporation accounts for approximately 10% of tear elimination in the young
    B) the contraction of the orbicularis muscle provides positive pressure in the tear sac, pulling tears in the nose
    C) when the eyelids open, negative pressure is produced in the sac and maintained by the valve of Rosenmüller
    D) the majority of tears drain through the lower lid punctum rather than the upper lid punctum

32. Which one of the following statements describing the adult orbit is FALSE?

    A) The volume of the orbit is 30 ml.
    B) The maximum width is 1 cm behind the anterior orbital margin.
    C) The depth of the orbit averages 50 mm from the orbital entrance to the apex.
    D) The medial walls are parallel and border the nasal cavity, ethmoid air cells, and sphenoid sinus posteriorly.

33. Which one of the following is NOT a branch of the ophthalmic division of the trigeminal nerve?

    A) Supratrochlear nerve
    B) Lacrimal nerve
    C) Long ciliary nerve
    D) Zygomaticofacial nerve

34. Within which bony structures is the nasolacrimal sac located?

    A) Lacrimal, ethmoid
    B) Maxillary, ethmoid
    C) Nasal, lacrimal
    D) Lacrimal, maxillary

35. Which type of epithelium lines the nasolacrimal sac, duct, and canaliculi?

    A) Stratified squamous epithelium
    B) Pseudostratified columnar epithelium
    C) Cuboidal epithelium
    D) Stratified columnar epithelium with goblet cell overlay

36. Where in the nose does the nasolacrimal duct open?

    A) Above the inferior turbinate
    B) Through the valve of Rosenmüller
    C) Through an ostium partially covered by a mucosal fold (valve of Hasner)
    D) Into the superior meatus

37. The "gray line" of the eyelid is:

    A) the mucocutaneous junction of the eyelid margin
    B) the location of the meibomian gland orifices
    C) the muscle of Riolan
    D) posterior to the tarsus

38. A full-thickness stab incision located 11 mm superior to the eyelid margin over the pupil in the caucasian upper eyelid would be close to each of the following structures EXCEPT:

A) superior tarsal muscle
B) peripheral arterial arcade
C) glands of Moll
D) orbital fat

39. Which one of the following is NOT a true basement membrane?

A) Descemet's membrane
B) Bruch's membrane
C) Lens capsule
D) Bowman's membrane

40. Which structure divides the lacrimal gland into two lobes?

A) Orbicularis oculi
B) Tarsus
C) Whitnall's ligament
D) Levator aponeurosis

41. Which muscle originates from the annulus of Zinn?

A) Superior oblique
B) Levator palpebrae
C) Lateral rectus
D) Inferior oblique

42. Which muscle inserts the farthest posterior to the limbus?

A) Medial rectus
B) Superior rectus
C) Inferior rectus
D) Superior oblique

43. Which statement regarding lens structure is FALSE?

A) The Y suture represents the ends of the lens fibers.
B) The lens nuclei are concentrated near the equator.
C) The lens fibers in the nucleus continue to divide throughout life.
D) The anterior Y suture is oriented upright.

44. Which statement regarding Müller cells is FALSE?

A) They are modified glial cells that provide structural framework supporting neural elements in the retina.
B) Their nuclei lie in the outer nuclear layer.
C) Their basal processes extend out to form the inner surface of the retina (inner limiting membrane).
D) The apical or outer cell processes extend beyond the outer nuclear layer, where they are connected to the photoreceptors by a system of terminal bars that comprise the external limiting membrane.

45. Which statement about the retinal pigment epithelium (RPE) is FALSE?

A) The RPE interdigitates with the apical processes of the rod and cone segments.
B) RPEs are densely adherent to Bruch's membrane.
C) RPEs comprise the inner blood–retinal barrier.
D) RPE cells are taller and contain a greater concentration of pigment in the macula.

46. All of the following statements about the choriocapillaris are correct EXCEPT:

A) it communicates freely with the optic disc capillaries
B) it is arranged in a segmental pattern that varies with location
C) the endothelium has a pore size sufficient to allow larger molecules, including proteins, to escape into the extravascular space
D) it is a major source of nutrition for RPE and outer retinal segments

47. Which one of the following is found in the inner plexiform layer?

A) Axons of the ganglion cells
B) Axons of the amacrine cells
C) Synapses of the photoreceptors
D) Footplates of the Müller cells

48. How many degrees is the fovea displaced from the optic nerve?

A) 15°
B) 23°
C) 10°
D) 6°

49. What is the diameter of the retinal vein as it crosses the edge of the optic nerve head?

A) 80 μm
B) 120 μm
C) 160 μm
D) 200 μm

50. The uvea is attached at all of the following sites EXCEPT:

A) ora serrata
B) vortex veins
C) scleral spur
D) long posterior ciliary vessels

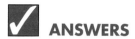 **ANSWERS**

1. B)   Day 23

2. D)   Day 33

The optic pits first appear on day 23 of gestation (Fig. 2-1). Evagination of the optic vesicle occurs on day 25 with induction of the lens on day 28. Closure of the optic fissure occurs on day 33 (Fig. 2-2). This closure allows pressurization of the globe.

   The optic fissure closes on approximately day 33 of gestation. It begins midway between the optic nerve and the iris and "zips up" in both anterior and posterior directions. The fissure is located inferiorly on the globe, and corresponding inferior iris (Fig. 2-3), choroidal, and optic nerve colobomas can be seen with failure of the fissure to close properly. Lid colobomas do not occur from failure of the fetal fissure to close (Table 2-1).

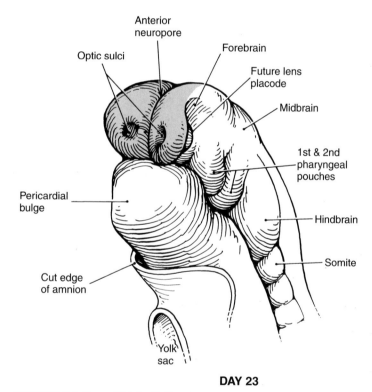

DAY 23

FIGURE 2-1. From Wright K. Textbook of ophthalmology. Baltimore: Williams & Wilkins, 1997.

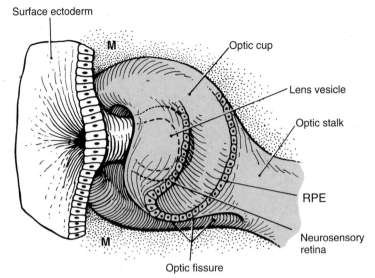

FIGURE 2-2. From Wright K. Textbook of ophthalmology. Baltimore: Williams & Wilkins, 1997.

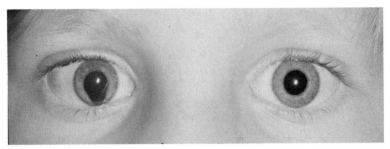

FIGURE 2-3

3. B) Lid coloboma

4. D) Surface ectoderm

5. B) Neural crest

6. A) Mesoderm

7. C) Neural ectoderm

8. D) Surface ectoderm

9. D) Surface ectoderm

10. A) Mesoderm

11. B) Neural crest

12. C) Neural ectoderm

13. C) Neural ectoderm

TABLE 2-1. Embryonic Derivation of Ocular Structures

Embryonic tissue	Structures
Mesoderm	Extraocular muscles Sclera (small area temporally) Vascular endothelium Schlemm's canal Blood
Neural crest	Corneal stroma and endothelium Trabecular meshwork Iris stroma Ciliary body stroma Ciliary muscles Sclera Orbital cartilage and bone Connective tisue of extraocular muscles
Neural ectoderm	Posterior iris epithelium Sphincter and dilator pupillae Ciliary epithelium Neural retina Retinal pigment epithelium Optic nerve
Surface ectoderm	Lacrimal gland Lids, lashes, and epidermal structures Conjunctival epithelium Corneal epithelium

[Handwritten margin notes: Mesoderm / Muscles / Schlemm's Canal ... Surface]

14. **D)** Surface ectoderm

At the 6-week stage, an ectodermal cord is buried in mesoderm between the maxillary and lateral nasal processes. This cord canalizes to the lid margin and inferior meatus during the third embryonic month. Defects in this process may result in an imperforate valve of Hasner or, more rarely, canaliculi or puncta.

15. **B)** Hyaloid canal remnants

16. **C)** Vitreous body

17. **A)** Zonules

Remnants of the hyaloidal system, including the hyaloidal canal, the hyaloidal vessels, and the posterior portions of the tunica vasculosa lentis, are all part of the primary vitreous (Fig. 2-4). The secondary vitreous eventually becomes the main vitreous body. The tertiary vitreous is the portion of the vitreous most peripherally located that is involved with the development of the zonular apparatus.

18. **B)** corneal leukoma

Remnants of the hyaloid vasculature system include the Mittendorf dot on the posterior aspect of the lens, the Bergmeister's papilla at the optic nerve head, and persistent pupillary membrane. A corneal leukoma may be seen with Peter's anomaly, but this represents an abnormality in anterior segment cleavage.

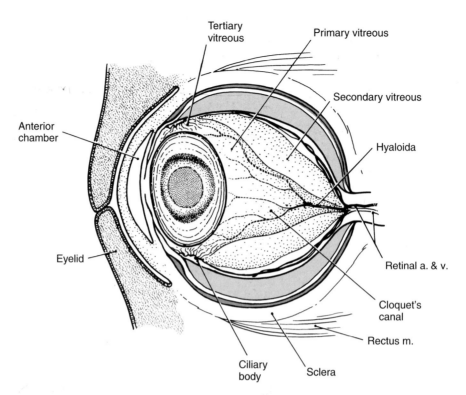

FIGURE 2-4. From Wright K. Textbook of ophthalmology. Baltimore: Williams & Wilkins, 1997.

19.   D)   All of the above

The vitreous is made up of 98% water and 0.1% colloids. The remainder of the solid matter consists of ions and low-molecular-weight solutes. The two major structural components are collagen and hyaluronic acid. Its strongest attachments are at the vitreous base (straddling the ora serrata), optic nerve, and retinal vessels. The collapse and contraction of collagen fibers, which occurs with age, causes pockets of fluid to form within the vitreous and the vitreous to reorganize and form posterior vitreous detachments (floaters).

20.   C)   Myelination progresses posteriorly from the lamina cribrosa.

Myelination of the optic nerve starts in the seventh month of gestation and is completed about 1 month after birth. Myelination starts at the chiasm and progresses toward the lamina cribrosa.

21.   D)   All of the above

The optic canal contains the optic nerve, ophthalmic artery, and sympathetic nerves. The superior orbital fissure is separated from the optic canal by the bony optic strut. The canal ranges between 8 and 10 mm in length. It typically measures less than 6.5 mm in diameter at the optic foramen.

22.   B)   Lacrimal

The orbital floor is composed of contributions from three bones: maxillary, zygomatic, and palatine (Fig. 2-5). The lacrimal bone is part of the medial orbital wall.

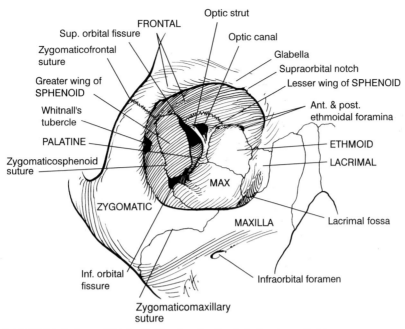

FIGURE 2-5. From Wright K. Textbook of ophthalmology. Baltimore: Williams & Wilkins, 1997.

23. C) the frontoethmoidal suture line, the posterior ethmoidal foramen, the posterior lacrimal crest

The infraorbital foramen is on the anterior face of the maxilla; the zygomaticotemporal foramen is in the lateral orbital rim; the supraorbital foramen is in the frontal bone; the superior orbital fissure separates the roof and the lateral walls of the orbit.

24. D) Attachments between the lateral rectus and the tubercle serve as a check ligament of the lateral rectus.

Whitnall's orbital tubercle is located entirely on the zygomatic bone approximately 2 mm inferior to the frontozygomatic suture line. Lockwood's ligament acts as a suspensory system for the globe. It attaches medially to the medial orbital wall behind the posterior lacrimal crest. It attaches laterally to the lateral retinaculum, which attaches to the lateral orbital tubercle. Whitnall's ligament is the superior transverse ligament that arises from the compacted sheath of the anterior portion of the levator muscle. Laterally, Whitnall's ligament attaches approximately 10 mm superior to the lateral orbital tubercle to the frontal bone and to the lacrimal gland capsule. Whitnall's ligament does send some extensions to the medial and lateral retinacula.

The check ligament of the lateral rectus, the lateral canthal tendon, the lateral horn of the levator aponeurosis, and Lockwood's ligament attach to the lateral retinaculum, which attaches to the lateral orbital tubercle.

25. D) None of the above

26. A) Superior orbital fissure

27. B) Inferior orbital fissure

28.   C)   Optic canal

29.   A)   Superior orbital fissure

Figure 2-6 shows the posterior orbit. The labeled bones are as follows: E = ethmoid, F = frontal, L = lacrimal, M = maxillary, S = sphenoid, Z = zygomatic.

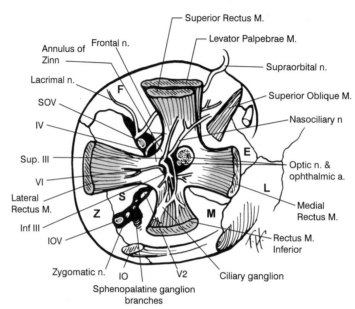

FIGURE 2-6. From Wright K. Textbook of ophthalmology. Baltimore: Williams & Wilkins, 1997.

30.   A)   Lateral rectus

The inferior or superior muscular branches of the ophthalmic artery provide all or part of the blood supply to all the extraocular muscles except the lateral rectus. The lateral rectus blood is supplied by a single vessel derived from the lacrimal artery. Each rectus muscle, except the lateral rectus, receives two anterior ciliary arteries that communicate with the major arteriole circle of the ciliary body.

31.   C)   when the eyelids open, negative pressure is produced in the sac and maintained by the valve of Rosenmüller

According to the tear pump action described by Rosengren-Doane, contraction of the orbicularis muscle provides a positive pressure in the tear sac, forcing tears into the nose through the valve of Hasner. Once the eyelids open and move laterally, a negative pressure is produced in the tear sac, which is maintained by the valve of Hasner. Once the eyelids are fully open, the puncta pop open and the negative pressure draws tears into the ampullae and canaliculi. Evaporation accounts for 10% and 20% of tear elimination in the young and older adults, respectively. Approximately 60% of the tears drain through the inferior punctum.

32.   C)   Depth of the orbit averages 50 mm from the orbital entrance to the apex.

The depth of the orbit varies from 40 to 45 mm from the orbital entrance to the orbital apex. The distance to the apex becomes important in the dissection or excision of a tumor in the posterior orbit or in the repair of an extensive blowout fracture.

33. D) Zygomaticofacial nerve

The trigeminal nerve divides into three segments: ophthalmic (V_1), maxillary (V_2), and mandibular (V_3). The ophthalmic nerve is divided into three branches: nasociliary, frontal, and lacrimal. The frontal nerve, a branch of the ophthalmic (V_1) segment, divides into the supraorbital and supratrochlear nerves. The maxillary (V_2) segment divides into the infraorbital, zygomatic, and superior alveolar nerves. The zygomaticofacial and zygomaticotemporal nerves are branches of the zygomatic nerve (V_2). Figure 2-7 diagrams the three segments of the trigeminal nerve and the various nerve branches.

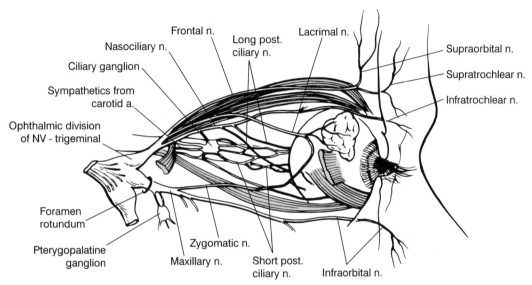

FIGURE 2-7. From Wright K. Textbook of ophthalmology. Baltimore: Williams & Wilkins, 1997.

34. D) Lacrimal, maxillary

The lacrimal sac fossa is bordered by the anterior lacrimal crest of the maxillary bone and the posterior lacrimal crest of the lacrimal bone. In a dacryocystorhinostomy (DCR), the ostomy is created at the maxillolacrimal suture line located in the lacrimal sac fossa.

35. B) Pseudostratified columnar epithelium

This pseudostratified columnar epithelium is similar to that found in the upper respiratory system. Additionally, the walls of the nasolacrimal system contain significant amounts of collagen, elastic tissue, and lymphoid tissue.

36. C) Through an ostium partially covered by a mucosal fold (valve of Hasner)

The lacrimal duct extends into the inferior meatus 3 to 5 mm before opening at the membranous valve of Hasner (Fig. 2-8). The maxillary sinus, middle ethmoid air cells, and anterior ethmoid air cells enter the nose at the level of the middle meatus. The posterior ethmoid air cells drain into the nose via the superior meatus. The sphenoethmoidal recess receives the openings of the sphenoid sinus.

37. C) the muscle of Riolan

The gray line corresponds to the lid's orbicularis muscle layer, the muscle of Riolan.

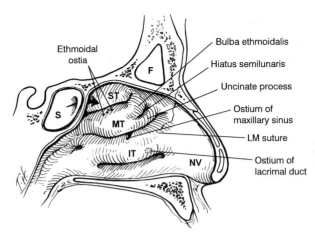

FIGURE 2-8. F = frontal sinus; IT = inferior turbinate; MT = middle turbinate; S = sphenoid sinus; ST = superior turbinate. From Wright K. Textbook of ophthalmology. Baltimore: Williams & Wilkins, 1997.

38.   C)   glands of Moll

A full-thickness incision in the upper eyelid 11 mm superior to the eyelid margin would involve the skin, orbicularis, orbital fat, and levator aponeurosis. The incision may also pass through the peripheral arterial arcade, the superior tarsal muscle, and the conjunctiva. The accessory glands of Wolfring are located along the orbital margin of each tarsus. The accessory lacrimal glands of Krause are located in the fornices, and most reside in the lateral part of the upper fornix. The glands of Moll would be located the farthest distance from this incision because they are located at the lid margin (Fig. 2-9).

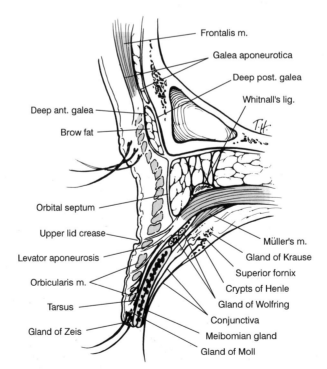

FIGURE 2-9. From Wright K. Textbook of ophthalmology. Baltimore: Williams & Wilkins, 1997.

39. D) Bowman's membrane

Bowman's membrane represents a compact collagen layer at the anterior aspect of the corneal stroma (Fig. 2-10). It is not a true basement membrane.

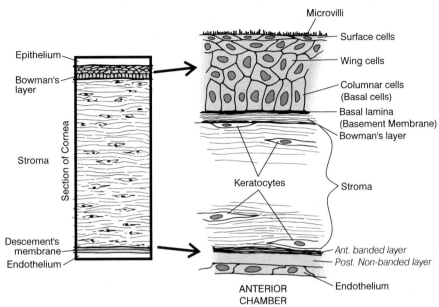

FIGURE 2-10. From Wright K. Textbook of ophthalmology. Baltimore: Williams & Wilkins, 1997.

40. D) Levator aponeurosis

The lacrimal gland is split into two lobes by the lateral extent of the levator aponeurosis.

41. C) Lateral rectus

All of the recti muscles originate from the annulus of Zinn (Fig. 2-11). The superior oblique and levator palpebrae originate superior to the annulus. The inferior oblique has its insertion medially on the maxilla.

42. D) Superior oblique

The recti muscles insert along the spiral of Tillaux with the medial rectus being the closest to the limbus (5.5 mm) and the superior rectus being the farthest (7.9 mm). The superior and inferior oblique muscles insert posterior to the equator. The superior oblique inserts on the globe in a long arc, with the anterior fibers near the insertion of the superior rectus.

43. C) The lens fibers in the nucleus continue to divide throughout life.

The lens (Fig. 2-12) is formed by the successive division and elongation of lens fibers from embryonic surface ectoderm. The nuclei are found in a lens bow near the equator of the lens. Dividing lens epithelium on the periphery continually adds fibers to the nucleus throughout life. The ends of the elongated lens fibers meet anteriorly and posteriorly, forming the Y sutures. The anterior suture is upright, whereas the posterior is inverted (Fig. 2-13).

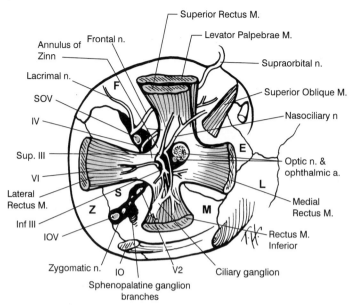

FIGURE 2-11. From Wright K. Textbook of ophthalmology. Baltimore: Williams & Wilkins, 1997.

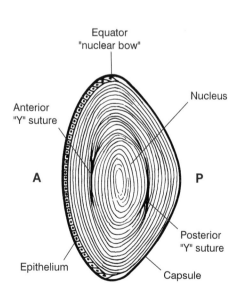

FIGURE 2-12. From Wright K. Textbook of ophthalmology. Baltimore: Williams & Wilkins, 1997.

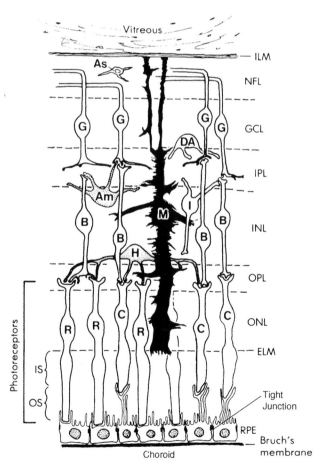

FIGURE 2-13. From Wright K. Textbook of ophthalmology. Baltimore: Williams & Wilkins, 1997.

44. B) Their nuclei lie in the outer nuclear layer.

The nuclei of the Müller cells lie in the inner nuclear layer, whereas the nuclei of the photoreceptors lie in the outer nuclear layer.

45. C) They comprise the inner blood–retinal barrier.

RPE cells comprise the outer blood–retinal barrier; the inner blood–retinal barrier consists of the endothelium lining the retinal blood vessels.

46. A) It communicates freely with the optic disc capillaries.

The choriocapillaris does not communicate freely with the optic disc capillaries. The choroidal circulation is from the posterior ciliary arteries; the optic disc and retinal arterioles are branches of the ophthalmic artery.

47. B) Axons of the amacrine cells

The nerve fiber layer contains the axons of the ganglion cells. The inner plexiform layer has axons of the bipolar and amacrine cells and the synapses of the ganglion cells. The outer plexiform layer has connections between the photoreceptors, horizontal cells, and bipolar cells. The footplates of the Müller cells form the internal limiting membrane.

48. A) 15°

This information is helpful when locating the blind spot on visual fields.

49. B) 120 μm

50. A) ora serrata

The retina is attached at the ora serrata and the optic nerve. The uvea has attachments at the optic nerve, scleral spur, vortex veins, and long and short posterior ciliary vessels. This anatomic difference helps to separate choroidal detachments from retinal detachments on ultrasonography.

Notes

3

Optics

QUESTIONS

1. At 20 feet, the smallest letters that a child can read is the 20/60 line. You have the child walk toward the eye chart. How far does she walk before she can see the 20/20 line?

    A)   15 feet
    B)   7 feet
    C)   13 feet
    D)   5 feet

2. An adult has diplopia and a left hypertropia of 6Δ. Which combination of prisms in his glasses would help to align the two images for him?

	OD	**OS**
A)	3Δ base-up	3Δ base-up
B)	6Δ base-down	Nothing
C)	4Δ base-down	2Δ base-down
D)	3Δ base-up	3Δ base-down

3. You measure a patient with a cranial VI nerve palsy to have an 8Δ distance esotropia. How far apart do the images of a fixation light at 6 m appear to the patient?

    A)   48 cm
    B)   8 cm
    C)   24 cm
    D)   36 cm

4. A 6Δ base-out and an 8Δ base-down prism are replaced by a single prism. What is the power of this prism?

    A)   10Δ
    B)   14Δ
    C)   7Δ
    D)   2Δ

5. A +10.00 D lens is positioned as in Figure 3-1. Two laser beams are aimed parallel to the axis of the lens: one 8 mm above the axis and the other 11 mm below the axis. At what distance past the lens do the beams cross?

    A)   10 cm
    B)   8 cm
    C)   9.5 cm
    D)   19 cm

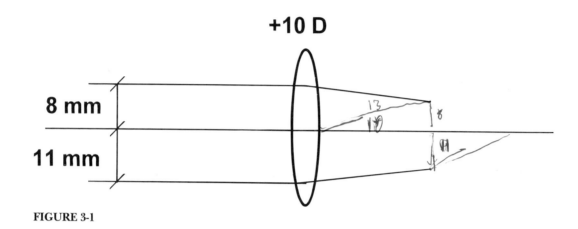

+10 D

8 mm

11 mm

FIGURE 3-1

Questions 6–7

6. An object is located 20 cm to the left of a −2.00 D lens. Where is the image located?

    A)   20 cm to the right of the lens
    B)   50 cm to the right of the lens
    C)   33 cm to the left of the lens
    D)   14 cm to the left of the lens

7. What type and orientation does this image have?

    A)   Virtual, inverted
    B)   Real, inverted
    C)   Virtual, upright
    D)   Real, upright

Questions 8–9

The light source and screens shown in Figure 3-2 are used to determine the power of an unknown lens. When the screen is 16 cm from the lens, a line at 45° is seen. When the screen is moved to 50 cm, the line is at 135°.

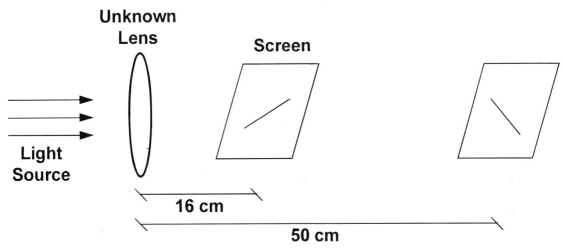

FIGURE 3-2

8. At what distance from the lens is a circle seen on the screen?

   A)   20 cm
   B)   25 cm
   C)   33 cm
   D)   37 cm

9. What is the prescription of this lens?

   A)   + 2.00 + 4.00 × 135°
   B)   + 6.00 − 4.00 × 135°
   C)   + 2.00 + 6.00 × 45°
   D)   + 6.00 − 2.00 × 45°

10. You have two +2.00 D lenses. How far apart are the two lenses so that an object at infinity is focused 1 m to the right of the second lens?

    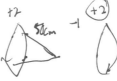

    A)   1.0 m
    B)   0.5 m
    C)   1.5 m
    D)   0.75 m

11. An object 25 cm from a +12.00 D lens is moved 15 cm toward the lens. How far does the image move away from the lens?

    A) 12.5 cm
    B) 37.5 cm
    C) 20 cm
    D) 7.5 cm

12. A 15-cm object is 25 cm to the left of a −2.00 D lens. How large is the resulting image?

    A) 17 cm
    B) 10 cm
    C) 7.5 cm
    D) 25 cm

13. Without correction, a child complains that objects closer than 33 cm are blurry. Cycloplegic refraction measured + 6.00 D sphere OU. How much accommodation does this child have?

    A) 6.00 D
    B) 12.00 D
    C) 3.00 D
    D) 9.00 D

Questions 14–15

14. What is the accommodative amplitude of a patient with a far point 20 cm behind the eye and a near point at infinity?

    A) 5 D
    B) 1 D
    C) 4 D
    D) 2.5 D

15. What reading add is needed to his corrected distance prescription so that at 40 cm this patient uses half of his accommodative amplitude?

    A) +2.50 D
    B) +1.75 D
    C) +2.00 D
    D) No reading add needed

16. When looking at an object at 25 cm, a patient has an esotropia of 30Δ. With + 3.00 D glasses, his esotropia decreases to 15Δ. What is his distance esodeviation without glasses?

    A) 6Δ
    B) 10Δ
    C) 18Δ
    D) 36Δ

17. A Galilean telescope is constructed with a +5.00 D objective and a −10.00 D eyepiece. What is the magnification of this telescope?

   A) ½×
   B) 50×
   C) 2×
   D) 5×

Questions 18–19

18. You have a +10 D lens and a +20 D lens. You want to make a 2× magnifier. What is the distance between the lenses to produce this magnification?

   A) 10 cm
   B) 15 cm
   C) 5 cm
   D) 25 cm

19. How much accommodation is required to view an object 1 m in front of the +10 D lens?

   A) 2 D
   B) 10 D
   C) 5 D
   D) 8 D

20. A 10Δ plastic prism and a 10Δ crown glass prism are placed under water. Under water, how much do the plastic and glass prisms deviate light?

	Plastic	Glass
A)	<10Δ	<10Δ
B)	<10Δ	>10Δ
C)	>10Δ	<10Δ
D)	10Δ	10Δ

21. Prescription swimming goggles are constructed from plastic (n = 1.45) plano-concave lenses. They measure −2.00 D in air. What is the power of the goggles when worn underwater (n_{water} = 1.33)?

   A) −1.50 D
   B) −2.25 D
   C) −2.00 D
   D) −3.33 D

22. An aquarium is 25 cm deep. A rock is viewed from above the aquarium. The water (n = 1.33) is then removed and replaced with silicone oil (n = 1.40). How does the location of the rock appear when viewed through the air, water, and oil?

	Appears closest	Appears farthest
A)	Oil	Water	Air
B)	Air	Water	Oil
C)	Air	Oil	Water
D)	Water	Oil	Air

23. A 2-cm object is 10 cm from an 8.00 D concave mirror. What is the size of the resulting image?

   A)   10 cm
   B)   20 cm
   C)   50 cm
   D)   80 cm

24. A PMMA IOL (n = 1.48) has a power of +25 D when measured under water. What is the power of this lens in the air?

   A)   80 D
   B)   48 D
   C)   29 D
   D)   23 D

25. A phakic patient undergoes a vitrectomy with replacement of his vitreous fluid (n = 1.34) with silicone oil (n=1.40). What change occurs in his prescription?

   A)   Myopic shift
   B)   Hyperopic shift
   C)   No significant change in prescription
   D)   Cannot be determined with the information given

Questions 26–27

26. An object is 100 cm from a +4 D concave mirror. What type and orientation of image is formed?

   A)   Virtual, inverted
   B)   Real, inverted
   C)   Virtual, erect
   D)   Real, erect

27. Where is the image located?

   A)   20 cm to the right of the mirror
   B)   20 cm to the left of the mirror
   C)   33 cm to the right of the mirror
   D)   33 cm to the left of the mirror

28. An object is 12.5 cm from a +3 D lens that is 10 cm from a plane mirror. How far apart are the image and object?

   A)   187.5 cm
   B)   100 cm
   C)   52.5 cm
   D)   22.5 cm

29. You use the duochrome test to refine the refraction of a patient. The patient says the red letters are much clearer than the green letters. The patient:

    A) is overplussed
    B) is overminused
    C) is anisometropic
    D) is presbyopic

30. You see the following reflex (Fig. 3-3) when performing streak retinoscopy on a patient. What needs to be done to neutralize this reflex?

    A) Rotate axis 15° clockwise, add positive sphere
    B) Rotate axis 15° counterclockwise, add negative sphere
    C) Rotate axis 15° counterclockwise, add positive sphere
    D) Rotate axis 15° clockwise, add negative sphere

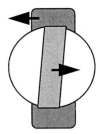

FIGURE 3-3

31. You hold a +1.00 D lens in front of a patient. At a working distance of 67 cm, you see against motion with the streak oriented at 90° and less against movement with the streak oriented at 180°. Which situation exists for this patient?

    A) Simple myopic astigmatism
    B) Compound myopic astigmatism
    C) Simple hyperopic astigmatism
    D) Compound hyperopic astigmatism

32. You perform streak retinoscopy on a cyclopleged infant. With the streak oriented vertically at 90°, you neutralize the reflex with a −2.00 D lens (after subtracting the working distance), and with the horizontal streak, +3.00 D lens. What is the cycloplegic refraction?

    A) +3.00 − 2.00 × 180°
    B) −2.00 + 3.00 × 90°
    C) −2.00 + 5.00 × 180°
    D) +3.00 − 5.00 × 180°

33. A patient wears +3.00 + 2.25 × 60°. If all of her astigmatism is corneal, what could her keratometry measure?

    A) 38.50 D at 120°, 43.75 D at 30°
    B) 40.00 D at 60°, 42.25 D at 150°
    C) 45.75 D at 30°, 48.00 D at 120°
    D) 41.25 D at 150°, 43.50 D at 60°

34. An uncorrected, cycloplegic patient looks at an Amsler grid 40 cm away. The vertical lines are focused sharply when a +4.75 D sphere is held in front of this eye. The horizontal lines are sharpest with a +6.00 D sphere. What is her distance correction?

A) +4.75 + 1.25 × 180°
B) +2.25 + 3.75 × 90°
C) +2.25 + 1.25 × 180°
D) +1.25 + 2.50 × 90°

35. A −4.00 D myopic patient has +2.00 D reading adds ground into his lenses. Which type of bifocal segment will minimize image displacement?

A) Round-top
B) Slab-off
C) Flat-top
D) Franklin

36. A 65-year-old hyperopic patient undergoes cataract surgery in his left eye. Following surgery his refraction measures:

$$+4.00 + 0.50 \times 90$$

$$-2.25 + 1.00 \times 90$$

Progressive bifocal, +2.50 add

He complains of difficulty adjusting to his new glasses. With each eye tested individually, his acuity is 20/20. Which of the following would best solve his problem?

A) Slab-off prism
B) Contact lenses
C) Flat-top bifocal
D) Cycloplegic refraction

37. A patient wears the following prescription:

$$- 1.00 + 2.00 \times 180°$$

$$- 2.50 + 1.00 \times 90° \qquad \text{Add} + 3.00 \text{ OU}$$

His bifocal segment is located 10 mm inferior to the optical center of the glasses. How much relative prism is induced when he looks through the top of his bifocal?

A) 1.50Δ right base-up
B) 2.00Δ left base-up
C) 2.50Δ right base-up
D) 3.50Δ right base-up

38. An aphakic patient wears +10.00 D glasses at a vertex distance of 10 mm. What power of contact lens should be ordered to fit on K's?

A) +9.0 D
B) +10.0 D
C) +11.0 D
D) +9.5 D

39. A patient has K's of 42.00 D at 90°/40.00 D at 180° and refraction of − 1.50 + 0.50 × 90°. A plano hard contact lens is fit on the flatter K. What over-refraction is measured?

    A)   −1.00 + 1.50 × 180°
    B)   +1.50 − 0.50 × 90°
    C)   −0.50 + 0.50 × 180°
    D)   +0.50 + 1.50 × 90°

40. Which change would allow a hard contact lens to fit more tightly to a cornea?

    A)   Decreasing the diameter from 8.80 mm to 8.40 mm
    B)   Decreasing the base curve from 8.20 mm to 8.00 mm
    C)   Increasing the optical zone from 8.20 mm to 8.40 mm
    D)   Increasing the power from −3.00 D to −3.50 D

41. Which one of the following single changes results in the selection of a lens more powerful than intended?

    A)   Using an A-constant of 116.8 instead of 117.3
    B)   Axial length measured as 20.5 mm rather than 20.2 mm
    C)   Average keratometry of 44.50 D in place of 44.00 D
    D)   Placing the lens in the anterior chamber instead of in the capsular bag

42. A patient wears aspheric bifocal contact lenses in both eyes. All of the following could be expected with these lenses EXCEPT:

    A)   multiple images
    B)   difficulty in dim light
    C)   glare with headlights
    D)   different image sizes between the eyes

43. What strength of lens is needed so that a patient with 20/160 visual acuity can read newsprint without accommodation?

    A)   +5.00 D
    B)   +8.00 D
    C)   +10.00 D
    D)   +12.50 D

44. Which optical principle is the basis for antireflective coatings on glasses and lenses?

    A)   Coherence
    B)   Diffraction
    C)   Interference
    D)   Polarization

45. A polarized lens is oriented so that it eliminates the vertical component of white light. Light polarized at 45° is projected through the lens. What percentage of the light is transmitted through the lens?

A) 0%
B) 45%
C) 50%
D) 71%

46. A patient purchased a pair of sunglasses with a dark blue tint. Which of these colors would be the hardest to see?

A) Red
B) Blue
C) Green
D) Purple

47. A patient who had bilateral LASIK is complaining of haloes and starbursts while driving at night. Which of the following measures could improve his symptoms?

A) Wear polarized glasses
B) Constrict pupil
C) Turn on the interior reading light in car
D) Treat with a larger ablation zone

48. Looking through the inferior prism of a Zeiss 4-mirror goniolens, you see the following in the slit lamp (Fig. 3-4):

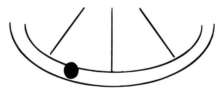

FIGURE 3-4

Where is the foreign body located in the trabecular meshwork.
A) 11 o'clock
B) 1 o'clock
C) 7 o'clock
D) 5 o'clock

49. A lesion is located supertemporal to the fovea of the right eye. What would the observer see through a Rodenstock panretinal lens (Fig. 3-5)?

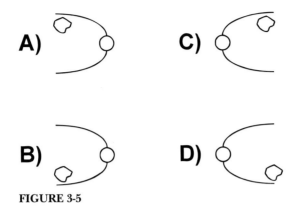

FIGURE 3-5

50. A patient has a red Maddox rod with the cylinders oriented horizontally placed over her left eye. What does she see when she views a distant white fixation light?

  A)   Red light, horizontal white line
  B)   Red light, vertical white line
  C)   White light, horizontal red line
  D)   White light, vertical red line

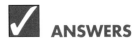 **ANSWERS**

The following formulas are essential for solving many of the optics questions:

- Lens power calculation:

    D = lens power (diopters), f = focal length (cm)

$$D = \frac{100\ cm}{f}$$

- Prentice's Rule:

$$PD = h \times D$$

    PD = prism deviation (Δ), h = distance from optical center (cm), D = lens power (diopters)

- Vergence formula:

$$U + D = V$$

    U = object vergence, D = lens power, V = image vergence

- Lens effectivity formula:

$$D_2 = \frac{D_1}{1 - s \times D_1}$$

    D_1 = old lens power (diopters), D_2 = lens powers (diopters), s = distance the lens is moved (meters) toward the eye

- Power of a spherical refracting surface:

$$D = \frac{n_2 - n_1}{r}$$

    D = power (diopters), n_1, n_2 = refractive indices, r = radius of curvature

- Transverse magnification:

$$M = \frac{image\ height}{object\ height} = \frac{image\ distance}{object\ distance} = \frac{U}{V}$$

    M = magnification, U = object vergence, V = image vergence

- Angular magnification: (reference distance = 25 cm)

$$M = \frac{D}{4}$$

    M = magnification, D = lens power

- Magnification of telescope:

$$M = \frac{D_{eyepiece}}{D_{objective}}$$

    M = magnification, $D_{eyepiece}$ = power of eyepiece, $D_{objective}$ = power of objective

- Reflecting power of spherical mirror:

$$D = \frac{100}{f} = \frac{200}{r}$$

D = lens power (diopters), f = focal length (cm), r = radius of curvature (cm)

- IOL power calculation:

$$D = A - 2.5 \,(\text{axial length}) - 0.9 \,(\text{average K reading})$$

D = IOL power, A = constant

1. C)   13 feet

A 20/20 letter subtends a visual angle of 5 minutes of arc when viewed at 20 feet. As you move close to an object, it subtends a larger visual angle. A 20/60 letter subtends 3× the visual angle of a 20/20 letter. Using similar triangles,

$$\frac{15 \; arc \; min}{5 \; arc \; min} = \frac{20 \; feet}{6.7 \; feet}$$

Therefore, the child must advance 13 feet to be 7 feet from the eye chart to see the letters (Fig. 3-6).

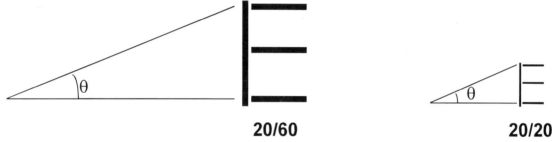

20/60   **20/20**

FIGURE 3-6

2. D)   3Δ base-up   3Δbase-down

A strabismic deviation can be neutralized by orienting an appropriate power prism with the apex in the same direction as the deviation. A 6Δ left hypertropia can be corrected with a 6Δ base-down prism in front of this eye. The prism can be divided between the eyes with 3Δ base-up in front of the right eye and a 3Δ base-down in front of the left (Fig. 3-7).

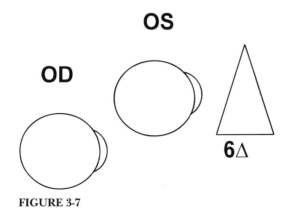

OS

OD

6Δ

FIGURE 3-7

3. A)   48 cm

A *prism diopter* is defined as the amount of deviation of a light by the prism measured at 100 cm. For every 100 cm, light is deviated 8 cm (Fig. 3-8). At 6 meters, 8Δ represents a deviation of 48 cm.

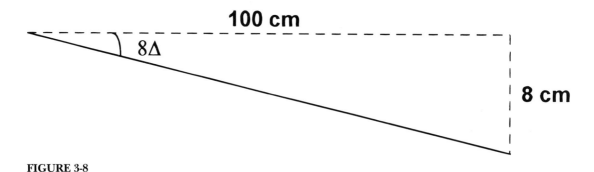

FIGURE 3-8

4. A)   10Δ

Prism power can be represented by vectors and added as this mathematical entity. The resultant vector is the hypotenuse of a right triangle with legs of 6 and 8, which is 10Δ base-down and out at 53° (Fig. 3-9).

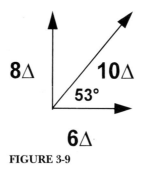

FIGURE 3-9

5. A)   10 cm

All rays parallel to the lens axis will converge on the secondary focal point whose location can be calculated as 100 cm/10 D = 10 cm. The result can also be obtained using Prentice's rule and ray tracing (Fig. 3-10).

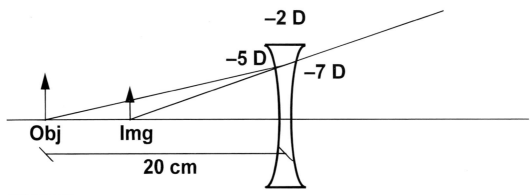

FIGURE 3-10

6. D)   14 cm to the left of the lens

Vergences are indicated in Figure 3-10.

Vergence of light entering the lens:

$$U = \frac{100}{20 \text{ cm}} = -5D$$

A negative sign indicates diverging rays of light.

Using the lens equation:

$$U + D = V$$
$$-5 + (-2) = -7$$

The location of the resulting image can be calculated:

$$\frac{100}{v} = -7$$
$$v = -14 \text{ cm}$$

The resulting image is 14 cm to the left of the lens.

7. C)   Virtual, upright

Three principal rays of light can be used to locate the position and orientation of images. These rays are described here and are shown in Figure 3-11 with the convex lens:

1)   A ray through the primary focal point will exit the lens parallel to the axis.
2)   A ray parallel to the axis will travel through the secondary focal point.
3)   A ray through the optical center of the lens will not be deviated.

For the concave lens in this question, the image is virtual and upright. By ray tracing, the image can be found on the left side of lens, thus creating a virtual image. By drawing the other principle rays, the image can be shown to be upright.

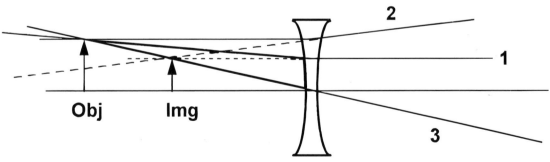

FIGURE 3-11

8. B)   25 cm

9. B) $+ 6.00 - 4.00 \times 135°$

In the apparatus, parallel rays of light are focused by the lens onto the screen. The lens focuses light into a 45° line at 16 cm; therefore, the power of the lens in the 45° axis (and 135° meridian) is $+ 6.00$ D. Similarly, the 135° axis has a power of $+ 2.00$ D. These lines represent each end of the conoid of Sturm. The circle of least confusion falls halfway (dioptrically) between each of these lines, or at $+ 4.00$ D. This corresponds to an image on the screen at 25 cm.

Figure 3-12 shows the power cross corresponding to the lens and thus the prescription: $+ 6.00 - 4.00 \times 135°$.

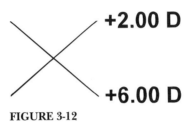

+2.00 D

+6.00 D

FIGURE 3-12

10. C)   1.5 m

The best way to approach this problem is to use vergences and work from both ends toward the center. The vergence of the light entering the first lens is 0 (coming from infinity). Light leaving the second lens is focused at 1 m ($+1$ D vergence). Using the lens equation, the vergences of light leaving the first lens and entering the second can be calculated to be $+2$ D and -1 D, respectively. Because they share the same intermediate image plane, the distance between the lenses is the sum of the two image distances (Fig. 3-13).

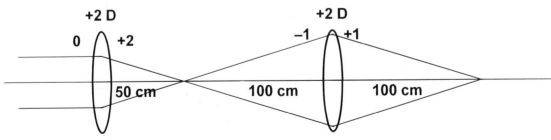

+2 D

+2 D

0   +2

−1   +1

50 cm

100 cm

100 cm

FIGURE 3-13

11. B) 37.5 cm

The amount of image movement can be calculated by measuring the difference between the image location at each position of the object (Fig. 3-14).
    The image moves $50.0 - 12.5$ cm $= 37.5$ cm

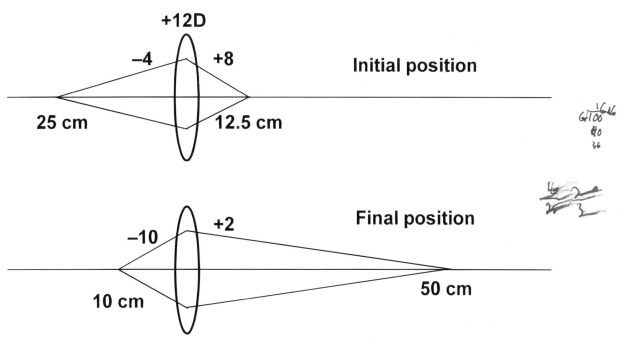

+12D

−4 **+8**

Initial position

25 cm **12.5 cm**

−10 **+2**

Final position

10 cm

50 cm

FIGURE 3-14

12. B) 10 cm

The vergences of light entering and leaving the lens are indicated in Figure 3-15. The magnification can be calculated as a ratio of the vergence entering the lens to that leaving the lens:

$$M = \frac{U}{V} = \frac{-4}{-6} = \frac{2}{3}$$

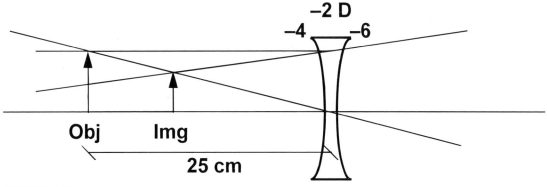

−2 D

−4 **−6**

Obj **Img**

25 cm

FIGURE 3-15

13. D)   9.00 D

With maximum accommodation, this child is able to focus at objects at 33 cm (3 D). Being an uncorrected hyperope, the child must accommodate through the 6.00 D of hyperopia to see clearly in the distance. An additional 3.00 D of accommodation are needed to focus at 33 cm. The total accommodation is 9.00 D.

14. A)   5 D

15. D)   No reading add needed

The far point and near points correspond to + 5.00 D and plano; thus, the patient has 5 D of accommodation. With a + 5.00 D distance prescription, he has the required 2.50 D of accommodation to focus at 40 cm (Fig. 3-16).

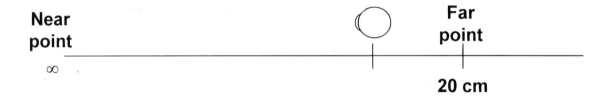

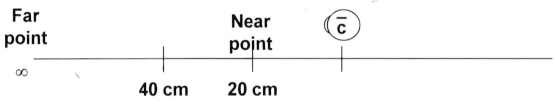

FIGURE 3-16

16. B)   10Δ

Using the gradient method for calculating the AC/A ratio:

$$\frac{AC}{A} = \frac{\Delta_{sc} - \Delta_{cc}}{D_{sc} - D_{cc}} = \frac{30 - 15}{3 - 0} = 5\frac{\Delta}{D}$$

For every diopter of accommodation, the patient increases his esotropia by 5Δ. At a distance, he accommodates 4 D less than at 25 cm; therefore, his uncorrected distance deviation will be 30 − (4 × 5) = 10Δ.

17. C)   2×

A Galilean telescope is constructed with converging and diverging lenses such that the primary focal point of the objective lens corresponds to the secondary focal point of the eyepiece lens. As a result, parallel rays from infinity entering the objective emerge as parallel rays from the eyepiece. Angular magnification occurs, which corresponds to the ratio of the power of the eyepiece:objective.

$$M_{angular} = \frac{Power\ of\ Eyepiece}{Power\ of\ Objective} = \frac{10}{5} = 2$$

18. B) 15 cm

An astronomical telescope is constructed of two convex (plus) lenses (Fig. 3-17). The secondary focal point of the first lens (objective) corresponds to the primary focal point of the second lens (eyepiece). The corresponding focal points of each lens in this case are 10 and 5 cm for a total of 15 cm. Incidentally, the astronomical telescope forms an inverted image.

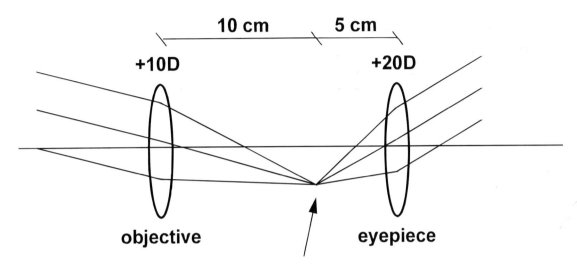

FIGURE 3-17

19. C) 5 D

The vergences can be calculated in Figure 3-18.

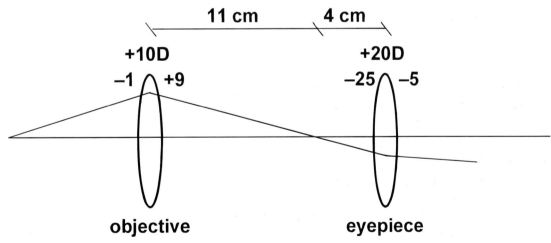

FIGURE 3-18

Plastic   Glass

20. A) $<10\Delta$ $<10\Delta$

Consider the situation when one surface of the prism is perpendicular to the beam of light (Prentice's position) as shown in Figure 3-19. The refraction of light only occurs at the second surface.

The refraction at this interface obeys Snell's Law:

$$n_{plastic} \sin \theta_1 = n_{water} \sin \theta_2$$

Because $n_{water} > n_{air}$, less bending of light will occur at the plastic–water interface than the plastic–air interface, effectively reducing the prismatic power of the lens. A glass lens will have a similar decrease in prismatic power.

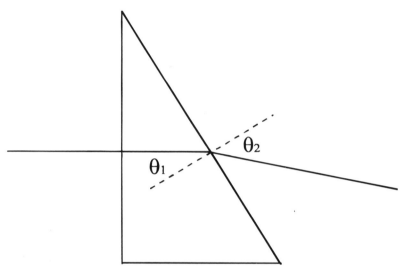

FIGURE 3-19

21. C) -2.00 D

When worn properly, the goggles (Fig. 3-20) have a plano surface at the water–plastic interface and thus no deviation of light. The power of the prescription is ground into the plastic–air interface. Underwater, this compartment should still contain air; therefore, no change in prescription power results.

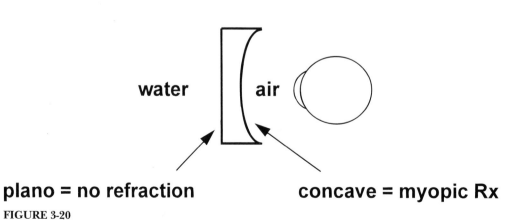

FIGURE 3-20

Appears Closest   *Appears Farthest*

22. A) Oil   Water   Air

Consider the three scenarios:

1. air (n = 1.00)
    No refraction occurs.
2. water (n = 1.33)
    Refraction occurs at air-water interface. The stone appears closer than it
    actually is.
3. oil (n = 1.40)

Higher index of refraction increases degree of bending of light, making the stone
seem even closer (Fig. 3-21).

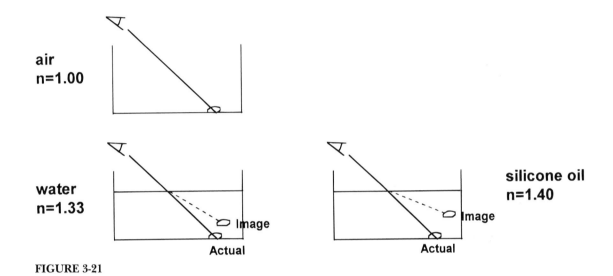

FIGURE 3-21

23. A) 10 cm

A concave mirror adds plus vergence to oncoming light in addition to reversing object and image space. The vergences are indicated on Figure 3-22. Similar to a lens, the magnification can be calculated using the vergences entering and leaving the mirror.

$$M = \frac{U}{V} = \frac{-10}{-2} = 5$$

Therefore, the image is 5× larger than the 2 cm object, or 10 cm tall.

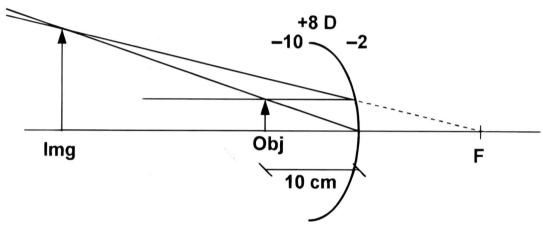

FIGURE 3-22

24. A) 80 D

$$\frac{D_{air}}{D_{water}} = \frac{n_{IOL} - n_{air}}{n_{IOL} - n_{water}} = \frac{1.48 - 1.00}{1.48 - 1.33} = \frac{0.48}{0.15}$$

$$D_{air} = \frac{0.48}{0.15} \times D_{water} = \frac{0.48}{0.15} \times 25 = 80 \ D$$

25. A) Myopic shift

Silicone oil has a higher index of refraction than vitreous so more refraction occurs at the posterior lens interface. This is similar to having a lens with a much higher dioptric power within the eye. The resultant prescription for the eye becomes more myopic.

26. B) Real, inverted

27. D)   33 cm to the left of the mirror

Using the vergence formula:

$$U + D = V$$

$$-1 + 4 = +3$$

Because V is positive, a real image located on the same side of the mirror as the object is formed. Because U and V have opposite signs, the image is inverted compared to the object.

The location of the image is $1/V = 1/3$ $m = 0.33$ m to the left of the mirror (Fig. 3-23).

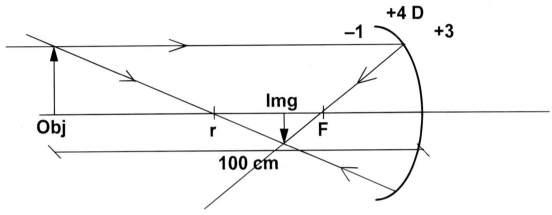

FIGURE 3-23

Ray tracing and vergence calculations also allow determination of the answer to these questions. Remember that mirrors flip object and image space. Therefore, the plus vergence "leaving" the mirror actually converges toward the left.

28. A)   187.5 cm

This problem can be separated into each optical component and they can be considered independently from each other.

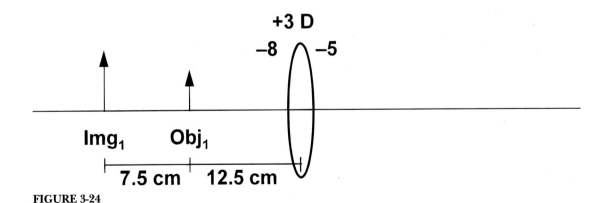

FIGURE 3-24

The first lens (Fig. 3-24) produces a virtual image (Img₁) 20 cm to the left of the lens (and 30 cm to the left of the mirror). This image becomes the object (Obj₂) of the mirror (Fig. 3-25).

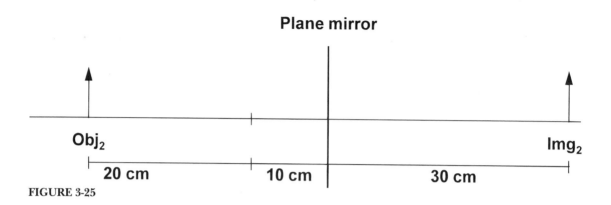

FIGURE 3-25

The image (Img₂) of the mirror becomes the object (Obj₃) of the lens again (Fig. 3-26). Note that the light is now traveling from right to left because object space is to the right of the lens.

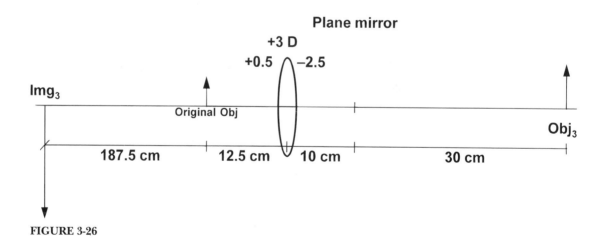

FIGURE 3-26

The final image (Img₃) is 200 cm to the left of the lens and 187.5 cm from the initial object.

29. A)   is overplussed

The duochrome test relies on the differential degree of refraction experienced by shorter and longer wavelengths of light. Shorter wavelengths (violet, blue, green) are bent more than longer wavelengths (orange, red) (Fig. 3-27). The difference in refraction between red and green is approximately 0.50 D.

In this case, the red portion of the spectrum is focused sharply on the retina. The endpoint of the duochrome test is to straddle the spectrum on the retina with red wavelengths posterior and green wavelengths anterior. This can be accomplished by adding diverging lenses (or removing converging lenses) to move the spectrum more posteriorly. The patient is therefore overplussed.

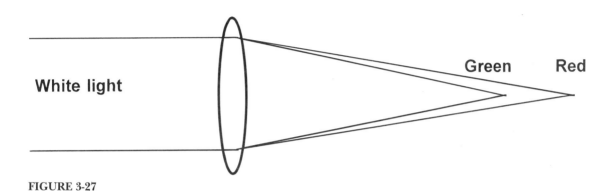

FIGURE 3-27

30. D)   Rotate axis 15° clockwise, add negative sphere

Among the phenomena seen with streak retinoscopy, the break phenomenon is demonstrated here. It occurs when the streak and reflex are off axis. The streak should be rotated 15° clockwise so that it is parallel to the reflex. As neutrality is approached, the reflex becomes wider until it fills the whole pupil. In this case of against movement, negative sphere is needed to neutralize the reflex.

31. B)   Compound myopic astigmatism

Against motion requires minus lenses to neutralize the reflex. The myopia is greater in the 180° meridian, which is measured with the streak oriented at 90°. The working distance of 67 cm corresponds to 1.50 D that needs to be subtracted from the lens in front of the eye. The + 1.00 D lens only partially compensates for the working distance. Removing this lens still leaves the prescription myopic.

32. C) $- 2.00 + 5.00 \times 180°$

With the streak oriented vertically and by moving it left and right, the power in the 180° meridian (and the power in the 90° axis) is actually being evaluated—likewise, when the beam is rotated 90°. This evaluation can be represented on the power cross in Figure 3-28.

The astigmatism is the difference between the two lenses, or $+ 5.00$ D. The final prescription is $- 2.00 + 5.00 \times 180°$.

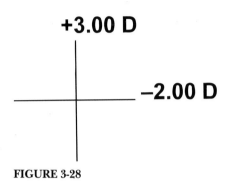

FIGURE 3-28

33. D)   41.25 D at 150°, 43.50 D at 60°

The power cross for the patient's prescription is drawn in Figure 3-29. Remember that the power of the cylinder is 90° from its axis.

The 2.25 D of astigmatic power of the glasses is oriented in the 150° meridian to correspond to the cornea's steeper meridian. The only K reading that is oriented properly with the correct amount of astigmatism is 41.25 D at 150°, 43.50 D at 60°.

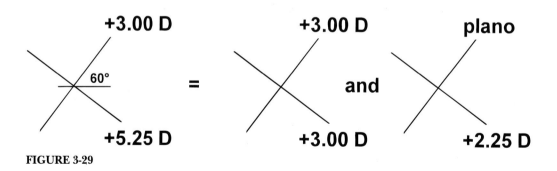

FIGURE 3-29

34. C) $+ 2.25 + 1.25 \times 180°$

When looking at an object at 40 cm, 2.5 D of accommodation is needed. The distance lenses would be $+ 2.25$ D and $+ 3.50$ D, respectively. The power of a lens in the horizontal meridian is responsible for focusing the vertical lines. This corresponds to the $+ 3.50$ D cylinder with axis at 90°. The cylinder power with axis 180° is $+ 2.25$ D.

35. A) Round-top

Image displacement is the difference in location of the image of an object seen through the bifocal compared with its actual position. It is particularly troublesome for patients. Bifocal types are selected to minimize this phenomenon. Image displacement is due to the total prismatic effect of the lens and bifocal when looking through the reading segment. With the round-top segment, the base-up prism induced by the minus lens is increased by the base-down prism of the bifocal. The other bifocal types (flat-top and Franklin) have the optical centers near the top of the segment and counteract the base-down prism.

Slab-off is a method of removing vertical prism from lenses for patients with anisometropia (Fig. 3-30).

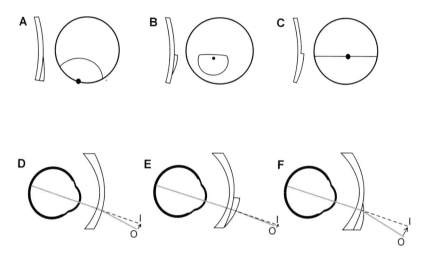

FIGURE 3-30. A = round-top bifocal; B = flat-top bifocal; C = executive (Franklin) bifocal; D = prism induced by looking off axis; E = reduction in prism with a flat-top or executive bifocal; F = increase in prism with a round-

36. B) Contact lenses

This patient is experiencing *aniseikonia* (difference in image size) due to the large difference in the prescriptions between his lenses. Wearing a contact lens would decrease the image size difference, which is greater at the vertex distance of spectacles. Slab-off prism would be helpful if there was induced prism causing difficulty using the bifocal segment. Changing the type of bifocal segment might be helpful if the patient is having trouble finding the correct zone to use; however, for distance, the bifocal should not interfere.

37. D)   3.50Δ right base-up

The power crosses pictured in Figure 3-31 correspond to the lenses in his glasses. The prisms induced by the bifocals are equal in each eye and cancel each other. When one looks downward, only the power in the 90° meridian is deviating light. Prentice's rule is used to calculate the prismatic effect of the lenses:

OD: $(+ 1.00 \text{ D}) \times (1.0 \text{ cm}) = 1.00Δ$ Base-up

OS: $(- 2.50 \text{ D}) \times (1.0 \text{ cm}) = 2.50Δ$ Base-down

Combining the prisms results in 3.50Δ base-up over the right eye.

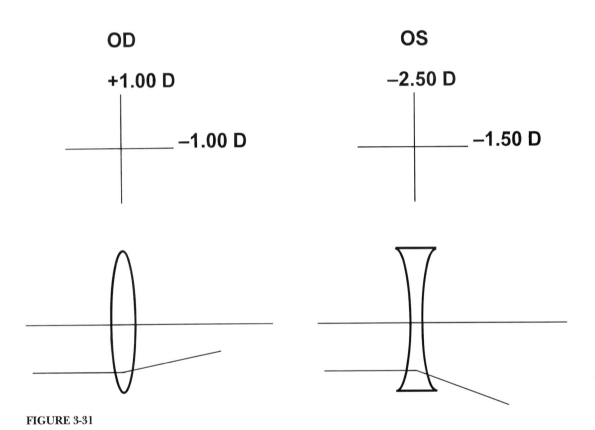

FIGURE 3-31

38. C)   + 11.0 D

The far point of the eye is located 10 cm behind the spectacle plane (9 cm behind the cornea) (Fig. 3-32). A lens placed on the cornea would need a power of 100/9 cm = + 11.1 D to focus light at this same point.
The lens affectivity formula may also be used to determine the same result:

$$D_2 = \frac{D_1}{1 - s \times D_1} = \frac{10}{1 - (0.01)\,(10)} = \frac{10}{0.9} = 11$$

where D_1 and D_2 are the old and new lens powers (diopters), respectively, s is the distance the lens is moved (meters) toward the eye.

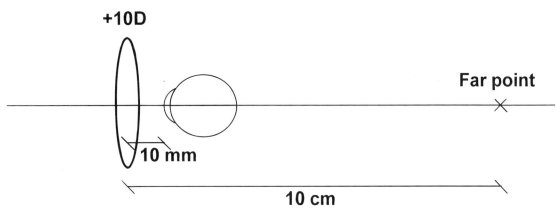

FIGURE 3-32

39. A)   − 1.00 + 1.50 × 180°

The cornea is steeper along the 90° meridian as pictured in Figure 3-33 (with-the-rule astigmatism). A contact lens fit on the flatter K would create a concave tear lens with 2 D of power along the 90° meridian.

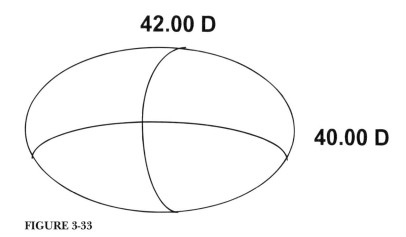

FIGURE 3-33

Looking at the power crosses for the tear lens and over-refraction, the answer can be calculated to be − 1.00 + 1.50 × 180° (Fig. 3-34).

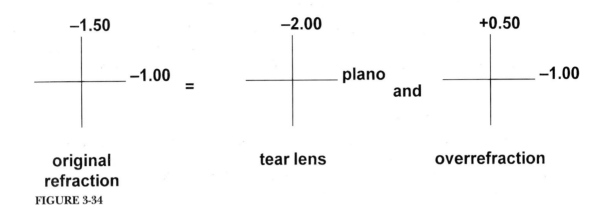

original refraction

tear lens

overrefraction

FIGURE 3-34

40.   B)   Decreasing the base curve from 8.20 mm to 8.00 mm

Decreasing the base curve makes the lens steeper and thus causes a tighter fit. Decreasing the lens diameter increases the mobility of the lens and thus causes a looser fit. The size of the optical zone and power of the lens do not affect the fit of a lens (Fig. 3-35).

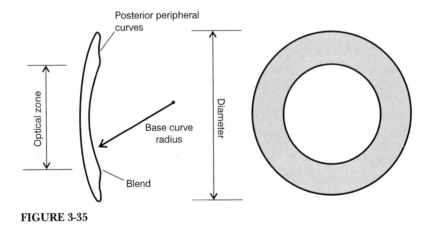

FIGURE 3-35

41. D) Placing the lens in the anterior chamber instead of in the capsular bag

The lens power formula is dependent on axial length (in millimeters) and keratometry (in diopters) as follows:

$$\text{Lens power} = A - 2.5 \, (\text{axial length}) - 0.9 \, (\text{average keratometry})$$

A higher A-constant, decreased axial length, or decreased keratometry readings would result in the calculation of a stronger lens. Moving a convex (plus) lens more anteriorly in the eye and away from the nodal point also effectively increases its power.

42. D) different image sizes between the eyes

Aspheric bifocal contact lenses have concentric zones that alternate between near and distance prescriptions (Fig. 3-36). Both the near and distance images are projected on the retina simultaneously. Because the light is split into two images, each is slightly dimmer. Glare can result from the transition region between the circular zones. No image size disparity is expected with the use of a contact lens.

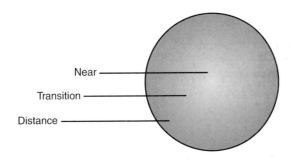

FIGURE 3-36

43. B) + 8.00 D

Kestenbaum's rule dictates the power of a lens needed to allow a patient with low vision to read newsprint. The power of lens is equal to the reciprocal of the visual acuity, that is, 160/20 = 8 D.

44.   C)   Interference

Antireflective coatings are based on interference of light to eliminate the reflection of certain wavelengths (Fig. 3-37). Thin coatings of plastic are placed on the surface of a lens such that certain wavelengths are reflected and are one-half wavelength out of phase with light reflected at the first interface. The destructive interference effectively negates these waveforms.

Diffraction is the bending of light rays when they pass through a thin grating or pinhole. *Polarization* is the elimination of light energy not vibrating along a particular axis. *Coherence* is a measure of the degree of the uniformity of a wavelength.

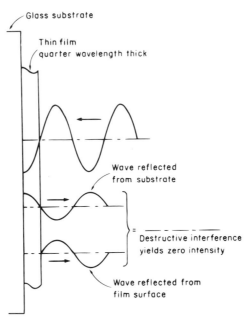

FIGURE 3-37. Reprinted with permission of the American Academy of Ophthalmology, *Basic Clinical and Science Course, Section 3, Optics, Refraction and Contact Lens*, San Francisco, 1993–1994.

45. D) 71%

Using a vector to represent the light (Fig. 3-38), a polarizing filter can eliminate the vertical vector component. The light intensity corresponds to the magnitude of the vector. Thus 71% of the light is transmitted through the lens. This may seem counterintuitive, but vectors do not add algebraically (unless they are both oriented in the same direction). Polarizing filters that are oriented perpendicular to each other do not let any light through.

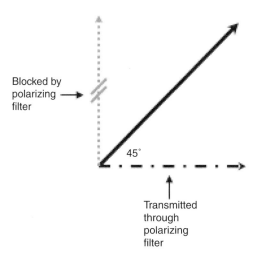

Blocked by polarizing filter

45°

Transmitted through polarizing filter

FIGURE 3-38

46. B) Blue

A blue lens would block to the greatest extent the blue wavelengths of light and permit transmission of the other wavelengths. This property is utilized in fundus photography where blue light is projected into the eye. A filter in the camera blocks the reflected blue wavelengths but permits the fluorescent green light to be transmitted and recorded on film.

47. A) Wear polarized glasses

The symptoms this patient is experiencing are common after LASIK. These side effects are more frequent with small ablation zones and large pupils. The reading light will cause a small amount of pupil constriction. Polarized glasses reduce reflected glare but are not recommended at night because they reduce the amount of light entering the eye and may result in greater pupillary dilation.

48. A)   11 o'clock

The Zeiss goniolens allows a view of the angle by using a mirror to direct light obliquely across the cornea (Fig. 3-39). The mirror in this view reverses superior and inferior but not left and right.

Looking through the interior gonioprism, the superior angle is visualized. The foreign body corresponds to the 11 o'clock position.

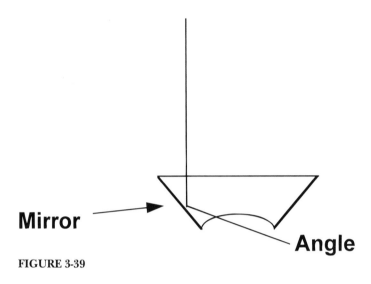

FIGURE 3-39

49. D)

The Rodenstock lens is a panretinal contact lens. The curved surface is in contact with the cornea using a coupling agent such as methylcellulose (Fig. 3-40). Refraction at this interface is minimal. A convex lens provides magnification and results in an inverted and reversed image.

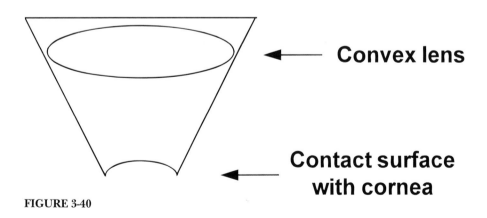

FIGURE 3-40

50. D)   White light, vertical red line

Maddox rods are cylinders of high plus power (Fig. 3-41). Light is focused very close to the rods (too close to actually see); instead, a virtual image perpendicular to these lights is visible. The left eye sees a vertical red line produced by the Maddox rod. The right eye sees a single white light.

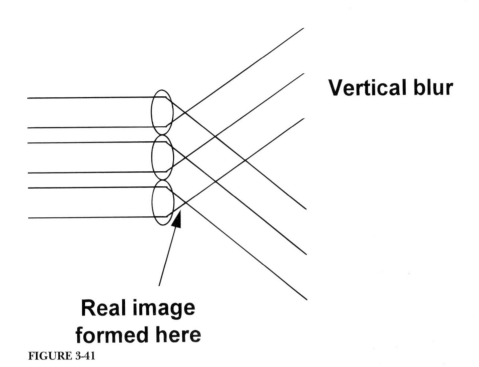

Vertical blur

Real image formed here

FIGURE 3-41

Notes

4

Neuro-
ophthalmology

QUESTIONS

1. On a T2-weighted MRI, which would appear hyperintense?

   A) Fat
   B) Blood in the carotid
   C) Bone
   D) Vitreous

2. A 30-year-old man was hit in his left eye at work and complains of sudden visual loss. You measure his best acuity to be light perception in this eye. Ophthalmic examination is normal. Which test does not rely on patient's interpretation of visual information?

   A) Red/green spectacle
   B) OKN drum
   C) Stereo acuity
   D) Color vision

3. A 15-year-old girl presented with 20/30 vision OD. Her CT scan showed an abnormality (Fig. 4-1). The most UNLIKELY finding would be:

   A) pigmented iris lesions
   B) a brother with the same problem
   C) good vision after surgical resection of the lesion
   D) propensity to develop CNS tumors

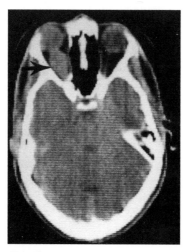

FIGURE 4-1

4. Which of the following DOES NOT distinguish optic neuropathy from amblyopia?

    A)   Brightness test
    B)   Color vision testing
    C)   Neutral density filters
    D)   Visual acuity with linear letters

Questions 5–10 (Figs. 4-2 to 4-6)

5. In which condition can psammoma bodies be found?

    A)   Figure 4-2
    B)   Figure 4-6
    C)   Figure 4-3
    D)   Figure 4-4

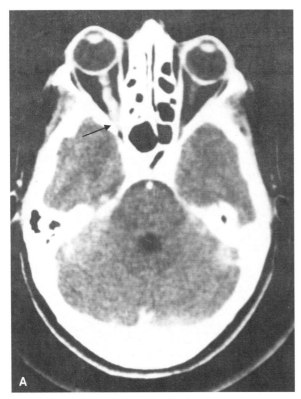

FIGURE 4-2. From K. Wright: Textbook of ophthalmology. Baltimore: Williams & Wilkins, 1997.

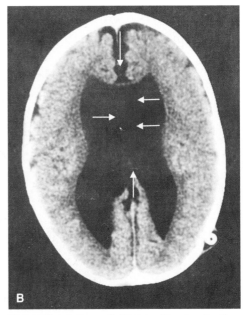

FIGURE 4-3. From K. Wright: Textbook of ophthalmology. Baltimore: Williams & Wilkins, 1997.

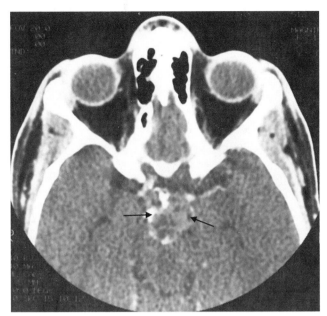

FIGURE 4-4. From K. Wright: Textbook of ophthalmology. Baltimore: Williams & Wilkins, 1997.

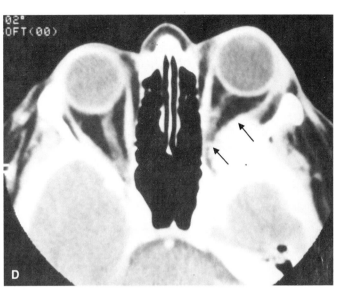

FIGURE 4-5. From K. Wright: Textbook of ophthalmology. Baltimore: Williams & Wilkins, 1997.

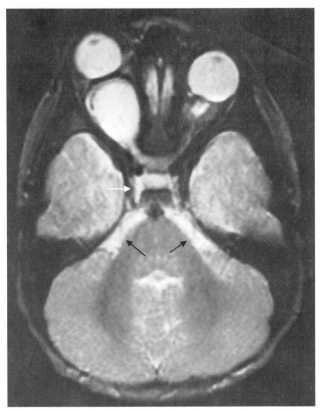

FIGURE 4-6. From K. Wright: Textbook of ophthalmology. Baltimore: Williams & Wilkins, 1997.

6. Which lesion may be found in association with the optic nerve shown in Figure 4-7?

    A) Figure 4-4
    B) Figure 4-3
    C) Figure 4-5
    D) Figure 4-2

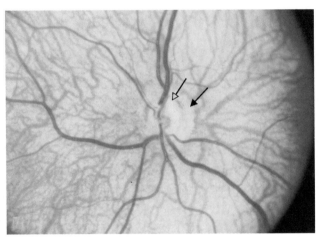

FIGURE 4-7. From K. Wright: Textbook of ophthalmology. Baltimore: Williams & Wilkins, 1997.

7. Which lesion caused the visual field defect shown in Figure 4-8?

    A) Figure 4-6
    B) Figure 4-2
    C) Figure 4-4
    D) Figure 4-3

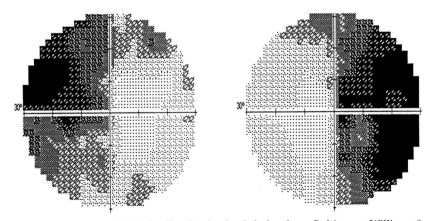

FIGURE 4-8. From K. Wright: Textbook of ophthalmology. Baltimore: Williams & Wilkins, 1997.

8. Figure 4-6 and the iris lesions shown in Figure 4-9 are found in the same patient. What syndrome does this patient have?

    A) DeMorsier's syndrome
    B) von Recklinghausen's disease
    C) Down's syndrome
    D) Gradenigo's syndrome

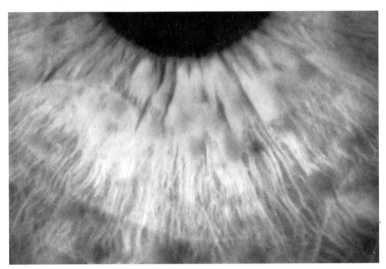

FIGURE 4-9

9. Which one of these conditions may need supplementation of pituitary hormones?

    A) Figure 4-2
    B) Figure 4-5
    C) Figure 4-6
    D) Figure 4-3

10. The optic nerve changes in Figure 4-10 are most frequently seen with which condition?

A) Figure 4-6
B) Figure 4-4
C) Figure 4-2
D) Figure 4-3

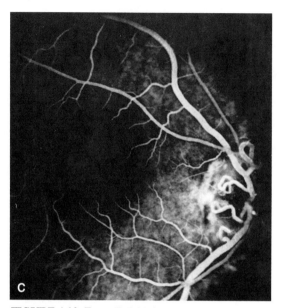

FIGURE 4-10. From K. Wright: Textbook of ophthalmology. Baltimore: Williams & Wilkins, 1997.

Questions 11–14

A 22-year-old white student presents with decreased visual acuity to 20/80 OU. He states that the vision in his left eye started to decline gradually over the past 3 months. His right eye has just recently become affected. His visual fields are shown in Figure 4-11.

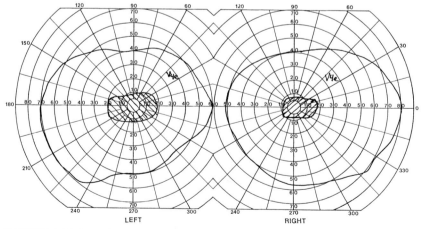

FIGURE 4-11. From K. Wright: Textbook of ophthalmology. Baltimore: Williams & Wilkins, 1997.

11. All of the following are possible causes for this condition EXCEPT:

   A)   alcohol-tobacco amblyopia
   B)   Leber's hereditary optic neuropathy
   C)   macular toxoplasmosis
   D)   bilateral occipital infarcts

12. You suspect Leber's hereditary optic neuropathy. What would be the best test to confirm your suspicion?

   A)   MRI scan of brain
   B)   Lumbar puncture
   C)   Serum electrophoresis
   D)   DNA analysis

13. Which fundus finding would be most suggestive of Leber's?

   A)   Sectoral optic atrophy
   B)   Optic nerve drusen
   C)   Hyperemic optic nerve with telangiectatic capillaries
   D)   Papilledema and a macular star

14. What percentage of his children will also be affected?

   A)   40%
   B)   None
   C)   100%
   D)   16%

15. Ingestion of all of the following can cause optic neuropathy EXCEPT:

   A)   isoniazid
   B)   methanol
   C)   ethambutol
   D)   ganciclovir

16. Where is a lesion that produces the visual field defect shown in Figure 4-12?

   A)   Right temporal lobe
   B)   Right parietal lobe
   C)   Right optic tract
   D)   Right optic nerve

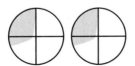

FIGURE 4-12. From K. Wright: Textbook of ophthalmology. Baltimore: Williams & Wilkins, 1997.

17. A 69-year-old man complains of intermittent diplopia for the past 3 years and denies
     any other systemic difficulties. Initially, the examination seems normal. The patient
     is asked to sustain left gaze (Fig. 4-13A), but has difficulty as shown at 30 seconds
     (Fig. 4-13B) and at 60 seconds (Fig. 4-13C). All of the following statements are true
     EXCEPT:

     A) he is more likely to develop dysthyroidism than an otherwise normal person his
         age
     B) the lack of acetylcholine receptor antibody in his blood makes myasthenia
         gravis an unlikely diagnosis
     C) cerebral MRI is unnecessary
     D) he is unlikely (<20% chance) to develop systemic muscular weakness

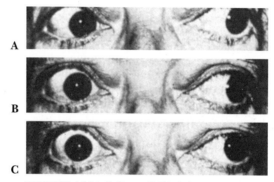

FIGURE 4-13A-C. From R.H. Osher and J.S.
Glaser. Am J Ophthalmol 1980;89;443–445.

18. A 35-year-old woman was referred for evaluation of ptosis and abnormal eye movements (Fig. 4-14). You might expect her to have any of the following EXCEPT:

    A) polychromatic lenticular deposits
    B) sluggishly reactive pupils
    C) 10-year-old photos showing bilateral ptosis
    D) French-Canadian ancestry

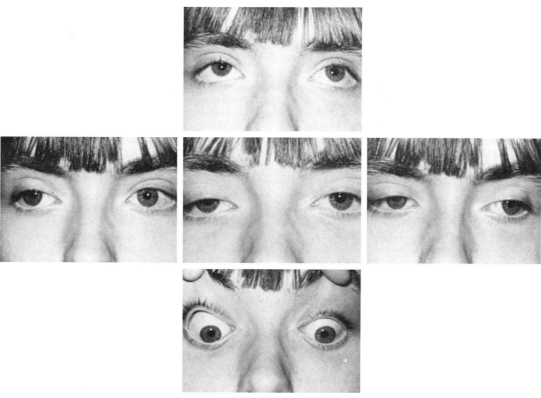

FIGURE 4-14. From N.R. Miller: Walsh and Hoyt's clinical neuro-ophthalmology. Volume 2: Autonomic nervous and ocular motor systems. Fourth Edition. Baltimore: Williams & Wilkins, 1985.

19. A 47-year-old woman develops headache and double vision. One of her midline sagittal MRIs is shown in Figure 4-15. On examination, she may have all of the following EXCEPT:

A) sixth nerve palsy
B) skew deviation
C) lid retraction
D) pupils that react well to a near stimulus but not to light

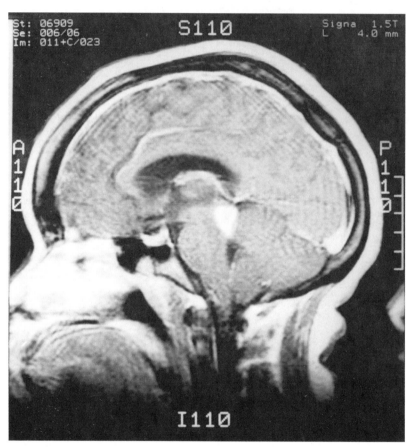

FIGURE 4-15. From N.R. Miller: Walsh and Hoyt's clinical neuro-ophthalmology. Volume 2: Autonomic nervous and ocular motor systems. Fourth Edition. Baltimore: Williams & Wilkins, 1985.

20. The patient shown in Figure 4-16 has normal vertical eye movements. The left eye developed left jerk nystagmus on attempted left gaze. Where is the most likely location of the causative lesion?

A) Left paramedian pontine reticular formation
B) Right third nerve nucleus
C) Left medial longitudinal fasciculus
D) Right medial longitudinal fasciculus

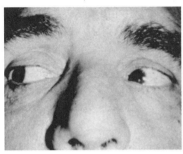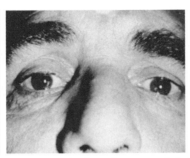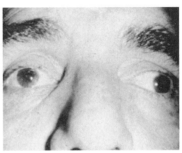

FIGURE 4-16. From N.R. Miller: Walsh and Hoyt's clinical neuro-ophthalmology. Volume 2: Autonomic nervous and ocular motor systems. Fourth Edition. Baltimore: Williams & Wilkins, 1985.

21. The patient in Figures 4-17, 4-18, and 4-19 has normal vertical eye movements. Where can her problem be localized?

A) Right sixth nerve nucleus
B) Left paramedian pontine reticular formation
C) Both medial longitudinal fasciculi
D) Right sixth nerve fascicle

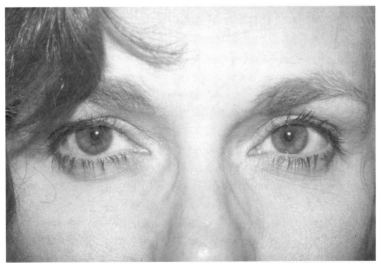

FIGURE 4-17. Attempted right gaze.

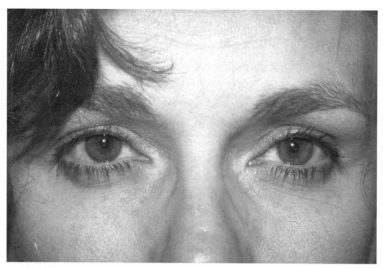

FIGURE 4-18. Primary position.

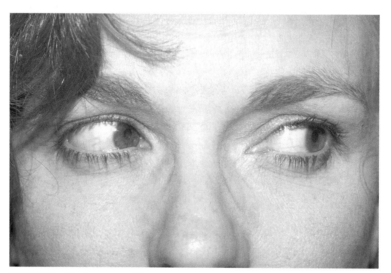

FIGURE 4-19. Attempted left gaze.

22. Which statement regarding the innervation of the extraocular muscles is FALSE?

    A)   The levator palpebrae is innervated by a fused central nucleus.
    B)   The superior oblique is innervated by the ipsilateral IV nucleus.
    C)   The inferior oblique is innervated by the ipsilateral III nucleus.
    D)   The superior rectus is innervated by the contralateral III nucleus.

23. Which one of the following conditions could be treated effectively with botulinum toxin (Botox)?

    A)   Bell's palsy
    B)   Hemifacial spasm
    C)   Myasthenia gravis
    D)   Strabismus in thyroid eye disease

Questions 24–26

A 55-year-old man who was in a car accident several days ago complains of intermittent vertical diplopia since the accident. His monocular acuity is 20/20 in each eye. His motility is diagramed in Figure 4-20.

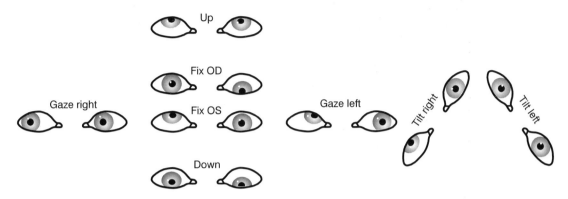

FIGURE 4-20. From K. Wright: Textbook of ophthalmology. Baltimore: Williams & Wilkins, 1997.

24. If only a single muscle is involved, which muscle is palsied?

   A)   Left superior rectus
   B)   Right inferior oblique
   C)   Right superior oblique
   D)   Left inferior rectus

25. What could be used to measure the amount of torsion that this patient has?

   A)   Double Maddox rods
   B)   Alternate cover test with prisms
   C)   Red filter and a light
   D)   Neutral density filters

26. Cover-uncover testing shows no shift (*orthotropia*), but alternate cover test shows a deviation neutralized with 12 PD base down prism in front of his right eye. What can this patient be told about his condition?

   A)   The injury from the accident is temporary and will resolve with time.
   B)   His symptoms and findings do not correspond to any organic neurologic condition.
   C)   This condition has been present for many years but has just recently been uncovered.
   D)   The accident has caused damage to nerves bilaterally.

Questions 27–35 Match each description with the corresponding structure from Figure 4-21.

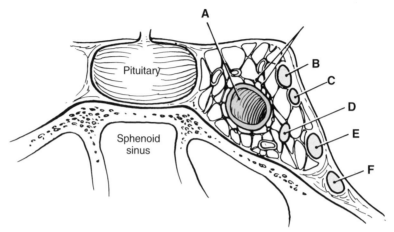

FIGURE 4-21. From K. Wright: Textbook of ophthalmology. Baltimore: Williams & Wilkins, 1997.

27. Innervates the primary abductor of the eye:

   A)   structure A
   B)   structure B
   C)   structure D
   D)   structure F

28. Efferent pupil constrictor fibers:

   A)   structure B
   B)   structure A
   C)   structure E
   D)   none of the above

29. Visual information from the retina:

   A)   structure A
   B)   structure B
   C)   structure C
   D)   none of the above

30. Corneal sensation:

   A)   structure E
   B)   structure D
   C)   structure F
   D)   structure A

31. Innervates the inferior oblique muscle:

    A) structure A
    B) structure C
    C) structure D
    D) structure B

32. Closes eyelid:

    A) structure F
    B) structure B
    C) structure A
    D) none of the above

33. Efferent fibers controlling lacrimation:

    A) structure A
    B) structure F
    C) structure E
    D) none of the above

34. Enters the orbit through the inferior orbital fissure

    A) structure B
    B) structure F
    C) structure E
    D) structure D

35. Which one of the following conditions would have positive forced ductions?

    A) Myasthenia gravis
    B) Thyroid eye disease
    C) Comitant strabismus
    D) Chronic progressive external ophthalmoplegia

Questions 36–37

A 63-year-old male diabetic patient has diplopia worse on upgaze. Ductions are full; however, on upgaze, the left eye only elevates halfway up (Fig. 4-22). His pupils and the remainder of the ocular examination are normal.

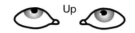

FIGURE 4-22. From K. Wright: Textbook of ophthalmology. Baltimore: Williams & Wilkins, 1997.

36. What finding would most likely accompany this examination?

    A) Right upper lid retraction
    B) Left nystagmus on upgaze
    C) Miotic left pupil
    D) Chin-down posturing

37. The patient is given a CT scan. Where would the lesion be located to cause this condition?

    A) Brainstem
    B) Orbital apex
    C) Cavernous sinus
    D) Juncture of the posterior communicating and internal carotid arteries

Questions 38–40 Match each condition to the location causing muscle weakness.

    A) Primary myopathy
    B) Neuromuscular junction
    C) Nerve axon
    D) Motor nucleus

38. Eaton-Lambert syndrome

39. Kearns-Sayre syndrome

40. Multiple sclerosis

41. Which syndrome includes cranial nerve III palsy, contralateral decreased sensation, and contralateral tremor in the extremities?

    A) Benedikt's syndrome
    B) Weber's syndrome
    C) Nothnagel's syndrome
    D) Tolosa-Hunt syndrome

42. Which one of the following is NOT an example of aberrant regeneration?

    A) Duane's retraction syndrome
    B) Crocodile tears
    C) Superior oblique myokymia
    D) Marcus Gunn jaw wink

43. Aberrant regeneration does NOT occur after injury to the oculomotor nerve with which one of the following conditions?

    A) Trauma
    B) Ischemia secondary to diabetes
    C) Tumor compression
    D) Aneurysm

44. Which cranial nerve is traumatized most commonly with a closed head injury?

    A) Cranial nerve III
    B) Cranial nerve II
    C) Cranial nerve IV
    D) Cranial nerve VI

Questions 45–48

Select the answer below that corresponds to the finding indicated.

    A) Diabetic cranial nerve III palsy
    B) Aneurysm
    C) Both
    D) Neither

45. Pupil commonly involved

46. Painful cranial nerve III palsy

47. Spontaneous resolution

48. Inability to abduct or adduct eye

49. A 74-year-old man developed difficulty reading and mild left arm weakness yesterday. Visual acuity is 20/20 OU and his visual fields are shown in Figures 4-23 and 4-24. What else would he be likely to have?

    A) Poor optokinetic nystagmus with the drum rotating left
    B) Poor optokinetic nystagmus with the drum rotating right
    C) Unformed visual hallucinations
    D) Formed visual hallucinations

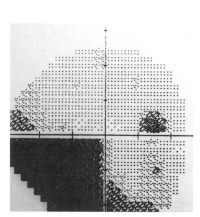

FIGURE 4-23   FIGURE 4-24

50. Supranuclear vertical gaze abnormalities can be seen in all of the following conditions EXCEPT:

    A) myasthenia gravis
    B) Parkinson's disease
    C) pineal region tumors
    D) ataxia-telangiectasia

51. Downbeat nystagmus may be a result of all of the following EXCEPT:

    A) normal lithium use
    B) a paraneoplastic syndrome
    C) craniocervical junction abnormalities
    D) pinealoma

52. A patient presents with irritation and conjunctival injection of the right eye. You find right orbicularis weakness, decreased ability to wrinkle the right forehead, slight right corneal anesthesia, and a small angle esodeviation develops on right gaze. What test would be most helpful?

    A) Tensilon test
    B) CT to rule out a left parietal lesion
    C) Thyroid function tests
    D) MRI to evaluate right cerebellopontine angle

53. What is the usual cause of hemifacial spasm?

A) Stroke

B) Dry eye

C) Facial nerve irritation by an adjacent blood vessel

D) Aberrant regeneration following Bell's palsy

54. All of the following statements are true of relative afferent pupillary defects (APD) EXCEPT:

A) In general, media opacities do not cause a relative APD.

B) Optic tract damage can result in an ipsilateral relative APD because of an asymmetric decussation in the chiasm.

C) The presence of a relative APD without any visual loss localizes damage to the contralateral brainstem.

D) Anisocoria is never associated directly with a relative APD.

55. A patient seeks ophthalmologic evaluation because a friend said his eyes "don't look right" (Fig. 4-25). More anisocoria was present in the dark than in the light. All of the following statements are true EXCEPT:

A) Neither pupil should constrict to pilocarpine 0.1%.

B) The responsible lesion could be interrupting the neural impulse as the neurons synapse in the ciliary ganglion.

C) The presence of a right abduction deficit would localize the lesion to the right cavernous sinus.

D) The right pupil would dilate poorly after cocaine 10% instillation.

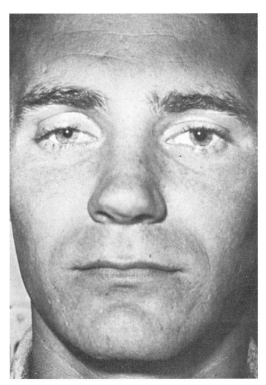

FIGURE 4-25. From N.R. Miller: Walsh and Hoyt's clinical neuro-ophthalmology. Volume 2: Autonomic nervous and ocular motor systems. Fourth Edition. Baltimore: Williams & Wilkins, 1985.

Questions 56–57

A 33-year-old recovery room nurse discovers her right pupil to be several millimeters larger than her left pupil. She denies diplopia, but she has had several headaches in the past week.

56. Findings helpful in diagnosing the etiology of her anisocoria include all of the following EXCEPT:

    A) 2 mm of right upper eyelid ptosis
    B) a right relative afferent pupillary defect
    C) a small right hypertropia develops on downgaze
    D) segmental contraction of the right iris

57. Her right pupil does not react to light, but otherwise the examination is normal. The next diagnostic step would be:

    A) 1 drop of 1% pilocarpine OU
    B) 1 drop of 0.1% pilocarpine OU
    C) cerebral arteriogram
    D) review of old photographs

58. The parasympathetic fibers to the lacrimal gland synapse in which ganglion?

    A) Geniculate
    B) Sphenopalatine
    C) Ciliary
    D) Superior cervical

59. Where is the cell body of the second order neuron in the sympathetic pathway for the pupil?

    A) Hypothalamus
    B) Superior cervical ganglion
    C) Ciliospinal center of Budge (C8–T2)
    D) Ciliary ganglion

Questions 60–64

Select the answer below that corresponds to the finding indicated.

    A)   First-order Horner's
    B)   Second-order Horner's
    C)   Third-order Horner's
    D)   All of the above

60. No dilation of the pupil after instillation of cocaine 10%

61. No dilation of the pupil after instillation of hydroxyamphetamine 1% (Paredrine)

62. Affected pupil smaller

63. Carotid dissection

64. Pancoast tumor

65. Which one of the following is a sign of congenital Horner's syndrome?

    A)   Iris heterochromia
    B)   Miotic pupil
    C)   Facial asymmetry
    D)   Unilateral epiphora

Questions 66–68

You see a patient in the ICU after cardiac bypass surgery. His right pupil is dilated and unreactive to light. You swing a light back and forth between his eyes.

66. What would be observed if he has a right afferent pupillary defect?

    A) When the light shines on the left eye, the left pupil dilates.
    B) When the light shines on the right eye, the left pupil dilates.
    C) When the light shines on the right eye, the left pupil constricts.
    D) Cannot be determined because the right eye is dilated.

67. No afferent pupillary defect is present. The ocular examination is unremarkable. Which drop placed in both eyes would provide the most additional information?

    A) Cocaine 10%
    B) Hydroxyamphetamine 1%
    C) Pilocarpine 0.1%
    D) Phenylephrine 2.5%

68. You decide to test the caloric response. Cold water is irrigated in the left ear. In what direction is the slow phase of the nystagmus?

    A) Left
    B) Right
    C) Up
    D) Down

69. What is the mechanism of action for edrophonium (Tensilon)?

    A) Inhibits acetylcholinesterase
    B) Releases acetylcholine (ACh) from the presynaptic terminal
    C) Directly binds to ACh sites on the receptor
    D) Prevents reuptake of ACh

70. What is the mechanism of action for cocaine?

    A) Inhibits Catechol-O-Methyl Transferase (COMT)
    B) Releases norepinephrine from the presynaptic terminal
    C) Directly binds to norepinephrine sites on the receptor
    D) Prevents reuptake of norepinephrine

71. What is the mechanism of action for hydroxyamphetamine (Paredrine)?

    A) Inhibits COMT
    B) Releases norepinephrine from the presynaptic terminal
    C) Directly binds to norepinephrine sites on the receptor
    D) Prevents reuptake of norepinephrine

72. What is the antidote for the crisis caused by an overdose of edrophonium (Tensilon)?

    A) Atropine
    B) Dantrolene
    C) Epinephrine
    D) Verapamil

73. Which one of the following is NOT a feature of Adie's pupil?

A) Vermiform movement of iris border
B) Hypersensitivity to parasympathomimetic drugs
C) Light-near dissociation
D) Anisocoria greater in the dark

Questions 74–75

A 44-year-old black woman noticed a change in vision yesterday. Today, visual acuity is 20/20 OD and 20/200 OS. There is a left relative afferent pupillary defect and a swollen left optic nerve head. The remainder of the examination is normal.

74. Of the following, which is the LEAST helpful historical factor?

A) Hyperthyroidism treated 1 year ago
B) Recent 1-month episode of left arm numbness
C) Hilar adenopathy on recent chest radiograph
D) Hypertension treated for 5 years

75. Additionally, she notes pain on eye movement. What is the best next step?

A) MRI
B) Oral prednisone
C) IV methylprednisolone
D) Observation and repeat examination in 1 month

Questions 76–77

A 72-year-old woman experienced three 10- to 15-minute episodes of "blurred vision" in the right eye over the past week. Her eye examination is normal.

76. The presence of which one of the following signs should elicit the most prompt attention to prevent permanent visual loss?

A) Right carotid bruit
B) Scalp tenderness
C) Blood pressure of 170/95
D) A cardiac murmur

77. This woman did not have any of the findings listed in the previous question. She also denied headache and numbness or weakness of her extremities. She did remember a 10-minute episode of double vision and recently has had difficulty chewing her breakfast because her jaw becomes tired. What would be the next step in the evaluation?

A) Carotid Dopplers
B) Antiphospholipid antibody levels
C) Erythrocyte sedimentation rate
D) Acetylcholine receptor antibody level

Questions 78–79

A 28-year-old woman developed diplopia on upgaze (Fig. 4-26). MRI of the brain was normal.

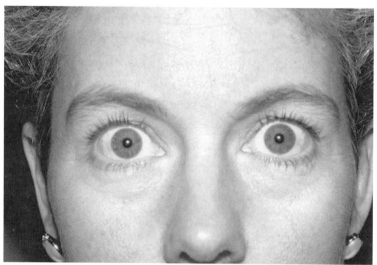

FIGURE 4-26

78. Compared with the normal population, she is more likely to develop:

    A) proptosis
    B) fatigable ptosis
    C) nonfatigable ophthalmoplegia
    D) all of the above

79. She was found to be hyperthyroid and was treated with radioactive iodine. Subsequently, she became hypothyroid and was treated with levothyroxine sodium (Synthroid). Now, 6 months later, she develops bilateral conjunctival injection and a right relative afferent pupillary defect. What is the most appropriate next step in management?

    A) Direct coronal CT scan of the orbits
    B) Thyroid function tests
    C) Oral prednisone
    D) Follow-up in 2 months

80. Neuroimaging would most likely be normal in an individual with which of the following syndromes?

    A) von Recklinghausen's disease
    B) Louis-Bar syndrome
    C) Bourneville's syndrome
    D) Sturge-Weber syndrome

Questions 81–86 Select the phakomatosis that matches the condition listed.

81. Seizures

    A) von Hippel-Lindau syndrome
    B) von Recklinghausen disease
    C) Louis-Bar syndrome
    D) Bourneville's syndrome

82. Glaucoma

    A) Wyburn-Mason syndrome
    B) Sturge-Weber syndrome
    C) Bourneville's syndrome
    D) von Hippel-Lindau syndrome

83. Retinal detachment

    A) von Hippel-Lindau syndrome
    B) Louis-Bar syndrome
    C) Wyburn-Mason syndrome
    D) von Recklinghausen disease

84. Astrocytic hamartomas

    A) Louis-Bar syndrome
    B) von Recklinghausen disease
    C) Sturge-Weber syndrome
    D) von Hippel-Lindau syndrome

85. Increased incidence of pheochromocytomas

    A) Louis-Bar syndrome
    B) von Hippel-Lindau syndrome
    C) Sturge-Weber syndrome
    D) Bourneville's syndrome

86. Thymic aplasia

    A) Wyburn-Mason syndrome
    B) Sturge-Weber syndrome
    C) von Hippel-Lindau syndrome
    D) Louis-Bar syndrome

87. Ocular pulsations may be seen in all of the following EXCEPT:

    A) neurofibromatosis
    B) carotid-cavernous sinus fistulas
    C) orbitoencephaloceles
    D) capillary hemangioma

88. A patient with multiple sclerosis could have all of the following EXCEPT:

    A) bitemporal visual field deficit
    B) retinal venous sheathing
    C) skew deviation
    D) amaurosis

89. Uhthoff's symptom describes:

    A) the decrease in vision with an increase in body temperature
    B) an electric shock sensation with neck flexion
    C) the inability to distinguish faces
    D) the ability to see moving objects but not stationary ones

90. A 29-year-old woman has had "migraine" headaches for several years. She recently developed episodes of "flashing lights off to the right" that affect her peripheral vision. Her automated perimetry is shown in Figures 4-27 and 4-28. The next step would be:

    A) cerebral MRI
    B) discontinue oral contraceptives
    C) sumatriptan (Imitrex)
    D) tangent screen

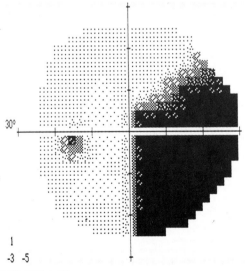

FIGURE 4-27

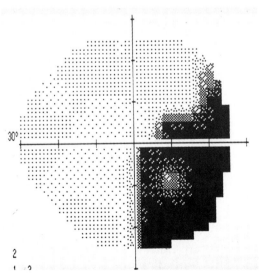

FIGURE 4-28

91. Which one of the following signs would NOT be expected with a classic migraine?

A) Premonitory aura
B) Scintillating lights
C) Headache
D) Persistent leg tingling and weakness

92. Which one of the following is NOT a criterion for the diagnosis of pseudotumor cerebri (idiopathic intracranial hypertension)?

A) Normal cerebrospinal fluid composition
B) Elevated opening pressure on lumbar puncture
C) Bilateral papilledema
D) Normal neuroimaging studies

93. Which one of the following describes the stereotypic patient with pseudotumor cerebri?

A) 75-year-old woman with history of TIAs
B) 58-year-old man with a type A personality
C) 35-year-old overweight woman
D) 15-year-old black man with a poor diet

94. A 68-year-old man developed a sudden onset of vomiting, imbalance, and double vision. On examination, he had a concomitant 10 PD left hypertropia and ataxia. What test should be ordered?

A) Cerebral arteriogram
B) Cerebral MRI and arteriography
C) Tensilon test
D) Carotid ultrasonography

95. Myasthenia patients are at higher risk for all of the following EXCEPT:

A) thymoma
B) Graves' disease
C) systemic lupus erythematosus
D) multiple sclerosis

96. Which muscles are affected most commonly in thyroid eye disease?

A) Medial rectus, inferior rectus
B) Superior rectus, inferior oblique
C) Lateral rectus, superior oblique
D) Inferior oblique, inferior rectus

97. A patient with thyroid eye disease has progressive loss of visual field. All of the following are possible treatments EXCEPT:

A) radiotherapy
B) surgical decompression of the orbit
C) optic nerve sheath decompression
D) steroids

98. Which one of the following statements is a conclusion of the Ischemic Optic Neuropathy Decompression Trial (IONDT)?

    A)   One third of the patients with optic nerve sheath decompression experienced improvement in acuity of three or more lines at 6 months.
    B)   The natural course of untreated Non-Arteritic Ischemic Optic Neuropathy (NAION) is progressive visual field loss.
    C)   The efficacy of optic nerve sheath decompression is equivocal and further study is needed.
    D)   Patients with optic nerve sheath decompression had better visual acuity at 6 months compared with the observation cohort.

99. Which treatment in the Optic Neuritis Treatment Trial had the highest rate of recurrence?

    A)   Oral prednisone alone
    B)   IV methylprednisolone alone
    C)   IV methylprednisolone and oral prednisone
    D)   Observation

100. Which one of the following is NOT involved with vertical eye movements?

    A)   Frontal eye fields
    B)   Paramedian pontine reticular formation
    C)   Interstitial nucleus of Cajal
    D)   Trochlear nucleus

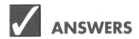 **ANSWERS**

1. D) Vitreous

MRIs allow excellent soft tissue definition by varying radiofrequency pulse sequences and measuring the resulting signal produced by the tissue. T1- and T2-weighted MRIs are able to highlight structures by the intensity of the signal generated after the magnetic pulse. Table 4-1 lists some of the differences between T1- and T2-weighted images. Air, fast moving blood, and bone generally produce no signal and are thus hypointense on the MRI. Fat and vitreous are opposite to one another in both the T1- and T2-weightings.

TABLE 4-1. Relative Signal Intensity on T1- and T2-weighted MRI Scan

Tissue	T1-weighted	T2-weighted
Brain		
white matter	Bright	Mod. Dark
gray matter	Mod. Dark	Bright
CSF	Very Dark	Very Bright
MS plaque	Dark	Bright
Infarct	Dark	Bright
Tumor	Dark	Bright
Abscess	Dark	Bright
Water	Very Dark	Very Bright
Fat	Bright	Dark
Cortical Bone	Dark	Dark
Air Dark	Dark	
Cyst	Very Dark	Very Bright
Tissue enhanced with gadolinium		
Low concentration	Very Bright	Bright
High concentration	Mod. Dark	Very Dark
Muscle	Dark	Dark
Hematoma		
Acute	Mod. dark	Dark
Subacute	Bright rim	Bright
Chronic	Dark rim +/− bright center	Dark rim +/− bright center

From Wright K. Textbook of ophthalmology. Baltimore: Williams & Wilkins, 1997.

2. B) OKN drum

A number of tests can be used to determine whether a patient has functional visual loss. Direct tests do not require the patient to verbally respond or interpret the visual information. Tests such as the swinging light test, optokinetic nystagmus response, and mirror test make it very difficult for a patient to feign disease. Indirect tests rely on the patient's cooperation and allow more definite measurement of visual acuity in the "injured" eye.

3. C) good vision after surgical resection of the lesion

This girl has an optic nerve glioma. Optic nerve gliomas have a fusiform appearance on CT scan. Optic nerve meningiomas, conversely, appear as parallel thickening of the optic nerve sheath (*railroad track sign*) and may have associated calcification. The only way to remove an optic nerve glioma is to remove the optic nerve. Optic nerve gliomas, Lisch nodules, and CNS tumors are often seen in association with neurofibromatosis type 1 (NF-1). NF-1 is inherited in an autosomal dominant manner, so this girl's brother could have the same problem.

4. D) Visual acuity with linear letters

Optic neuropathy and amblyopia may both occur in children. Several tests may help to distinguish between these entities. Brightness sense is diminished in optic neuropathy, not amblyopia. Color vision testing helps differentiate because color vision is not affected by amblyopia but decreased with optic neuritis. Neutral density filters would reduce visual acuity with optic neuropathy, but in amblyopia, acuity actually improves. Visual acuity tested by linear letters is reduced in both amblyopia and optic neuritis.

5. A) Figure 4-2

6. B) Figure 4-3

7. C) Figure 4-4

8. B) von Recklinghausen's disease

9. D) Figure 4-3

10. C) Figure 4-2

   Figure 4-2 = nerve sheath meningioma
   Figure 4-3 = absence of the septum pellucidum
   Figure 4-4 = suprasellar craniopharyngioma
   Figure 4-5 = sphenoid wing meningioma
   Figure 4-6 = optic nerve glioma

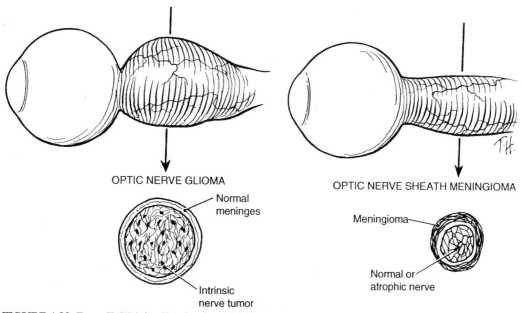

FIGURE 4-29. From K. Wright: Textbook of ophthalmology. Baltimore: Williams & Wilkins, 1997.

Optic nerve sheath gliomas and meningiomas can readily be distinguished on CT because of their appearance (Fig. 4-29). The glioma produces fusiform enlargement, whereas the meningioma produces the railroad track sign on CT. Gliomas, Lisch nodules (see Fig. 4-9), absence of the sphenoid wing, plexiform neurofibromas, and café-au-lait skin lesions are all manifestations of neurofibromatosis, or *von Recklinghausen's disease.*

Meningiomas have proliferation of benign meningothelial cells in whorls. Calcified psammoma bodies are commonly found. They cause damage by compression of adjacent structures. Lesions of the sphenoid wing can compress the optic nerve and cause visual field loss. Optic atrophy, proptosis, and optociliary shunt vessels (see Fig. 4-10) can be found with this condition.

Suprasellar craniopharyngiomas are found more commonly in children and young adults and are derived from remnants of Rathke's pouch. They are located near the pituitary and optic chiasm and, with growth, compress these structures. A bitemporal hemianopsia (see Fig. 4-8) has resulted from such a lesion. These lesions are often calcified and can be seen readily on CT scan.

Absence of the septum pellucidum can be found as part of DeMorsier's syndrome (septo-optic dysplasia) along with optic nerve hypoplasia (see Fig. 4-7) and pituitary abnormalities. These patients should have pituitary hormone studies because they may require supplementation.

11. C)   macular toxoplasmosis

Macular toxoplasmosis is a congenital infection that affects central vision from birth. All of the other conditions may cause acquired bilateral central scotomas. Bilateral occipital infarcts would be extremely rare in such a young patient.

12. D)   DNA analysis

13. C)   Hyperemic optic nerve with telangiectatic capillaries

14. B)   None

Leber's hereditary optic neuropathy (LHON) is caused by an abnormality in mitochondrial DNA. Several mutations have been identified, including a nucleotide substitution at position 11,778 of the mitochondrial DNA coding for subunit 4 of NADH dehydrogenase. Because mitochondrial DNA is only transmitted along the maternal line, men cannot pass this disease to their offspring.

In the acute phase, the optic nerve in LHON is hyperemic and swollen with telangiectatic capillaries. The nerve does not leak on fluorescein angiography. Later stages may only manifest optic atrophy.

15. D)   ganciclovir

A large number of medications have been associated with optic neuropathy. Among them are the antituberculous drugs isoniazid and ethambutol. Ganciclovir has not been described to cause an optic neuropathy.

16. A) Right temporal lobe

A homonymous visual field defect is caused by a lesion posterior to the chiasm. The homonymous left superotemporal quadrantanopia in Figure 4-30 is caused by injury to the inferior fibers that must detour through the temporal lobe to avoid the ventricles (Meyer's loop).

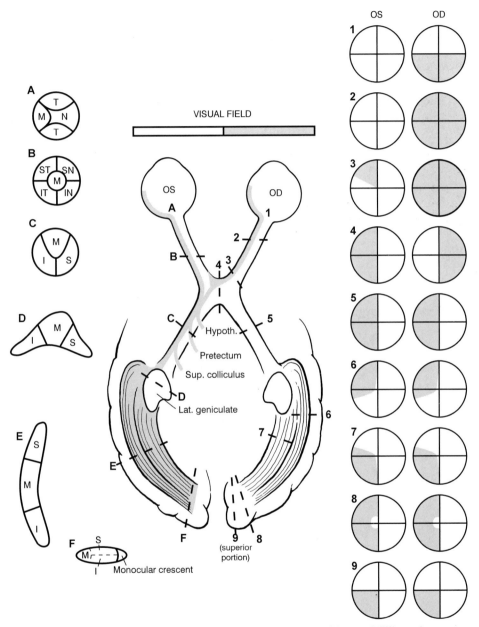

FIGURE 4-30. From K. Wright: Textbook of ophthalmology. Baltimore: Williams & Wilkins, 1997.

17. B) the lack of acetylcholine receptor antibody in his blood makes myasthenia gravis an unlikely diagnosis

Figure 4-13 demonstrates fatigable ophthalmoplegia, a sign virtually pathognomonic for myasthenia gravis. The patient has no systemic weakness and thus has ocular myasthenia gravis. Acetylcholine receptor antibodies with no systemic involvement are only found in about 60% of patients. Dysthyroidism is more common in patients with myasthenia gravis. Tensilon testing, not MRI, should be obtained. When a patient has isolated ocular myasthenia gravis for more than 2 years, there is a less than 20% chance that he or she will develop systemic disease.

18.   B)   sluggishly reactive pupils

Figure 4-14 shows generalized ophthalmoplegia and ptosis, findings compatible with either chronic progressive external ophthalmoplegia (CPEO) or myasthenia gravis. Neither of these conditions affect pupillary reactivity. Polychromatic lenticular deposits are seen in myotonic dystrophy, and patients with oculopharyngeal dystrophy often have a French-Canadian ancestry. CPEO can be seen in both of these conditions. Patients with CPEO typically have a long history of gradually worsening ptosis that can be documented in old photographs. This patient could also have cardiac conduction abnormalities and pigmentary retinopathy (Kearns-Sayre).

19.   A)   sixth nerve palsy

The MRI shows abnormal signal in the area of the dorsal midbrain (Fig. 4-31, *arrow*). Skew deviation, lid retraction (Collier's sign), and pupillary light-near dissociation are all signs of Parinaud's dorsal midbrain syndrome. The sixth nerve arises in the pons (Fig. 4-31, *curved arrow*) and should not be affected by this lesion.

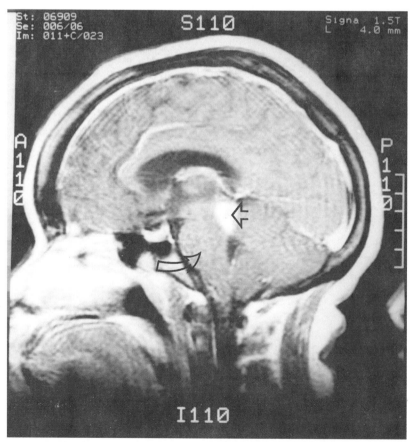

FIGURE 4-31

20. D)   Right medial longitudinal fasciculus

Figure 4-32 shows normal horizontal movement of the left eye and poor adduction of the right eye. The combination of abnormal adduction and contralateral abducting nystagmus represents an internuclear ophthalmoplegia. Damage has occurred to the interneurons connecting the left sixth nerve nucleus and the right third nerve nucleus (medial rectus subdivision) traveling in the right medial longitudinal fasciculus. Poor adduction could also occur from third nerve dysfunction, but this patient has no ptosis, mydriasis, or involvement of the superior rectus, inferior rectus, or inferior oblique muscles. Damage to the left paramedian pontine reticular formation results in a left gaze palsy.

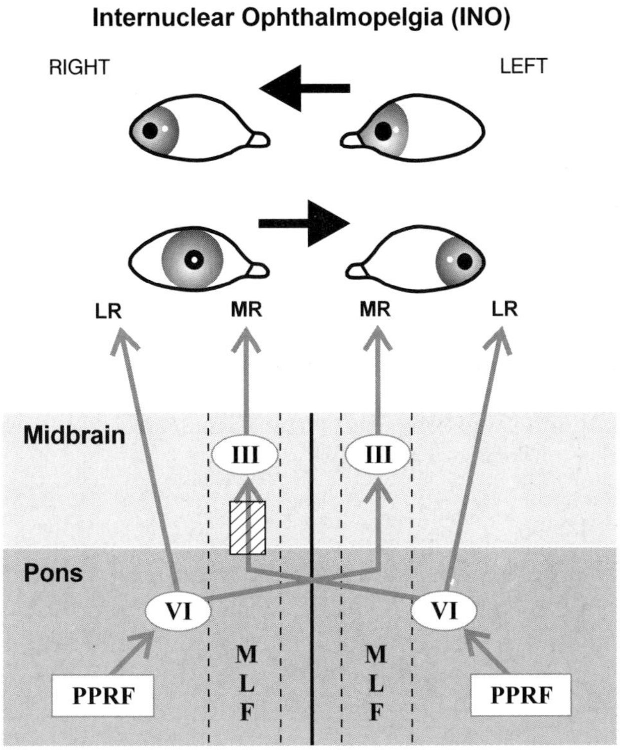

Internuclear Ophthalmopelgia (INO)

FIGURE 4-32. From K. Wright: Textbook of ophthalmology. Baltimore: Williams & Wilkins, 1997.

21. A)   Right sixth nerve nucleus

Figures 4-17, 4-18, and 4-19 show a right gaze palsy. The sixth nerve nucleus contains both sixth nerve axons and interneurons destined for the contralateral medial rectus subnucleus via the medial longitudinal fasciculus. Thus, a lesion of the sixth nerve nucleus would produce an ipsilateral gaze palsy. Left paramedian pontine reticular formation damage would result in a left gaze palsy. Damage to both medial longitudinal fasciculi would cause a bilateral internuclear ophthalmoplegia. A lesion of the right sixth nerve fascicle would produce a right abduction deficit.

22. B)   The superior oblique is innervated by the ipsilateral IV nucleus.

As shown in Figure 4-33, the levator palpebrae are innervated by a fused central nucleus. Therefore, unilateral ptosis as a result of a nuclear lesion is not possible. Ipsilateral nuclei innervate the inferior rectus, medial rectus, inferior oblique, and lateral rectus muscles. The nuclei controlling the superior rectus and superior oblique muscles have crossed projections. The superior oblique muscle is innervated by the *contralateral* IV nucleus.

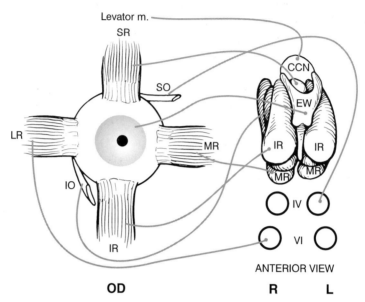

FIGURE 4-33. From K. Wright: Textbook of ophthalmology. Baltimore: Williams & Wilkins, 1997.

23. B)   Hemifacial spasm

Botulinum toxin produces a temporary blockade of acetylcholine release at the motor nerve terminal. This treatment has been used for nonrestrictive strabismus and for reducing muscle spasms such as in essential blepharospasm and hemifacial spasm. In Bell's palsy, the muscle is already weak, thus injection of botulinum toxin would have no benefit. Variable weakness (myasthenia gravis) would not be helped by paralyzing a muscle with botulinum toxin.

24. C)   Right superior oblique

The Park's three-step test can be used to determine which muscle is palsied. The patient has a right hypertropia in primary position, which is worse on left gaze. The hypertropia also worsens on right head tilt. This pattern indicates a right superior oblique palsy.

25. A)   Double Maddox rods

The Maddox rod takes a point source of light and converts it into a straight line. With a Maddox rod in front of each eye (in a trial frame), the patient can rotate one of the rods until the lines he sees in each eye are parallel. The difference in the axes of the two Maddox rods is the degree of torsion. The alternate cover test allows the measurement of horizontal and vertical tropias, but it cannot be used for torsion.

Red filter and a muscle light will diagnose vertical and horizontal diplopia not torsion. Neutral density filters reduce overall luminance and may be helpful for assessing afferent pupillary defects.

26. C) This condition has been present for many years but has just recently uncovered.

Vertical fusion amplitudes are useful for distinguishing congenital from acquired fourth nerve palsies. Normal vertical fusion amplitudes are 3 to 5 PD. In congenital IV palsy, patient can develop amplitudes of 10 to 25 PD, and large vertical fusion amplitudes are an indication of a longstanding vertical deviation usually since childhood. If the cover-uncover test shows no deviation but the alternate cover test discloses a deviation, this means a phoria and indicates fusion amplitude. In this case the patient has a right hyperphoria of 12 PD; this means that the vertical fusion amplitude is at least 12 PD (much more than normal), indicating a longstanding deviation. Although trauma is the most common cause of acquired IV palsy, it is also (often coincidentally) the trigger that allows congenital palsies to be manifest. In addition to increased vertical fusion amplitudes, these patients may have a head tilt to the contralateral side to reduce the hypertropia. Old photographs may be helpful in demonstrating this feature.

27. C) structure D (Fig. 4-34)

The primary abductor of the eye is the lateral rectus, innervated by cranial nerve VI.

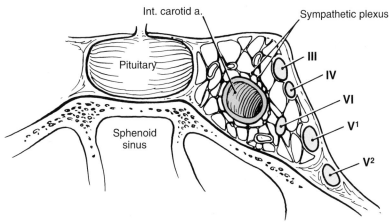

FIGURE 4-34. From K. Wright: Textbook of ophthalmology. Baltimore: Williams & Wilkins, 1997.

28. A) structure B

Parasympathetic neurons to the pupil constrictor travel with cranial nerve III to the ciliary ganglion where they synapse and then join the short ciliary nerves.

29. D) none of the above

The optic nerve carries visual information from the retina. Cranial nerve II is not pictured on this section.

30. A) structure E

Corneal sensation is subserved by branches of V1.

31. D)   structure B

The inferior oblique receives innervation from the inferior division of cranial nerve III.

32. D)   none of the above

Eyelid closure is caused by action of the orbicularis muscles controlled by cranial nerve VII. Eyelid opening results from the levator palpebrae (cranial nerve III) and Müller's muscle (sympathetics).

33. D)   none of the above

Lacrimation is controlled by parasympathetic neurons that travel from the superior salivatory nucleus along the nervus intermedius through the greater petrosal canal. At the pterygopalatine ganglion, the nerves synapse and postganglionic branches join cranial nerve V2 to travel to the lacrimal gland.

34. B)   structure F

The superior orbital fissure transmits the branches of cranial nerve V1, III, IV, and VI. Cranial nerve V2 enters the orbit through the inferior orbital fissure.

35. B)   Thyroid eye disease

Positive forced ductions indicate a restrictive process that may be caused by thyroid eye disease, blow-out fractures, fat adherence syndrome, and Brown's syndrome, among others. Disorders of the neuromuscular junction (myasthenia) and of the muscle itself (CPEO) do not cause restriction.

36. A)   Right upper lid retraction

This patient has an isolated superior division of cranial nerve III paresis affecting the left superior rectus and levator palpebrae. The most likely cause for this condition is a diabetic ischemic neuropathy. The weakened levator would cause a left ptosis. He can compensate for this by overstimulating the levator to raise the left lid, consequently raising the right lid higher. Mechanically lifting the left lid will produce a paradoxic right ptosis.

37. B)   Orbital apex

The only location at which an oculomotor superior division nerve palsy could occur without affecting additional cranial nerves or the inferior division of cranial nerve III is in the orbital apex. Posterior to the orbital apex, the superior and inferior divisions are joined, and a compressive lesion selective to one division would be very improbable. A unilateral ptosis does not occur with a nuclear lesion.

38. B)   Neuromuscular junction

Eaton-Lambert syndrome is thought to be an autoimmune disease similar to myasthenia gravis. Abnormalities of conduction at the neuromuscular junction lead to muscle weakness and fatigue. Ocular manifestations are less common with Eaton-Lambert than with myasthenia.

39. A)   Primary myopathy

CPEO and related conditions such as Kearns-Sayre syndrome have abnormalities caused by mutations in mitochondrial DNA. Biopsies of the muscles of these patients demonstrate "ragged red fibers." Kearns-Sayre syndrome also includes pigmentary retinopathy, cardiac conduction abnormalities, and other systemic findings.

40. C)   Nerve axon

The primary pathologic process in multiple sclerosis is demyelination of axons. Multiple sclerosis should be considered when the signs and symptoms cannot be localized to a single lesion.

41. A)   Benedikt's syndrome

The location of a lesion affecting the oculomotor nerve can be determined by the associated neurologic deficits. An oculomotor nuclear lesion also involving the ipsilateral cerebral peduncle causes contralateral hemiparesis (*Weber's syndrome*). Cranial nerve III palsy with contralateral decreased sensation and contralateral tremor (red nucleus affected) is *Benedikt's syndrome. Nothnagel's syndrome* has involvement of the brachium conjunctivum and ipsilateral cerebellar ataxia.

Tolosa-Hunt syndrome, caused by inflammation of the cavernous sinus, involves multiple cranial nerves. Prompt resolution occurs with corticosteroid treatment.

42. C)   Superior oblique myokymia

Superior oblique myokymia is an episodic twitching of the superior oblique muscle. Patients may experience a slight rotatory sensation lasting from seconds to minutes. The exact cause is unknown, but carbamazepine or propranolol has been effective treatments.

43. B)   Ischemia secondary to diabetes

Damage to the oculomotor nerve with trauma or compressive lesions can cause aberrant regeneration. Ischemic neuropathy does not result in aberrant regeneration.

44. C)   Cranial nerve IV

The trochlear nerve has the longest intracranial course and is the most commonly injured nerve following closed head injury. Cranial nerve VI palsy can also be injured with head trauma. Any condition that causes increased intracranial pressure (pseudotumor cerebri, tumor, hydrocephalus) may result in cranial nerve VI palsy.

45. B)   Aneurysm

Aneurysms damage nerves by extrinsic compression. The parasympathetic pupillomotor fibers controlling the pupil are found on the outside of the oculomotor nerve and are the first to be injured with external pressure. Diabetic microvascular insults affect the central fibers of the nerve to a greater degree than the outer fibers, and as a result, pupil involvement is less common (<20%).

46. C)   Both

Cranial nerve III palsy caused by aneurysm is almost invariably painful; palsy from diabetes may be painful or painless.

47.   A)   Diabetic cranial nerve III palsy

Diabetic nerve palsies will usually resolve over 2 to 4 months. There may be some slight residual damage. If the palsy does not resolve spontaneously, the possibility of an aneurysm must be investigated.

48.   D)   Neither

This indicates involvement of both the medial rectus (cranial nerve III) and lateral rectus (cranial nerve VI). It would be very uncommon for either diabetic microvascular or aneurysmal compressive lesions to involve both of these nerves simultaneously.

49.   A)   Poor optokinetic nystagmus with the drum rotating left

The visual fields show a left, inferior, homonymous hemianopsia. This field deficit, in combination with a left hemiparesis, indicates damage to the right parietal lobe. Acutely, ipsilateral pursuit may be affected by parietal lesions. Thus, the patient could have difficulty pursuing the optokinetic drum as it rotates to the left, and poor optokinetic nystagmus would result. Unformed visual hallucinations typically occur with occipital lobe damage, whereas formed visual hallucinations are associated with temporal lobe lesions.

50.   A)   myasthenia gravis

Myasthenia gravis might produce ophthalmoplegia that mimics supranuclear vertical gaze abnormalities, but the pathophysiology is at the acetylcholine receptor. Parkinson's disease, pineal region tumors (dorsal midbrain syndrome), and ataxia-telangiectasia all can cause supranuclear gaze palsy.

51.   D)   pinealoma

Downbeat nystagmus has been associated with both therapeutic and toxic lithium levels. The nystagmus does not necessarily resolve after the lithium is stopped. It has been reported as a remote effect of cancer (paraneoplastic cerebellar degeneration); gynecologic malignancy and small cell carcinoma of the lung are implicated most frequently. Craniocervical junction abnormalities (tumor, syrinx, Arnold-Chiari malformations) can be ruled out with MRI. Pinealomas or other lesions in the dorsal midbrain result in Parinaud's dorsal midbrain syndrome. Features include contraction-retraction nystagmus, upgaze paralysis, and light-near dissociation.

52.   D)   MRI to evaluate right cerebellopontine angle

This patient has corneal exposure as a result of partial right facial nerve palsy (orbicularis weakness, inability to wrinkle forehead). Right corneal anesthesia indicates right trigeminal nerve dysfunction. A mild right abducens nerve palsy would produce an esodeviation on right gaze. These three cranial nerves are in close proximity in the cerebellopontine angle. Myasthenia gravis could produce facial weakness and ophthalmoplegia but not corneal anesthesia. Signs of Grave's disease would include conjunctival injection, irritation, and ophthalmoplegia but not facial weakness. A parietal lesion might cause contralateral facial anesthesia and lower facial weakness, but weakness of the forehead is a sign of peripheral facial nerve dysfunction.

53. C)   Facial nerve irritation by an adjacent blood vessel

Hemifacial spasm is typically caused by irritation of the facial nerve as it exits the brainstem. Rarely, compression by tumor may cause this condition. Dry eye may result in blepharospasm but not spasm of the lower facial musculature. Aberrant regeneration of the facial nerve may result in inappropriate muscle contraction, but this should follow a pattern (i.e., orbicularis contraction on attempted smiling).

54. B)   Optic tract damage can result in an ipsilateral relative APD because of an asymmetric decussation in the chiasm.

A contralateral relative APD would be present if the optic tract was damaged because relatively more nasal fibers from the contralateral eye cross in the chiasm. Approximately 52% of the optic nerve axons cross in the chiasm, whereas 48% remain ipsilateral.

Cataracts, vitreous hemorrhage, and hyphema generally do not produce relative APDs, although extremely dense opacities have been reported to produce small relative APDs. Damage to the pupillomotor fibers after they separate from the visual fibers in the midbrain can result in a small contralateral relative APD without visual loss because of the asymmetric decussation in the chiasm. Anisocoria is caused by asymmetric efferent pupillomotor input. Asymmetric afferent pupillomotor damage does not cause asymmetric input to the efferent pupillomotor system (Edinger-Westphal nuclei) because of its double decussation in the chiasm and posterior commissure.

55. B)   The responsible lesion could be interrupting the neural impulse as the neurons synapse in the ciliary ganglion.

The patient has right ptosis and miosis, or a right Horner's syndrome. The sympathetic axons travel through the ciliary ganglion but do not synapse. A right abduction deficit could represent a sixth nerve palsy. The postganglionic sympathetic chain and the sixth nerve travel together only in the cavernous sinus. Thus, a cavernous sinus lesion would be most likely if an abduction deficit were present. Parasympathetic denervation supersensitivity is not present in Horner's syndrome, so neither pupil should constrict to dilute pilocarpine. Cocaine inhibits the reuptake of norepinephrine and causes dilation if the sympathetic chain is intact. In Horner's syndrome, no norepinephrine is present; thus the pupil will not dilate.

56. B)   a right relative afferent pupillary defect

A relative afferent pupillary defect never causes anisocoria because the pupillary fiber decussations in the chiasm and posterior commissure ensure equal efferent input to both iris sphincter muscles. Right upper eyelid ptosis and a right hypertropia on downgaze could both be signs of third nerve dysfunction (levator palpebrae and inferior rectus weakness, respectively). Segmental iris contraction is a sign of Adie's tonic pupil.

57.   B)   1 drop of 0.1% pilocarpine OU

You suspect her anisocoria may be pharmacologic because of the lack of other findings. If so, her right pupil should not constrict to 1% pilocarpine. However, if you proceed with 1% pilocarpine and her pupils both constrict, she still could have either an Adie's tonic pupil or a partial oculomotor nerve palsy. At that point, it is too late to use the 0.1% pilocarpine drops. Thus, testing for denervation supersensitivity (0.1% pilocarpine) should be done first. Cerebral arteriogram is appropriate if testing indicates third nerve dysfunction. Old photographs are most helpful if physiologic anisocoria is suspected.

58.   B)   Sphenopalatine

The primary parasympathetic nerve cell bodies are located in the superior salivatory nucleus. Their axons leave the brain with the nervus intermedius (glossopalatine) nerve to travel with cranial nerve VII through the geniculate ganglion and then emerge from the petrous portion of the sphenoid bone as the greater superficial petrosal nerve. The greater superficial petrosal nerve is then joined by the secondary sympathetics from the deep petrosal nerve and enter the pterygoid canal (vidian canal). The vidian nerve emerges from the pterygoid canal and enters the sphenopalatine ganglion (pterygopalatine) where the primary parasympathetic fibers synapse and then exit as secondary parasympathetic fibers. These secretomotor fibers then join the zygomatic nerve (a branch of the maxillary division of cranial nerve V), which sends a communicating branch that enters the lacrimal gland. Most references state that this communicating branch joins and travels with the sensory lacrimal nerve to the lacrimal gland. However, our dissections have shown that the communicating branch usually enters the lacrimal gland directly.

The geniculate ganglion is transversed by cranial nerve VII and contains the cell bodies that provide the sense of taste from the anterior two-thirds of the tongue.

The ciliary ganglion is the intraorbital location where the primary parasympathetic fibers from the Edinger-Westphal nucleus synapse with the secondary parasympathetic nerves. The secondary parasympathetic fibers innervate the ciliary body and iris sphincter muscle to provide accommodation and constriction of the pupil.

The cell bodies of the secondary sympathetic fibers, which provide innervation to the superior tarsal muscle, the pupillary dilator muscle, facial blood vessels, skin and sweat glands, reside in the superior cervical ganglion.

59. C)   Ciliospinal center of Budge (C8–T2)

The sympathetic pathway consists of a chain of three neurons. The first neuron travels from the hypothalamus along the brainstem to synapse in the intermediolateral column of the spinal cord, the ciliospinal center of Budge. The second order neuron exits the brainstem about the level of T1 and joins the cervical sympathetic chain. At the superior cervical ganglion, the second order neuron synapses with the third order neuron, which travels along the carotid plexus. Branches join the ophthalmic division of the trigeminal nerve and pass through the ciliary ganglion to the nasociliary and short ciliary nerves (Fig. 4-35).

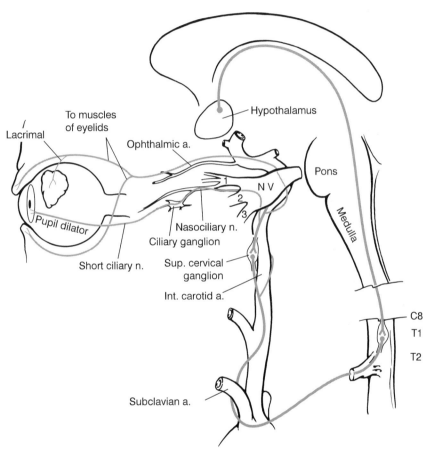

FIGURE 4-35. From K. Wright: Textbook of ophthalmology. Baltimore: Williams & Wilkins, 1997.

60. D)   All of the above

61. C)   Third-order Horner's

62. D)   All of the above

63. C)   Third-order Horner's

64.   B)   Second-order Horner's

Horner's syndrome is a result of interruption of sympathetic input to the eye. The classic triad consists of ptosis, miosis, and anhidrosis. Pharmacologic tests with cocaine and hydroxyamphetamine help to localize the specific interrupted neuron that causes the Horner's (Table 4-2). Cocaine prevents reuptake of norepinephrine into the presynaptic terminal from the synaptic cleft. With the sympathetics intact, cocaine increases the duration that norepinephrine remains in the synaptic cleft, causing pupillary dilation. In Horner's syndrome (first, second, and third order), there is little activity at the cleft and hence no dilation. Hydroxyamphetamine causes

TABLE 4-2. Evaluation of Anisocoria

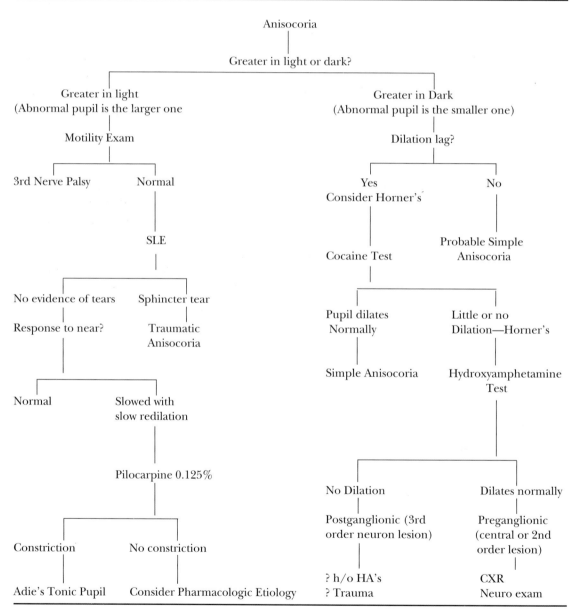

From Wright K. Textbook of ophthalmology. Baltimore: Williams & Wilkins, 1997.

the release of norepinephrine from the presynaptic terminal. In first or second order Horner's, this results in pupillary dilation. If the third order neuron is injured, it is unable to release norepinephrine and the pupil remains miotic.

Localization of the lesion in Horner's syndrome can also be made by the accompanying findings. A Pancoast tumor at the apex of the lung is in close proximity to the location at which the sympathetics exit the spinal column. Neck surgery can disrupt portions of the cervical sympathetic chain. Carotid dissection can damage the sympathetic plexus as it ascends along the artery.

65. A)   Iris heterochromia

Sympathetic innervation plays a role in the development of pigmentation of the iris. Congenital interruption of the sympathetics to one eye will result in the ipsilateral iris having less pigment than the fellow eye.

66. B)   When the light shines on the right eye, the left pupil dilates.

One dilated pupil does not preclude the detection of an afferent pupillary defect. Because the pupillary efferents are equal bilaterally, the consensual light response can be used instead of the direct response to detect an afferent defect. With damage to the right optic nerve, both pupils will dilate when the light swings from left to right.

67. C)   Pilocarpine 0.1%

The differential of a dilated pupil includes traumatic mydriasis, Adie's pupil, and pharmacologic dilation. Iris sphincter tears or a history of blunt trauma would be present with traumatic mydriasis. The other two possibilities can be differentiated by using dilute pilocarpine. Adie's tonic pupil is hypersensitive to parasympathomimetics and will constrict with pilocarpine 0.1%. Acute Adie's, however, may not constrict and can mimic pharmacologic dilation. Cocaine and hydroxyamphetamine drops are useful for the diagnosis of a Horner's syndrome. Phenylephrine binds directly to the postsynaptic receptor, causing dilation.

68. A)   Left

The mnemonic COWS—cold-opposite-warm-same (Fig. 4-36)—helps to give the direction of the fast phase of the nystagmus. In this case, the left eye is irrigated with cold water, so the fast phase will be toward the right. Consequently, the slow phase of the nystagmus is to the left. Bilateral cold water irrigation will produce nystagmus with fast phase upward (Table 4-3).

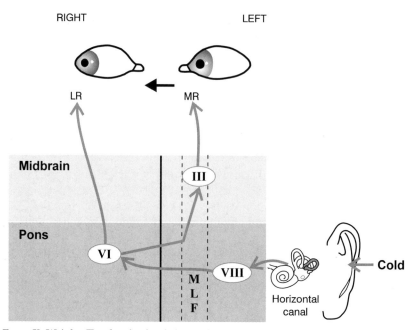

FIGURE 4-36. From K. Wright: Textbook of ophthalmology. Baltimore: Williams & Wilkins, 1997.

TABLE 4-3. Caloric Vestibular Stimulation

Eye Movement Direction Relative to Side Stimulated.

	Awake		Comatose	
	(Jerk nystagmus-FAST phase)		(Tonic deviation-no nystagmus)	
	Unilateral	Bilateral	Unilateral	Bilateral
Cold Water	Opposite	Upward	Same	Downward
Warm Water	Same	Downward	Opposite	Upward

From Wright K. Textbook of ophthalmology. Baltimore: William & Wilkins, 1997.

69. A)   Inhibits acetylcholinesterase

In myasthenia, there are fewer receptor sites on the postsynaptic terminal because of blockage of sites by immunologic complexes. Edrophonium is a short-acting anticholinesterase inhibitor. It prolongs the duration of acetylcholine in the synaptic cleft. As a result, the muscles contract with more force.

70. D)   Prevents reuptake of norepinephrine

71. B)   Releases norepinephrine from the presynaptic terminal

Cocaine and hydroxyamphetamine (Paredrine) are used in the test for Horner's syndrome. Cocaine blocks the reuptake of norepinephrine from the synaptic cleft, prolonging the effect of released neurotransmitter. In Horner's syndrome, little norepinephrine is released, and as a result, cocaine has little effect. Paredrine, in contrast, causes the release of norepinephrine from the presynaptic terminal. In first and second order Horner's, norepinephrine released from the third order neuron causes dilation of the pupil. In third order Horner's, this neuron is damaged and no norepinephrine is released by Paredrine.

72. A)   Atropine

Tensilon prolongs the effect of acetylcholine in the synaptic cleft, causing a cholinergic crisis (sweating, nausea and vomiting, salivation, fever). Atropine blocks acetylcholine receptor sites on the postsynaptic terminal.

73. D)   Anisocoria greater in the dark

An Adie's tonic pupil is dilated and poorly reactive to light. In the light, the fellow pupil constricts and the anisocoria is more pronounced. The cause of Adie's pupil is unknown, but it may be caused by a miswiring of the parasympathetics in the ciliary ganglion. The vermiform movement of the iris border occurs as mis-synchronized neural impulses cause segmental iris sphincter contraction. These pupils are hypersensitive to parasympathomimetics and will constrict with dilute pilocarpine. A normal pupil will have minimal miosis with dilute pilocarpine.

74. A)   Hyperthyroidism treated 1 year ago

This woman has a left optic neuropathy without any orbital signs. Compressive optic neuropathy associated with thyroid ophthalmopathy should be accompanied by the typical signs of proptosis, chemosis, and lid retraction.

Multiple sclerosis, sarcoidosis, and anterior ischemic optic neuropathy may cause isolated optic neuropathy and may be associated with arm numbness, hilar adenopathy, and hypertension, respectively.

75. A)   MRI

This patient most likely has optic neuritis. The presence of periventricular plaques on MRI increases her risk of developing multiple sclerosis. Treatment of higher risk patients with IV methylprednisolone (Solu-Medrol) decreases the rate of developing multiple sclerosis over the next 2 years. Thus, observation would not be appropriate. Treatment with oral prednisone alone increases the rate of recurrence of optic neuritis and is thus contraindicated.

76. B)   Scalp tenderness

Temporal arteritis must be considered in anyone with transient visual loss who is over 55 years of age. The presence of scalp tenderness should raise suspicions further. Permanent visual loss caused by ischemic optic neuropathy could occur at any moment, and prompt treatment with corticosteroids could be preventative. A carotid bruit or cardiac murmur may signify a potential embolic focus and should be evaluated. However, permanent visual loss would be much less likely. Similarly, hypertension is a risk factor for vascular disease and should be treated, but it need not be done urgently.

77.   C)   Erythrocyte sedimentation rate

Fatigue with chewing is a form of jaw claudication. Transient diplopia could be a result of ocular motor nerve ischemia. In combination, these symptoms are very suggestive of temporal arteritis.

Carotid Dopplers would be appropriate to evaluate transient visual loss if symptoms of temporal arteritis were not present. The antiphospholipid antibody syndrome (lupus anticoagulant, anticardiolipin antibody) can cause transient visual loss, typically in younger adults, and should be considered in the appropriate setting. Myasthenia gravis can cause transient diplopia and fatigue on chewing but not transient visual loss.

78.   D)   all of the above

Figure 4-26 shows bilateral eyelid retraction. This usually is a sign of thyroid orbitopathy, an overaction of Müller's muscle. Eyelid retraction can also be seen in Parinaud's dorsal midbrain syndrome (Collier's sign), but then neuroimaging would be abnormal. Patients with thyroid orbitopathy may develop proptosis and nonfatigable ophthalmoplegia from extraocular muscle involvement. Myasthenia gravis is associated with dysthyroidism, and thus fatigable ptosis could occur.

79.   A)   Direct coronal CT scan of the orbits

The patient now has an optic neuropathy. Patients with thyroid dysfunction can develop or experience worsening of ophthalmopathy at any time after appropriate systemic treatment. Thus, the first consideration should be to rule out optic nerve compression by enlarged extraocular muscles. CT scan with direct coronal views would be the best test. Visual fields would also be helpful. Once the diagnosis has been established, a short course of prednisone can be used to decrease optic nerve compression until definitive treatment (orbital radiation, orbital decompression) can be instituted. Thyroid function tests to ascertain appropriate systemic treatment should be obtained but are not the first consideration. One should never simply observe a patient with an unexplained optic neuropathy.

80.   B)   Louis-Bar syndrome

Individuals with von Recklinghausen's disease (neurofibromatosis) are prone to CNS tumors, including optic nerve glioma and meningioma, chiasmal glioma, and acoustic schwannoma. Bourneville's syndrome (tuberous sclerosis) is characterized by seizures, mental retardation, and calcified CNS lesions ("tubers"). Individuals with Sturge-Weber syndrome (encephalo-trigeminal angiomatosis) typically have intracranial calcification associated with pial angiomatosis. Louis-Bar syndrome (ataxia-telangiectasia) is not associated with any CNS abnormalities detectable with neuroimaging.

81. D)   Bourneville's syndrome

82. B)   Sturge-Weber syndrome

83. A)   von Hippel-Lindau syndrome

84. B)   von Recklinghausen disease

85. B)   von Hippel-Lindau syndrome

86. D)   Louis-Bar syndrome

The phakomatoses encompass a broad spectrum of diseases that have hamartomas affecting the eye, skin, CNS, and visceral organs.

Patients with Bourneville's syndrome, or tuberous sclerosis, typically have mental retardation, seizures, and adenoma sebaceum. Astrocytic hamartomas found in the retina or brain are often calcified. Skin findings include café-au-lait spots, ash leaf depigmentation (shagreen patches), and periungual fibromas.

von Recklinghausen's disease, or neurofibromatosis, describes a disorder with café-au-lait skin lesions, plexiform neurofibromas, CNS gliomas and meningiomas, pheochromocytomas, and acoustic schwannomas. Ocular manifestations include glaucoma, astrocytic hamartomas, and optic nerve gliomas. Absence of the sphenoid wing can give pulsatile proptosis.

Angiomatosis retinae (von Hippel-Lindau) presents with capillary angiomas of the retina and cerebellar hemangioblastomas. Cerebellar lesions may cause vertigo and ataxia. Associated visceral findings include pancreatic, hepatic, and renal cysts, renal cell carcinoma, and pheochromocytomas. Ocular manifestations of Wyburn-Mason are arteriovenous malformations with dilated tortuous vessels in the retina and brain. Louis-Bar, or ataxia-telangiectasia, presents with cutaneous and conjunctival telangiectasias, diffuse cerebellar atrophy, thymic aplasia, and recurrent sinopulmonary infections. Sturge-Weber (encephalotrigeminal angiomatosis) is characterized by the port wine stain, ipsilateral intracranial hemangioma, seizures, mental retardation, and glaucoma from elevated episcleral venous pressure.

87. D)   capillary hemangioma

Pulsations are either from a) abnormal vascular flow (arteriovenous malformations or carotid-cavernous sinus fistulas) or b) transmission of normal intracranial pulsations (mucocele encephalocoele), surgical removal of bone or sphenoid abnormalities in neurofibromatosis. Additionally, pulsation without bruits may be produced by neurofibromatosis meningoencephaloceles or as a result of the surgical removal of the orbital roof. Capillary hemangiomas consist of endothelial cells and small vascular spaces. Although primarily located periocular, a significant orbital component may be causing proptosis. However, the flow through these tumors is not high enough to cause pulsation.

88. D)   amaurosis

Bitemporal hemianopsia and skew deviation can occur if demyelination occurs in the optic chiasm or supranuclear vertical gaze pathway, respectively. Uveitis, including iritis, pars planitis, and retinal venous sheathing, has been reported in multiple sclerosis.

89. A)   the decrease in vision with an increase in body temperature

Uhthoff's symptom occurs with optic neuritis and is a decrease in vision with an increase in body temperature. Exercise or hot showers may trigger this symptom. *Lhermitte's sign* is the electric shock sensation with neck flexion and is found in patients with multiple sclerosis. A bilateral medial occipitotemporal lesion causes *prosopagnosia*, the inability to distinguish faces. The *Riddoch phenomenon* occurs in patients with cortical blindness who are able to perceive objects in motion, but cannot see stationary objects.

90. A)   cerebral MRI

Figures 4-27 and 4-28 show a partial right homonymous hemianopsia. Although migraine can cause persistent visual field deficit, it is unusual. Cerebral arteriovenous malformations and tumors can mimic migraine and cause visual field loss. Therefore, neuroimaging is essential. Oral contraceptives can exacerbate migraine, and sumatriptan (Imitrex) is an effective form of migraine treatment in about 80% of patients. Both of these measures would apply only if the appropriate evaluation was normal. A tangent screen can be used if malingering is suspected.

91. D)   Persistent leg tingling and weakness

The classic migraine has several components: a preceding aura, expanding scintillating scotoma, and throbbing headache. Neurologic deficits are not usually found, which may suggest alternate causes, such as a complex migraine, TIA, or stroke.

92. C)   Bilateral papilledema

Pseudotumor cerebri is a diagnosis of exclusion. Obstructive, compressive, and infiltrative CNS lesions must be excluded. Papilledema, although commonly present, is a result of the increased intracranial pressure and is not necessary for the diagnosis. The optic nerve swelling may be unilateral or asymmetric.

93. C)   35-year-old overweight woman

Patients with pseudotumor cerebri have a distinctive profile. They are typically obese women between the ages of 20 and 40 years. The exact etiology of this condition is unknown. A hormonal imbalance has been hypothesized because pseudotumor cerebri may be exacerbated with pregnancy.

94. B)   Cerebral MRI and arteriography

This elderly man has symptoms (vomiting, imbalance) and signs (skew deviation, ataxia) of vertebral-basilar insufficiency. Cerebral MRI and MRA would be the best tests because the brainstem, cerebellum, and arteries (vertebral, basilar) could be evaluated. Cerebral arteriography may be necessary depending on the MRI and MRA results, but it should not be the first step. Tensilon testing would be appropriate if the ocular misalignment were present without other signs and symptoms. Ultrasonography of the carotid arteries would not be appropriate because the patient has posterior circulation signs and symptoms.

95.   D)   multiple sclerosis

Patients with myasthenia gravis are at risk for other autoimmune diseases, including systemic lupus erythematosus, rheumatoid arthritis, and hyperthyroidism. Thymic hyperplasia and thymomas are also more common, and patients should have a chest CT to investigate this possibility.

96.   A)   Medial rectus, inferior rectus

The medial and inferior recti are enlarged most commonly with thyroid eye disease. The lateral and superior recti are affected less commonly. The oblique muscles are almost never involved.

97.   C)   optic nerve sheath decompression

Visual field loss from thyroid eye disease is usually the result of compression of the optic nerve from soft tissue swelling and enlargement of the extraocular muscles. Treatment options include radiotherapy, corticosteroids, and surgical decompression. Optic nerve sheath decompression does not relieve the orbital congestion and would not be effective in this condition.

98.   A)   One third of the patients with optic nerve sheath decompression had improvement in acuity of three or more lines at 6 months.

The Ischemic Optic Neuropathy Decompression Trial (IONDT) was an NIH-sponsored randomized, single-masked, multicenter trial comparing close observation with optic nerve sheath fenestration for nonarteritic anterior ischemic optic neuropathy. The study was terminated early by the Data and Safety Monitoring Committee. Patients in the surgery group did no better when compared with the observation group regarding improved visual acuity of three or more lines at 6 months. Approximately one third of the surgery patients had improvement in acuity, whereas over 40% of the observation patients improved. Moreover, surgery was associated with a higher risk of loss of three or more lines of acuity (surgery: 24%, observation: 12%). The IONDT conclusively states that optic nerve sheath decompression is not effective.

99.   A)   Oral prednisone alone

Patients in the Optic Neuritis Treatment Trial were randomized to one of three arms: placebo, oral prednisone alone, or combination IV methylprednisolone and oral prednisone. Oral steroids alone did not have a significant difference in visual recovery compared with the control group; however, the recurrence rate of optic neuritis was increased. The IV steroid group had faster recovery of visual acuity and a slight improvement in acuity over the control group.

100. B)   Paramedian pontine reticular formation

The supranuclear control of vertical saccades originates in the frontal eye fields or in the superior colliculus. They project to neurons in the rostral interstitial nucleus of the medial longitudinal fasciculus (riMLF) and on to the nuclei of cranial nerve III and IV. The interstitial nucleus of Cajal is involved with vertical pursuit control. The paramedian pontine reticular formation (PPRF) controls horizontal eye movements (Fig. 4-37).

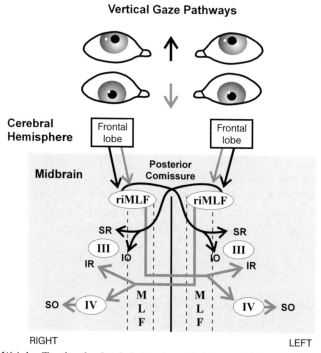

FIGURE 4-37. From K. Wright: Textbook of ophthalmology. Baltimore: Williams & Wilkins, 1997.

Notes

Notes

5

Pediatrics and Strabismus

QUESTIONS

1. Which statement is FALSE about patients with homocystinuria?

    A) Affected individuals have osteoporosis and progressive renal dysfunction.
    B) Patients are abnormal from birth, with seizures and mental retardation.
    C) Ectopia lentis may occur in over 30%.
    D) Patients may benefit from a diet low in methionine and high in cysteine.

2. Which statement about galactosemia is true?

    A) Disease effects are limited to the eye.
    B) Cataracts are inevitably progressive.
    C) It can result from a defect in galactokinase or galactose-1-P uridyl transferase.
    D) It can lead to an accumulation of galactose in the lens, forming a snowflake cataract.

3. All of the following are characteristics of patients with Lowe's syndrome EXCEPT:

    A) autosomal dominant inheritance
    B) renal tubular acidosis
    C) bilateral congenital cataracts
    D) infantile glaucoma

4. True statements concerning the conjunctivitis in the neonate pictured in Figure 5-1 include each of the following EXCEPT:

    A) Definitive diagnosis can be made by seeing intracytoplasmic inclusion bodies on Giemsa stain.
    B) Herpes simplex is not an important cause in infants under 4 weeks of age.
    C) Differential diagnosis includes both viral and bacterial diseases.
    D) Initial work-up should include particular attention to the corneal epithelium.

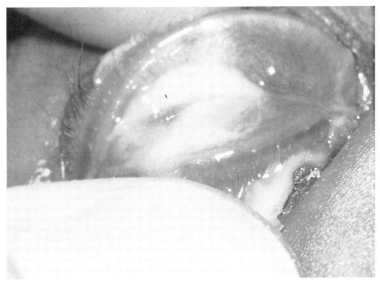

FIGURE 5-1

5. Which one of the following statements is LEAST accurate with regard to the condition in Figure 5-2?

    A) Differential diagnosis includes hemangioma, encephalocele, and dermoid cyst.
    B) Nasolacrimal duct (NLD) probing after 6 months of age.
    C) Definitive therapy includes NLD probing.
    D) If the condition is infected, IV antibiotics are needed.

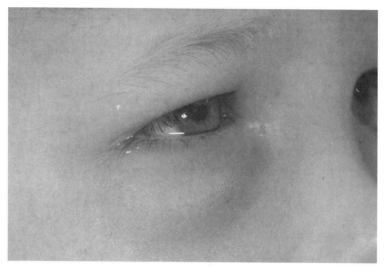

FIGURE 5-2

6. The left eye of a 2-year-old child is shown in Figure 5-3. The punctum is cannulated and fluorescein solution is irrigated (Fig. 5-4). Which one of the following statements is FALSE?

    A) This condition is associated with tear reflux and nasolacrimal duct obstruction.
    B) The anomaly involves an abnormality of neural ectoderm.
    C) If this condition is infected, topical antibiotics are usually sufficient to temporize the condition.
    D) These tracts are lined with epithelium.

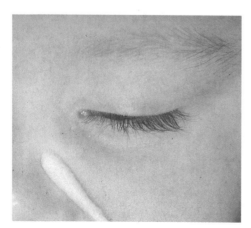

FIGURE 5-3

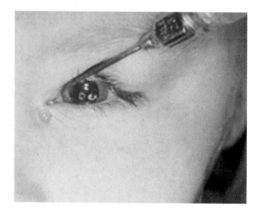

FIGURE 5-4

7. Which one of the following statements regarding megalocornea is FALSE?

    A) This condition is defined as a clear normal appearing cornea with a diameter measuring greater than 13 mm.
    B) This condition is often associated with anterior megalophthalmos, an autosomal dominant disorder.
    C) The simple form of megalocornea is usually seen as a bilateral condition.
    D) Tearing and IOP are important factors in the work-up.

8. Which one of the following statements concerning Figure 5-5 is FALSE?

    A) This developmental anomaly can demonstrate both lens and iris adhesions to the corneal endothelium.
    B) The condition has progressive corneal opacification.
    C) The peripheral cornea is unaffected.
    D) This condition results from a developmental problem with neural crest cells.

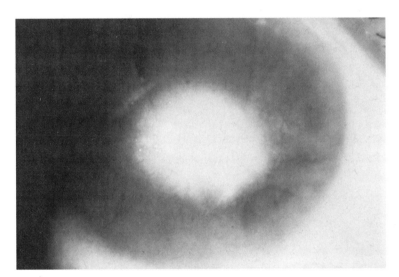

FIGURE 5-5. From Wright K. Textbook of ophthalmology. Baltimore: Williams & Wilkins, 1997.

9. A 3-year-old girl presents with the lesion shown in Figure 5-6. All of the following statements are true EXCEPT:

A) This lesion is anterior to Bowman's membrane and can be scraped off without concern of stromal involvement.

B) Associated findings include preauricular skin tags, upper eyelid coloboma, and vertebral anomalies.

C) Often there is an associated arc of lipid in the cornea in advance of the lesion.

D) These lesions may have hair follicles or sweat glands in them.

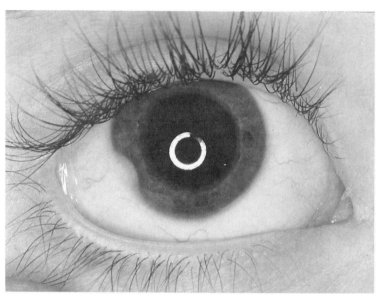

FIGURE 5-6. From Wright K. Textbook of ophthalmology. Baltimore: Williams & Wilkins, 1997.

10. The patient pictured in Figure 5-7 has congenital hereditary endothelial dystrophy (CHED). Which one of the following statements regarding this disease is TRUE?

A) CHED is primarily a unilateral disease.
B) CHED could be differentiated from congenital hereditary stromal dystrophy (CHSD) by pachymetry.
C) The dominant form is stationary and the recessive form is progressive.
D) Patients with the dominant form are more likely to demonstrate nystagmus than the recessive form.

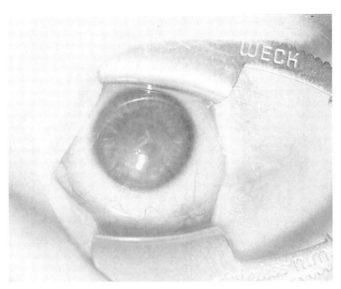

FIGURE 5-7

11. All of the following are causes of heterochromic irides EXCEPT:

A) Horner's syndrome
B) Albinism
C) Juvenile xanthogranuloma (JXG)
D) Waardenburg-Klein syndrome

12. Which one of the following ocular or systemic conditions is NOT associated with ectopia lentis (Fig. 5-8)?

   A) Homocystinuria
   B) Aniridia
   C) Microcornea
   D) Weill-Marchesani

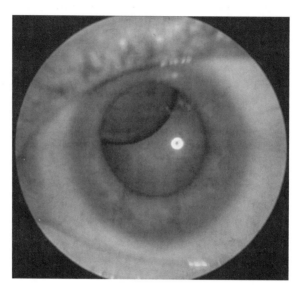

FIGURE 5-8

13. A 1-month-old infant presents with bilateral nuclear cataracts (Fig. 5-9). What is the most common identifiable cause for the cataracts?

   A) Hereditary autosomal dominant
   B) Persistent hyperplastic primary vitreous (PHPV)
   C) Galactosemia
   D) Intrauterine infection

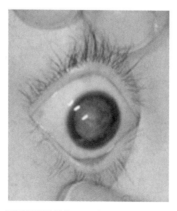

FIGURE 5-9

14. What is the optimum time to operate on a patient with bilateral dense congenital cataracts?

   A)   As soon as possible, even within the first few weeks of life
   B)   Between 2 months and 6 months of age
   C)   Between 6 months and 1 year of age
   D)   Between 1 and 2 years of age

15. Which one of the following is the preferred treatment for congenital cataracts in the 1-month-old infant with compliant parents?

   A)   Lensectomy, anterior vitrectomy, and fitting of contact lens
   B)   Intracapsular cataract extraction with contact lens fitting
   C)   Aspiration of lens and implantation of posterior chamber IOL
   D)   Lensectomy, anterior vitrectomy, and fitting with aphakic glasses

16. Each of the following statements regarding the disease depicted in Figure 5-10 is true EXCEPT:

   A)   photophobia and tearing may be the only presenting signs
   B)   although surgical therapy is usually indicated, medical therapy is often used initially
   C)   gonioscopy has clearly identifiable landmarks facilitating goniotomy as a first line therapy
   D)   horizontally oriented breaks in Descemet's membrane may be found in the buphthalmic eye

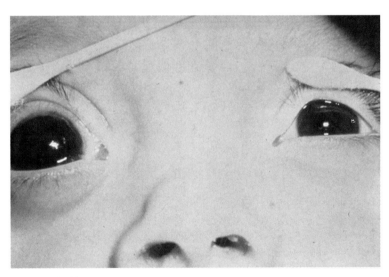

FIGURE 5-10

17. Iridocyclitis is associated most frequently with which form of juvenile rheumatoid arthritis (JRA)?

   A)   Pauciarticular antinuclear antibody (ANA) positive
   B)   Polyarticular, rheumatoid factor negative
   C)   Polyarticular, rheumatoid factor positive
   D)   Pauciarticular ANA negative

Questions 18–19

A 3-year-old child is referred by his pediatrician with a 7-day history of fever of unknown etiology and bilateral conjunctival infection. Other findings include a polymorphous rash, erythema and edema of the palms and soles, periungual desquamation, cervical lymphadenopathy, infected pharynx and tongue, and fissuring of the lips. Ophthalmic evaluation reveals a mild bilateral anterior uveitis.

18. Which one of the following studies is most appropriate?

    A) Electrocardiogram
    B) Two-dimensional echocardiography
    C) Chest radiograph
    D) HLA-B27

19. Which one of the following is the treatment of choice for this condition?

    A) Systemic corticosteroid therapy
    B) Parenteral penicillin
    C) Isoniazid
    D) Aspirin

Questions 20–21

An infant girl is born 4 weeks prematurely and manifests jaundice, an intractable rash, persistent rhinitis, pneumonia, anemia, generalized lymphadenopathy, and bony abnormalities on radiograph.

20. Which one of the following historical features is the most important when questioning the mother regarding the history of the pregnancy?

    A) Diet
    B) Alcohol or drug use
    C) Exposure to environmental toxins
    D) Sexual history

21. Which one of the following findings would most likely be present on ophthalmic examination of this newborn child?

    A) Interstitial keratitis
    B) Segmental pigmentation of the retinal periphery and chorioretinitis
    C) Scleritis
    D) Anterior uveitis

22. All of the following would be considered in the differential diagnosis of vitreous hemorrhage in an 8-year-old child EXCEPT:

    A) trauma
    B) juvenile X-linked retinoschisis
    C) pars planitis
    D) melanocytoma

23. An 8-year-old boy presents with 20/60 vision and exhibits the macular finding shown in Figure 5-11. Which one of the following is NOT true of this disorder?

    A) Spoke-wheel configuration of the macula
    B) Cleavage of the retina at the nerve fiber layer
    C) Attenuated b-wave on electroretinogram (ERG)
    D) Macular microcysts exhibit classic petalloid leakage on fluorescein angiography

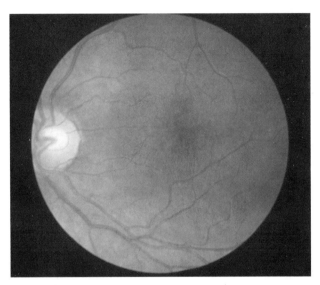

FIGURE 5-11

24. A 4-year-old girl presents for evaluation of poor vision. Ophthalmologic examination reveals translucent irides, hypopigmentation of the fundi, and foveal hypoplasia. Each one of the following may be an associated finding EXCEPT:

    A) bleeding diathesis
    B) recurrent sinopulmonary infections
    C) oculodigital massage
    D) sensory nystagmus

25. Figure 5-12 is representative of a child infected with a nematode that was contracted from a common house pet. Which one of the following statements regarding this process is FALSE?

A) This infection may present with either anterior or posterior segment involvement.
B) The infection often manifests as an eosinophilic granuloma.
C) On CT, calcification is frequently present.
D) This infection can present as an apparent exotropia in which there are no refixation movements on alternate cover testing.

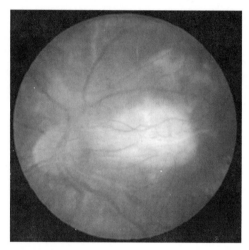

FIGURE 5-12

26. An infant is referred for poor tracking. On examination, the child does not fix or follow, there is searching nystagmus. The rest of the ocular exam is otherwise normal. Which one of the following is LEAST likely in the differential?

A) Achromatopsia
B) Congenital stationary night blindness
C) Leber's congenital amaurosis
D) Ocular albinism

27. An infant presents for evaluation of poor vision. Which one of the following signs is LEAST worrisome?

A) Eye-popping reflex
B) Gazing at bright lights
C) Eye rubbing
D) Paradoxic pupillary response to light

28. Which one of the following statements regarding ocular toxoplasmosis is FALSE?

A) Less than 10% of individuals younger than 5 years of age demonstrate antibodies against toxoplasmosis.
B) Toxoplasma oocysts shed by cats in their feces may remain infective for up to 1 year.
C) Maternal infection earlier in the course of pregnancy results in a greater risk of infection to the fetus.
D) Retinochoroiditis typically involves the retinal periphery and infrequently involves the macula.

29. An infant born prematurely at 27 weeks of gestation weighing 950 g has been admitted to the neonatal ICU. When should this infant have his initial retinal examination to screen for retinopathy of prematurity (ROP)?

    A) Immediately
    B) 1 to 2 weeks after birth
    C) 4 to 6 weeks after birth
    D) 8 to 10 weeks after birth

30. According to the guidelines from the Cryotherapy for ROP Cooperative Study, cryotherapy or laser therapy should be initiated in patients with which one of the following stages of ROP?

    A) 5 contiguous clock hours of stage 3 plus
    B) 8 cumulative clock hours of stage 2 plus
    C) 5 contiguous clock hours of stage 1
    D) 8 cumulative clock hours of stage 1

31. Which one of the following is the LEAST important risk factor for developing ROP?

    A) Hyperoxia
    B) Low birth weight (<1250 g)
    C) Twins
    D) Gestational age

32. Which one of the following statements regarding Coats' disease is TRUE?

    A) It has an autosomal dominant pattern of inheritance with variable penetrance.
    B) It is usually bilateral.
    C) Males are affected more frequently than females.
    D) It is usually diagnosed before 2 years of age.

33. Which one of the following statements regarding juvenile onset diabetes mellitus (JODM) is FALSE?

    A) Background diabetic retinopathy rarely occurs under the age of 20 years.
    B) Retinopathy rarely occurs less than 3 years after onset of diabetes mellitus.
    C) The prevalence of retinopathy in patients with JODM for more than 15 years approaches 90%.
    D) Teenage diabetics should be examined for the presence of retinopathy within 5 years of diagnosis.

34. A 5-year-old boy presents for evaluation of decreased vision. Ophthalmologic examination reveals degenerative changes involving the vitreous and retina and an optically empty vitreous. Which one of the following is the LEAST likely diagnosis?

    A) Wagner dystrophy
    B) Stickler syndrome
    C) Goldmann-Favre dystrophy
    D) Kearns-Sayre syndrome

35. Which one of the following statements regarding retinitis pigmentosa is true?

    A) The X-linked form is least common but most disabling.
    B) Signs and symptoms typically precede ERG abnormalities.
    C) Retinal pigmentary changes in the midperiphery are always present.
    D) The initial visual field defect is a ring scotoma.

36. Which one of the following statements regarding cone dystrophies is FALSE?

    A) Cone dystrophies are characterized by decreased central vision, color blindness, and photophobia.
    B) Night blindness and loss of peripheral vision frequently develop late in the course of the disease.
    C) Visual loss and photophobia usually precede clinically visible macular changes.
    D) Specific ERG findings include abnormal single-flash photopic response and flicker response.

37. A 10-year-old girl is referred for an ophthalmologic examination after failing her school eye exam. Her best-corrected visual acuity is 20/50 in her right eye and 20/40 in her left. Examination reveals a normal anterior segment with an abnormal fundus appearance bilaterally. Her left eye is shown in Figure 5-13. Which one of the following would be most useful in establishing the diagnosis?

    A) Electro-oculogram (EOG)
    B) ERG
    C) Visually evoked cortical potential
    D) Fluorescein angiogram

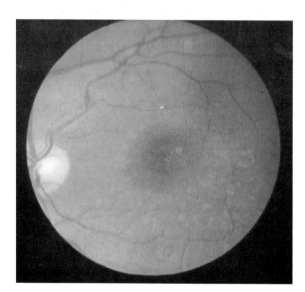

FIGURE 5-13

38.   A 10-year-old boy is referred for evaluation of decreased vision in his left eye. Examination reveals an uncorrected visual acuity of 20/20 in his right eye and 20/40 in his left, which is correctable to 20/20 with glasses. Examination of the left fundus reveals a yellow-orange cystic macular lesion (Fig. 5-14). The father of this child reports that several members of his family including himself and a sister have suffered from mild to moderate deterioration of vision since youth. Which one of the following would be most helpful in establishing the diagnosis?

A)   EOG
B)   Ultrasound
C)   Visual evoked cortical potential
D)   Fluorescein angiogram

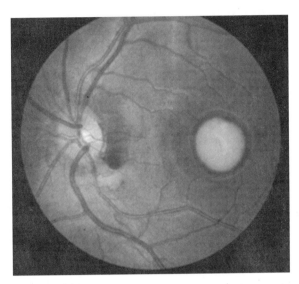

FIGURE 5-14

Questions 39–44 Optic nerve disorders (Fig. 5-15 to 5-20).

39.   Which figure is associated with glial proliferation and folding of the retina?

   A)   Figure 5-15
   B)   Figure 5-16
   C)   Figure 5-18
   D)   Figure 5-19

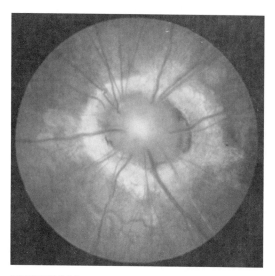

FIGURE 5-15

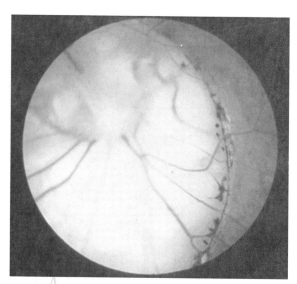

FIGURE 5-16

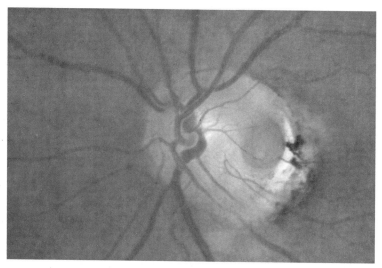

FIGURE 5-17

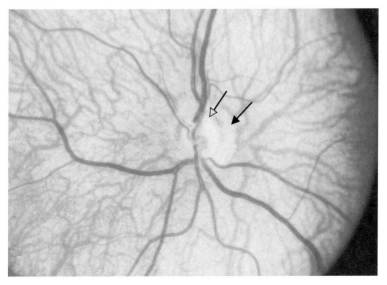

FIGURE 5-18

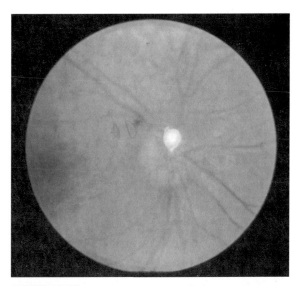

FIGURE 5-19

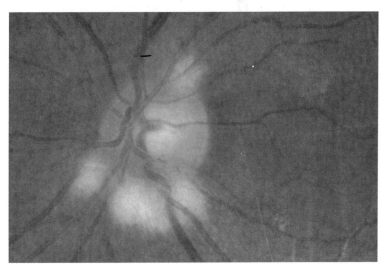

FIGURE 5-20

40. Which figure is a result of faulty closure of the fetal fissure?

A) Figure 5-16
B) Figure 5-18
C) Figure 5-19
D) Figure 5-20

41. Which condition requires an endocrine evaluation and neuroimaging studies?

A) Figure 5-16
B) Figure 5-17
C) Figure 5-18
D) Figure 5-20

42. Which patient is at risk for developing serous macular detachments?

A) Figure 5-15
B) Figure 5-17
C) Figure 5-18
D) Figure 5-19

43. Which condition can be found in conjunction with aniridia?

A) Figure 5-15
B) Figure 5-16
C) Figure 5-18
D) Figure 5-20

44. Which condition is found in conjunction with the posterior lens opacity shown in Figure 5-21?

A) Figure 5-15
B) Figure 5-16
C) Figure 5-19
D) Figure 5-20

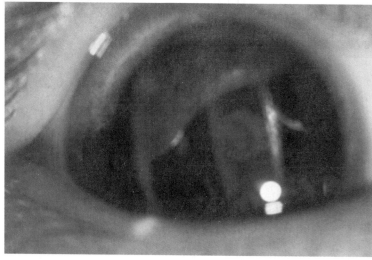

FIGURE 5-21

45. Which one of the following is NOT true of retinoblastoma?

A) There is an increased incidence of developing secondary malignant tumors later in life.

B) Two mutations in chromosome 13 are required to develop retinoblastoma.

C) Retinoblastoma may present as orbital cellulitis, strabismus, or hyphema.

D) The Reese-Ellsworth classification of retinoblastoma provides prognostic information about patient survival.

46. The patient in Figure 5-22 has:

A) *craniosynostosis*—this patient would likely demonstrate midfacial hypoplasia, V-pattern exotropia, proptosis, and telecanthus

B) *Pierre-Robin sequence*—this patient would likely demonstrate micrognathia, glossoptosis, and cleft palate

C) *mandibulofacial dysostosis*—this patient would likely demonstrate microstomia, coloboma, and malar and mandibular hypoplasia

D) *fetal alcohol syndrome*—this patient would likely demonstrate an antimongoloid slant, deficiency of meibomian glands in the lower lid, and absent lower lid puncta

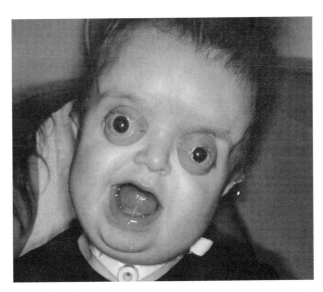

FIGURE 5-22

47. A 2-year-old child presents with unilateral periorbital inflammation. Which one of the following is the LEAST likely cause?

A) Dermoid cyst

B) Rhabdomyosarcoma

C) Orbital cellulitis

D) Toxoplasmosis

48. An infant presents with a hyphema with no history of trauma. Which one of the following is the LEAST likely cause?

A) JXG

B) Herpes simplex uveitis

C) Lymphoma

D) Retinoblastoma

49. A 2-year-old boy presents with periorbital ecchymosis. The differential diagnosis includes all of the following EXCEPT:

    A) neuroblastoma
    B) leukemia
    C) lymphangioma
    D) dermoid cyst

50. Neuroblastoma is characterized by all of the following EXCEPT:

    A) metastasis from the adrenal gland
    B) possible spontaneous regression
    C) poor prognosis if diagnosed before 1 year of age
    D) periorbital ecchymosis

51. Which one of the following phacomatoses has NO known mode of inheritance?

    A) Sturge-Weber syndrome
    B) Neurofibromatosis
    C) Tuberous sclerosis
    D) von Hippel-Lindau disease

52. Which one of the following statements regarding neurofibromatosis is FALSE?

    A) Café-au-lait spots appear in over 99% of patients with this disorder.
    B) Tumors of the CNS, including optic nerve gliomas, astrocytomas, acoustic neuromas, meningiomas, and neurofibromas, occur in 5% to 10% of patients with neurofibromatosis.
    C) Lisch nodules appear in over 90% of patients over the age of 6 years but are nondiagnostic because they may appear in normal patients as well.
    D) Up to 50% of patients with plexiform neurofibromas involving the upper eyelid develop ipsilateral glaucoma.

Questions 53–55

The child pictured in Figure 5-23 has a lesion on the right side of his face present since birth.

53. Characteristics of this lesion (see Fig. 5-23) include all of the following EXCEPT:

A) similar lesions can be found in the orbit
B) low flow lesion angiographically
C) spontaneous regression in most cases
D) usually presents within the first 6 months of age

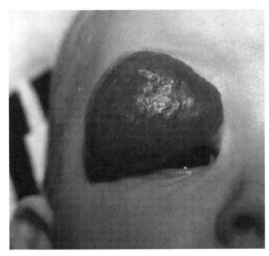

FIGURE 5-23

54. Which treatment approach is most appropriate for this child?

A) Radiotherapy
B) Incision and drainage
C) Corticosteroids
D) Observation

55. What complication may result in this child if the lesion is left untreated?

A) Hemorrhage
B) Orbital cellulitis
C) Amblyopia
D) Metastasis

56. Which muscle is a synergist to the lateral rectus?

A) Medial rectus
B) Inferior oblique
C) Superior rectus
D) Inferior rectus

57. Which muscle is most effective as a depressor of the eye when it is abducted 23° from the midline?

A) Medial rectus
B) Inferior oblique
C) Superior oblique
D) Inferior rectus

58. All of the statements regarding a pediatric ophthalmology evaluation are true EXCEPT:

A) A child demonstrates eccentric fixation. This indicates poor vision, usually 20/200 or worse.
B) The cover-uncover test is used to identify a tropia.
C) The deviation measured with the alternate cover test is the phoria plus the tropia.
D) Temporal displacement of the light reflex that does not shift during cover-uncover or alternate cover testing represents a positive angle kappa.

59. Which one of the following statements is FALSE about the Hirschberg or corneal light reflex test?

A) The corneal light reflex is a misnomer as the light reflex comes from behind the pupil.
B) The Krimsky test uses prisms in front of the fixing eye or the nonfixing eye to center the deviated light reflex.
C) The Bruckner test uses the red reflex to determine the presence of strabismus. If strabismus is present, the fixing eye will have the brighter reflex.
D) The Maddox rod can be used to help measure both cyclodeviations as well as horizontal or vertical deviations.

60. The child in Figure 5-24 was brought in by her observant mother for evaluation of crossed eyes, which the mother has noticed for the past month. Which one of the following statements is LEAST likely?

   A)   The cover-uncover test will demonstrate a tropia; when the fixing eye is covered, the other eye will display an abduction movement.

   B)   Both the cover-uncover test and the alternate cover test, even with excellent fixation on an accommodative target, will not demonstrate any deviation.

   C)   This child is unlikely to demonstrate inferior oblique overaction or dissociated vertical deviation. These findings generally develop after initial presentation of esotropia.

   D)   With time, this condition will spontaneously improve.

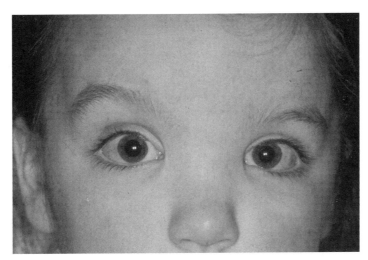

FIGURE 5-24

61. Which one of the following statements regarding optokinetic nystagmus (OKN) is FALSE?

   A)   The slow phase occurs in the same direction as that in which the repetitive visual stimulus is moved.

   B)   The frontal lobes control the slow pursuit movement.

   C)   In patients with congenital motor nystagmus, a reversal of the OKN response can occur.

   D)   An OKN response elicited in an infant indicates that some visual input is present.

62. A 32-year-old woman presents with insidious onset of diplopia. On alternate cover testing, the patient has a right hypertropia, worse on right head tilt and left gaze. A palsy of which muscle might cause her symptoms?

   A)   Right superior oblique

   B)   Left superior rectus

   C)   Left inferior oblique

   D)   Right inferior rectus

63. Which one of the following characteristics regarding the three-step test is TRUE?

A)   Able to differentiate between restrictive and paralytic palsies
B)   Distinguishes a palsy from an overactive muscle
C)   Separates congenital from acquired disorders
D)   Most applicable when a single muscle is involved

64. A 3-year-old child with esotropia since birth has the deviation shown in Figure 5-25. The incomitance of this deviation is most likely secondary to a muscle that:

A)   passes between the sclera and a rectus muscle
B)   elevates, intorts, and adducts
C)   passes below sclera and above an adjacent muscle
D)   has its insertion near the macula

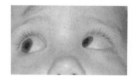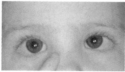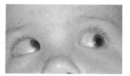

FIGURE 5-25

65. A 2-month-old boy (Fig. 5-26) with large angle esotropia and apparent cross-fixation presents to your office. The LEAST likely diagnosis on your differential is:

A)   congenital esotropia
B)   Möbius syndrome
C)   dense amblyopia
D)   congenital fibrosis syndrome

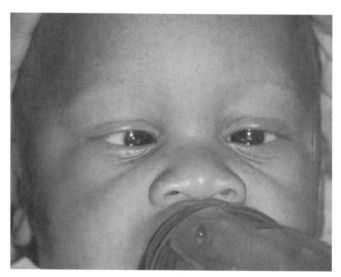

FIGURE 5-26

66. A child presents with both eyes in the adducted position. To best determine if this is the result of a bilateral lateral rectus palsy, you could try each of the following EXCEPT:

    A) doll's head movements
    B) saccadic eye movements generated by an OKN drum
    C) patching one eye and testing ductions
    D) forced duction testing

67. Each of the following is true regarding accommodative esotropia EXCEPT:

    A) always high AC/A ratio
    B) usually intermittent at onset and becoming constant
    C) amblyopia is very common (>95%)
    D) rarely develop diplopia

68. Bifocals are appropriate for a patient with which one of the following measurements?

    A) Dcc ET25 wearing the full distance correction of + 3.00 D OU
       Ncc ET40 wearing the full distance correction of + 3.00 D OU
    B) Dcc ortho wearing full distance correction of + 1.00 D OU
       Ncc ET15 wearing full distance correction of + 1.00 D OU
    C) Dsc ET20 first time visit, cycloplegic retinoscopy + 3.00 D OU
    D) Dcc ET10 wearing full cycloplegic correction of − 2.50 D OU
       Ncc ET13 wearing full cycloplegic correction of − 2.50 D OU

69. Which is most consistent with accommodative esotropia?

    A) Dissociated vertical deviation (DVD)
    B) Acquired onset from infancy to 4 years of age
    C) Poor to no binocular potential
    D) Cycloplegic refraction of + 8.00 D

70. A 2-year-old child presents with intermittent exotropia. All of the following would most likely describe her condition EXCEPT:

    A) suppression
    B) excellent stereopsis
    C) large convergence amplitudes
    D) amblyopia

71. An 8-year-old girl returns 1 day after bilateral lateral rectus recessions for intermittent exotropia. She measures 8 PD of consecutive esotropia and has diplopia. The parents are concerned. Your best course of action is:

    A) begin convergence exercises
    B) observe the child; tell the parents you are satisfied because this is the desired result postoperative day 1
    C) prescribe prism glasses to maintain fusion
    D) suggest that reoperation may be necessary

72. A 3-year-old boy measures XT35 distance and X(T)'15 at near fixation. How would this deviation be characterized?

A) True divergence excess
B) Pseudo-divergence excess
C) Basic exotropia
D) Cannot determine from the information provided

73. Which one of the following indications is the weakest for X(T) surgery?

A) Increasing degree of exodeviation in the tropia phase
B) Increasing ease of dissociation
C) Poor recovery of fusion once tropic
D) A deviation of greater than 15 PD

74. A 22-year-old emmetropic patient has difficulty reading. On alternate cover testing, she is orthophoric at distance and has an exodeviation of 15 PD at near. The best treatment option would be:

A) orthoptic therapy with a base out prism or pencil push-up exercises
B) + 2.00 D reading glasses
C) bilateral medial rectus recessions
D) unilateral recess-resect procedure

75. Which one of the following best illustrates an exception to Sherrington's law?

A) Dissociated vertical deviation
B) Duane's type I
C) Convergence
D) Alternating esotropia

Questions 76–79

A 5-year-old girl is referred by her pediatrician for evaluation of esotropia. Ophthalmologic examination reveals esotropia in the primary position with markedly limited abduction of the left eye, although there is minimal restriction of adduction of the left eye and lid fissure narrowing on attempted adduction. Right ocular motility and fissure height are normal.

76. This case most likely represents which one of the following syndromes?

A) Duane's retraction syndrome type I
B) Duane's retraction syndrome type II
C) Duane's retraction syndrome type III
D) Brown's syndrome

77. Electromyography in this patient would most likely reveal which one of the following patterns of electrical activity?

A) Electrical activity of the left lateral rectus muscle both in abduction and adduction
B) Electrical activity of the left lateral rectus muscle only in abduction

C)   Electrical activity of both the left medial and left lateral rectus muscles on both abduction and adduction

D)   Absence of electrical activity in the left lateral rectus muscle on abduction, with paradoxical activity on adduction

78.   Each of the following may be associated with Duane's retraction syndrome EXCEPT:

A)   thalidomide
B)   Marcus Gunn jaw winking
C)   Goldenhar's syndrome
D)   glaucoma

79.   Which one of the following statements regarding Duane's retraction syndrome is TRUE?

A)   The incidence of amblyopia is high.
B)   A Faden procedure may reduce the upshoot of the affected eye on adduction.
C)   The lid fissure narrowing is secondary to abnormal innervation of the levator muscle.
D)   The strabismus is comitant.

80.   All of the following are characteristics of congenital third nerve palsy EXCEPT:

A)   esodeviation
B)   abnormal pupillary function
C)   hypotropia
D)   ptosis

81.   A 4-year-old boy presents with the measurements in Figure 5-27. He is 25 PD exotropic at near. He has 1+ overacting inferior obliques. He has no evidence of amblyopia. The most reasonable surgical approach is:

A)   resection of both medial recti with supraplacement
B)   recession of both lateral recti with supraplacement
C)   recession of both lateral recti with inferior oblique weakening
D)   recess-resect with supraplacement of the lateral rectus and infraplacement of the medial rectus

	XT 45	
XT 30 RHT 2	XT 30	XT 30 LHT 2
	XT 20	

FIGURE 5-27

82. Which one of the following statements is true of DVD?

    A) It is rare in patients with congenital esotropia.
    B) It is usually a unilateral condition.
    C) The deviated eye extorts as it elevates.
    D) It violates Hering's law.

Questions 83–86

83. A 6-year-old boy presents with an exodeviation of 30 PD at distance and 10 PD at near on alternate cover testing. What is the next most appropriate step?

    A) Recess the lateral recti for 30 PD.
    B) Occlude one eye for 30 minutes and remeasure the deviation.
    C) Dispense glasses prescription with bifocal.
    D) Recess the lateral recti for an amount intermediate between the distance and near deviation.

84. A patch test is performed on this patient and he now measures 30 PD at distance and 15 PD at near. What is the next most appropriate step?

    A) Recess the lateral recti for 30 PD.
    B) Remeasure the deviation with a + 3.00 D add OU.
    C) Recess the lateral recti for an amount intermediate between the distance and near deviation.
    D) Dispense glasses prescription with bifocal.

85. This 6-year-old patient then undergoes a bilateral lateral rectus recession. One week later, he measures 15 PD consecutive esotropia. The child is complaining of diplopia. What is the next most appropriate step?

    A) Observe and have the patient return in 6 weeks.
    B) Start full-time patch OD.
    C) Start penalization OD.
    D) Start alternate patching.

86. At 3 weeks postoperative, the child is still 15 PD esotropic. What is the next most appropriate step?

    A) Operate for 15 PD esotropia.
    B) Prescribe enough base out prism to fully neutralize the esotropia.
    C) Prescribe enough base out prism to alleviate the diplopia but leave a small residual esophoria.
    D) Prescribe a miotic.

87. A 6-year-old child with 30 PD of intermittent exotropia and 40 seconds arc stereo acuity exhibits an A-pattern with superior oblique overaction and a small right hyperphoria in primary gaze, a left hyperphoria in left gaze, and a larger right hyperphoria in right gaze. The right hyperphoria significantly increases on downgaze. What would be the most reasonable surgical approach?

    A)   Lateral rectus recessions plus superior oblique tenotomies

    B)   Lateral rectus recessions plus infraplace the lateral recti

    C)   Lateral rectus recessions plus supraplace the lateral recti

    D)   Lateral rectus recessions plus superior oblique tuck

88. A 5-year-old girl presents with the ocular motility pattern shown in Figure 5-28. All of the following are true of this condition EXCEPT:

    A)   an inelastic superior oblique muscle tendon complex

    B)   down shoot in adduction

    C)   superior oblique overaction with A-pattern is common

    D)   forced ductions in this case will be positive

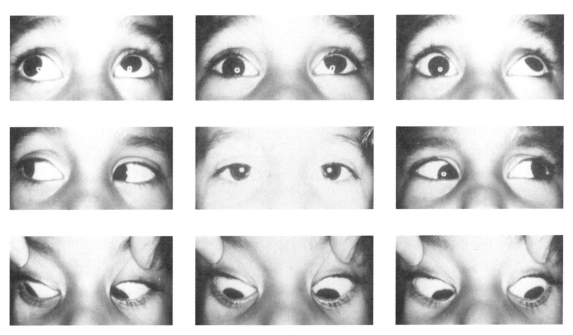

FIGURE 5-28. From Wright K. Textbook of ophthalmology. Baltimore: Williams & Wilkins, 1997.

89. An 8-year-old boy presents with the ocular motility shown in Figure 5-29. Which one of the following is NOT true of this condition?

A) Patients with this condition have normal vertical fusion amplitudes.
B) This condition often has inferior oblique overaction.
C) The patient has a compensatory head tilt away from the pathology
D) Early onset of this condition can result in facial asymmetry.

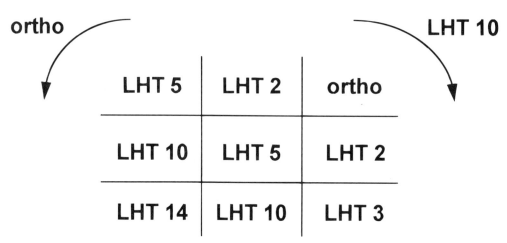

FIGURE 5-29

90. Which one of the following statements concerning Botulinum toxin (Botox) is FALSE?

A) The effect of Botox lasts clinically for 3 months in extraocular muscles.
B) Botox interferes with cholinergic receptors preventing release of acetylcholine (ACh).
C) Botox has been proven to be effective as the primary treatment of most types of strabismus.
D) Side effects include ptosis, diplopia, and, rarely, globe perforation.

91. Botulinum toxin injections have been found to be the treatment of choice in the following cases:

A) non resolving cranial nerve VI palsy
B) moderate or large angle strabismus
C) blepharospasm
D) Brown's syndrome

92. Latent nystagmus is characterized by all of the following statements EXCEPT:

A) null point in adduction
B) fast phase to the fixing eye
C) increases with monocular occlusion
D) is often associated with intermittent exotropia

Questions 93–94

A 2-year-old girl is referred by her pediatrician for evaluation of a residual small angle esotropia and face turn after strabismus surgery for infantile estropia. Examination reveals intermittent esotropia 15 PD with the fixing eye in adduction even when one eye is occluded. A horizontal nystagmus is present with the fast phase to the fixing eye and it increases when the fixing eye is abducted. Cycloplegic refraction shows + 3.00 OU.

93.   The most likely diagnosis is:

   A)   congenital nystagmus
   B)   spasmus nutans
   C)   latent nystagmus with face turn to place the fixing eye in the null point
   D)   dissociated nystagmus

94.   The most appropriate treatment for the patient in question 93 is:

   A)   Botox injection of both medial rectus muscles
   B)   bilateral medial rectus recessions
   C)   prescribe full hyperopic correction + 3.00 OU
   D)   convergence exercises

95.   Each of the following is a characteristic of spasmus nutans EXCEPT:

   A)   monocular or dissociated nystagmus, which is rapid and of small amplitude
   B)   usually disappears within 2 years
   C)   head bobbing
   D)   optic atrophy

96.   Characteristics of congenital motor nystagmus include each of the following EXCEPT:

   A)   oscillopsia is frequently present
   B)   affected patients typically have visual acuity ranging from 20/20 to 20/70
   C)   a null point may exist
   D)   the nystagmus does not occur while the patient is asleep

97.   Which one of the following is NOT a cause of congenital sensory nystagmus?

   A)   Congenital cataracts
   B)   Aniridia with foveal hypoplasia
   C)   Rod monochromatism
   D)   Arnold-Chiari malformation

98.   Which one of the following statements concerning dyslexia is NOT valid?

   A)   Children with dyslexia have the same incidence of ocular abnormalities as children without dyslexia.
   B)   Visual training, including muscle exercises, ocular pursuit, or tracking exercises, has been proven to improve academic abilities of dyslexic or learning disabled children.
   C)   Dyslexia is uncommon in countries such as Japan, which use one sound for each symbol.
   D)   Boys are three times more likely to develop dyslexia than girls.

99. All of the following are true of malignant hyperthermia (MH) EXCEPT:

A)   mortality rate from MH is less than 20%
B)   MH may be manifested by trismus and tachycardia during induction
C)   elevated body temperature is a late sign of MH
D)   MH can be triggered by succinylcholine, enflurane, and lidocaine

100. What is the treatment for malignant hyperthermia?

A)   Dantrolene
B)   Insulin and potassium
C)   Nitroglycerin
D)   Atropine

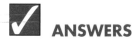

ANSWERS

---

1. **B)** Patients are abnormal from birth, with seizures and mental retardation.

   Homocystinuria is an autosomal recessive inborn error of methionine metabolism. Patients exhibit elevated serum levels of methionine and homocystine. Lens dislocation is bilateral, with 30% occurring in infancy and 80% occurring by age 15. Normal lens zonules have a high concentration of cysteine, and deficiency results in abnormal, brittle zonules. A diet low in methionine and high in cysteine can reduce lens dislocation. Patients are normal at birth and develop seizures, mental retardation, and osteoporosis. The patients are usually tall with light-colored hair.

2. **C)** It can result from a defect in galactokinase or galactose-1-P uridyl transferase.

   Galactosemia is an autosomal recessive inborn error of metabolism affecting the conversion of galactose to glucose caused by a defect in galactokinase, UDP-galactose-4-epimerase, or galactose-1-P uridyl transferase (most common). Excess galactose accumulation in body tissues with subsequent conversion to galactitol leads to the classic oil-droplet cataract, liver dysfunction, and mental deficiency within the first few weeks of life. If left untreated, it is fatal. Three quarters of patients develop cataracts because the nucleus and deep cortex become increasingly opacified. In some cases, early cataract formation can be reversed with dietary intervention.

3. **A)** autosomal dominant inheritance

   Lowe's syndrome is an X-linked recessive disorder characterized by renal tubular acidosis, bilateral congenital cataracts, glaucoma, mental retardation, muscular hypotonia, and failure to thrive.

4. **B)** Herpes simplex is not an important cause in infants under 4 weeks of age.

   Ophthalmia neonatorum can be the manifestation of several different infections or chemical conjunctivitis. The differential diagnosis includes Chlamydia, Neisseria gonorrhea, herpes simplex, and other bacteria. Chlamydia can be diagnosed with Giemsa stain, which reveals intracytoplasmic inclusion bodies. Although Chlamydia conjunctivitis can be treated with topical erythromycin, the patient must be treated with systemic therapy to prevent an associated Chlamydia pneumonitis. The pneumonia usually has its onset 3 to 13 weeks later. Neisseria gonorrhea is well known for its potential to penetrate an intact corneal epithelium and cause a corneal perforation. Herpes simplex type 2 is an important cause of neonatal conjunctivitis with keratitis with involvement of the corneal epithelium. Untreated neonatal herpes keratitis can cause corneal scarring and dense amblyopia. In infants with immature immune systems, the typical hyperacute purulent conjunctivitis may not be present. Both topical and IV antibiotics are needed for this severe infection. Chemical conjunctivitis caused by topical silver nitrate application has onset within 24 hours of birth, and conjunctival scraping shows few to no polymorphonuclear neutrophils (PMNs).

5. B)   NLD probing after 6 months of age.

    The photograph demonstrates a dacryocystocele. This presents at birth and is an enlargement of the lacrimal sac associated with a blockage at the valve of Hasner. Its appearance has been confused with hemangioma, encephalocele, and dermoid. If these cysts become infected, sepsis is possible; therefore early NLD probing in neonates and IV antibiotics are often necessary.

6. B)   The anomaly involves an abnormality of neuralectoderm.

    Pictured in Figure 5-3 is a congenital lacrimal fistula. Figure 5-4 shows fluorescein exiting from the fistula when the nasolacrimal duct is irrigated. This congenital anomaly represents an accessory epithelial-lined communication between the lacrimal system (usually the common canaliculus or the lacrimal sac) and the skin and is a problem of surface ectoderm not neuralectoderm. If it is associated with nasolacrimal duct obstruction, there is often discharge and reflux through the fistula. In this situation, topical antibiotics, probing of the nasolacrimal duct, and excision of the fistulas are appropriate therapy. There has been no association between this condition and a fistula to the maxillary sinus.

7. B)   This condition is often associated with anterior megalophthalmos, an autosomal dominant disorder.

    By 2 years of age, the cornea is approximately adult size. *Simple megalocornea* is defined as both corneas measuring greater than 13 mm in children older than 2 years, and greater than 12 mm in infants. Congenital glaucoma is associated with epiphora and increased IOP and must be ruled out of the differential diagnosis. The most common type of megalocornea is associated with anterior megalophthalmos, an X-linked recessive disorder.

8. B)   The condition has progressive corneal opacification.

    Peter's anomaly results from a developmental problem of faulty migration of neural crest cells. Neural crest cells usually migrate between the surface ectoderm of the cornea and the separating lens. As a result of faulty separation, both lens and iris may remain adherent to the central cornea, causing a central corneal opacity. Both Descemet's membrane and layers of the posterior stroma may be absent. The peripheral cornea is characteristically clear because Descemet's membrane and the endothelium are intact. In many cases, the corneal opacity will decrease over time.

9. A)   This lesion is anterior to Bowman's membrane and can be scraped off without concern of stromal involvement.

    Corneal/limbal dermoids are hamartomatous lesions consisting of fibrofatty tissue, surrounded by keratinized epithelium, often containing hair follicles, sebaceous glands, and sweat glands. They are usually located at the inferotemporal limbus, and they are associated with lipid in the corneal stroma surrounding the edge of the lesion. Large dermoids can cause astigmatism and amblyopia. Excision may be difficult because they may involve Bowman's layer and corneal stroma and, as a result, cause postoperative scarring, astigmatism, and amblyopia. Some require corneal patch grafts. Corneal dermoids can be found in association with Goldenhar's syndrome, which also includes preauricular appendages (Fig. 5-30), aural fistulas, maxillary or mandibular hypoplasia, hemifacial microsomia, vertebral deformities, notching of the upper eyelid, and Duane's syndrome.

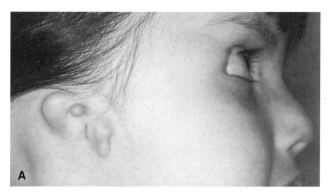

FIGURE 5-30. From Wright K. Textbook of ophthalmology. Baltimore: Williams & Wilkins, 1997.

10. B) CHED could be differentiated from congenital hereditary stromal dystrophy (CHSD) by pachymetry.

CHED is one of many diseases that causes cloudy corneas in children. It is a bilateral disease and comes in two forms, both having markedly thickened corneas. The *autosomal dominant form* is progressive and presents between 1 and 2 years of age with photophobia and tearing. Nystagmus is usually absent. The *autosomal recessive form* is present since birth and stationary. A sensory nystagmus is more commonly associated with the recessive form because vision is poor since birth. This disease must be differentiated from congenital glaucoma, which may present with buphthalmos and enlarged corneal diameters. CHSD usually presents with only central corneal involvement and a clear periphery. In CHSD, only the stroma is involved; there is no corneal edema, photophobia, or tearing. CHSD and CHED can also be differentiated on the basis of pachymetry; CHSD has normal corneal thickness.

11. B) Albinism

JXG is primarily a cutaneous disorder characterized by benign histiocytic proliferation. Iris involvement is seen as richly vascularized orange nodules or as diffusely infiltrative, leading to heterochromia. Congenital Horner's results in a hypochromic iris on the involved side. Waardenburg's syndrome is an autosomal dominant disorder characterized by developmental anomalies of the eyelids, nasal root, and eyebrows along with heterochromia iridis, white forelocks, and sensorineural deafness. Albinism results in bilateral loss of iris pigmentation and therefore does not result in heterochromia.

12. C) Microcornea

Microcornea is the only listed diagnosis not associated with ectopia lentis. Other conditions associated with ectopia lentis are Marfan's, hyperlysinemia, sulfite oxidase deficiency, trauma, syphilis, and Ehlers-Danlos.

13. A) Hereditary autosomal dominant

When determining the etiology of congenital cataracts, it is best to first determine whether they are unilateral or bilateral. Bilateral cataracts are often inherited in an autosomal dominant fashion. Bilateral disease may also indicate a metabolic or systemic disease such as diabetes mellitus, galactosemia, or Lowe's syndrome. In contrast, unilateral congenital cataracts are caused by local dysgenesis and are not inherited. PHPV, anterior polar, and posterior lenticonus are commonly unilateral.

14. A)   As soon as possible, even within the first few weeks of life

The critical period of visual development is the first few months of life. During this time, the visual areas of the brain are developing rapidly. Earlier treatment can result in better visual acuity. Bilateral visually significant cataracts can cause irreversible amblyopia and sensory nystagmus.

15. A)   Lensectomy, anterior vitrectomy, and fitting of contact lens

There are different views on the "best" treatment of congenital cataracts. Weigert's ligament, a connection between the peripheral posterior capsule and the anterior vitreous, is strong, and intracapsular surgery will most likely result in excessive vitreous loss and traction on the retina. IOL implantation has become a preferred method of treatment by many; however, most feel that an IOL should not be implanted in children younger than 2 years of age. This is partly a result of the increase in the size of the anterior segment during the first 2 years of life. Children also have high rates of capsular opacification. Contact lenses are preferred over aphakic glasses as the former reduces aniseikonia and astigmatism.

16. C)   gonioscopy has clearly identifiable landmarks facilitating goniotomy as a first line therapy.

Congenital glaucoma may present with corneal edema and enlargement, epiphora, and photophobia. Associated horizontal breaks in Descemet's membrane, Haab striae, are secondary to increased IOP. Vertical breaks in Descemet's are often the result of forceps delivery. Congenital glaucoma is bilateral in up to two-thirds of cases. Vision may be poor in the involved eye or eyes, and there may be a secondary myopic shift from globe enlargement. On initial visit, the cornea is often cloudy, obscuring gonioscopy and prohibiting a goniotomy. Carbonic anhydrase inhibitors and β-blockers are used to lower IOP initially, and after the cornea clears, a goniotomy or trabeculotomy may be performed. When gonioscopy is possible, the normal landmarks are poorly recognizable, and some feel that a "Barkan's membrane" overlies the angle. This membrane is incised at the time of goniotomy.

17. A)   Pauciarticular ANA positive

JRA is a disease process characterized by chronic synovitis associated with extra-articular manifestations (Table 5-1). The age of onset is variable but typically is after 2 years of age. It is more common in girls than in boys. Iridocyclitis is associated most commonly with the pauciarticular onset form of JRA as well as seronegativity for rheumatoid factor and positivity for antinuclear antibody. Approximately 80% of patients with JRA and a positive ANA will develop anterior uveitis. Patients with polyarticular or systemic forms of JRA rarely develop iridocyclitis. An important distinction is the pauciarticular onset, which is the important prognostic indicator. The progression to involvement of additional joints is not protective in terms of developing uveitis.

TABLE 5-1. Subgroups of Juvenile Rheumatoid Arthritis (JRA)

	Polyarticular[1] *RF-Negative*	Polyarticular *RF-Positive*	Pauciarticular[2] Early *Onset*	Pauciarticular Late *Onset*	Systematic Onset *(Still's Disease)*
% of JRA patients	30%	10%	25%	15%	20%
Sex	90% girls	80% girls	80% girls	90% boys	60% boys
Age at onset	throughout childhood	late childhood	early childhood	late childhood	throughout childhood
Joints involved	any	any	large joints	large joints	any
Iridocyclitis	rare	no	20–40% chronic	10–20% acute	rare
Serologic tests	RF negative	100% RF positive	RF negative	RF negative	RF negative
	25% ANA positive	75% ANA positive	60% ANA positive	ANA negative 75% HLA-B27 positive	ANA negative
Severity of Extraarticular Manifestations	intermediate	intermediate	mild	mild	severe

[1]Five or more joints involved
[2]Four or fewer joints involved
RF = rheumatoid factor
ANA = antinuclear antibody

18. B) Two-dimensional echocardiography

This patient presents with manifestations of Kawasaki syndrome, a systemic vasculitis of unknown etiology affecting the skin, mucous membranes, and heart. The most serious complication, vasculitis, involves the coronary arteries resulting in formation of coronary artery aneurysms. Two-dimensional echocardiography is indicated in these patients to evaluate ventricular function and to detect the presence of pericardial fluid and coronary artery aneurysms.

19. D) Aspirin

Aspirin is the treatment of choice for patients with Kawasaki syndrome. Systemic corticosteroid therapy use is associated with an increased rate of coronary artery aneurysm formation and is therefore contraindicated. Penicillin and isoniazid are not indicated because this is not an infectious process.

20. D) Sexual history

These are the classic features of an infant with congenital syphilis. Maternal spirochetemia with *Treponema pallidum* may lead to fetal infection. In cases of maternal primary or secondary syphilis, approximately half of the offspring will be infected. In cases of untreated late syphilis, about 30% of offspring will contract the disease.

21. B) Segmental pigmentation of the retinal periphery and chorioretinitis

Some patients may manifest active chorioretinitis, in most, the only evidence of chorioretinitis is segmental pigmentation of the retinal periphery with a salt-and-pepper appearance to the fundus.

Interstitial keratitis represents an inflammatory response to treponemal antigens and usually presents between 7 and 17 years of age. Anterior uveitis and glaucoma may develop, but these are less common manifestations and are usually not found in the newborn. Hutchinson's triad for syphilis includes interstitial keratitis; widely spaced, peg-shaped teeth; and deafness. Other systemic manifestations include saddle nose, saber shins, and rhagades (linear scars often found around the mouth).

22. D) melanocytoma

Causes of vitreous hemorrhage in children include conditions such as pars planitis, juvenile X-linked retinoschisis, and trauma. Melanocytomas are elevated, deeply pigmented lesions most often found at the optic nerve head. Histologically, they appear as a benign proliferation of melanocytic cells. They are not known to cause vitreous hemorrhage.

23. D) Macular microcysts exhibit classic petalloid leakage on fluorescein angiography

Juvenile X-linked retinoschisis is characterized by cleavage of the retina at the nerve fiber layer as opposed to senile retinoschisis where cleavage is in the outer plexiform layer. Because the photoreceptors are unaffected, the a-wave on the ERG is intact, but both the scotopic and photopic b-waves are reduced in proportion to the amount of retinal schisis. The EOG and dark adaptation test are normal or abnormal depending on the stage of disease. The macula is involved early, showing microcysts and radiating retinal folds, but fluorescein angiography exhibits no leakage. Peripheral schisis usually develops later. Vitreous veils and strands form. If a vessel is torn with these veils, vitreous hemorrhage results; this often is how children present. Typically, vision is reduced to the 20/50 to 20/100 level, but expressivity is variable.

24. C) oculodigital massage

This child has albinism. In addition to iris transillumination defects, patients have decreased fundus pigmentation and may have foveal hypoplasia and, consequently, a sensory nystagmus.

Chediak-Higashi and Hermansky-Pudlak syndromes are potentially lethal forms of albinism, both of which are inherited in an autosomal recessive fashion. Chediak-Higashi syndrome is characterized by neutropenia, lymphocytosis, anemia, and thrombocytopenia. Neutrophils and other lysosome-containing cells characteristically have large granules and have impaired chemotaxis and microbial killing caused by poor fusion of lysosomes to phagosomes. Patients suffer from recurrent infections and are at increased risk of developing lymphoreticular malignancies. Hermansky-Pudlak syndrome is more common in Puerto Ricans, and patients with this syndrome have abnormal platelets and a susceptibility to bleeding and bruising.

Oculodigital massage is characteristic of Leber's congenital amaurosis, another disease in the differential of sensory nystagmus but without iris transillumination defects.

25. C)   On CT, calcification is frequently present.

Toxocara canis is a nematode larva ingested by children playing in the dirt or from improperly cleaned lettuce or carrots. The typical lesion on pathologic examination is an eosinophilic granuloma. Often mistaken for retinoblastoma, Toxocara does not have calcification on CT. Peripheral Toxocara lesions can cause traction on the retina, dragging the macula temporally and causing an apparent exotropia. Although Toxocara predominantly affects the eye, it can also infect the lungs and liver.

26. B)   Congenital stationary night blindness

When an infant presents with poor vision, searching nystagmus, and an apparently normal examination, conditions to consider include albinism, achromatopsia, and Leber's congenital amaurosis. *Achromatopsia,* or rod monochromatism, is an autosomal recessive disorder with total lack of cones, with color blindness that results in 20/200 vision, photophobia, and nystagmus. The fundus is usually normal in infancy and the EOG is usually normal. In *albinism,* the signs in infancy are often subtle and may be missed. They would include iris transillumination defects, hypopigmented fundus, and foveal hypoplasia. *Congenital stationary night blindness* is marked by infantile onset of night blindness but not searching nystagmus. The ERG shows normal to near-normal photopic waveform but nearly nonrecordable scotopic waveform. Other diagnoses include optic nerve hypoplasia and aniridia but they are usually diagnosed by the ocular exam.

27. A)   Eye-popping reflex

The eye-popping reflex is a neonatal reflex described by Perez in 1972. It involves a pronounced widening of the palpebral fissures after an abrupt decrease in ambient illumination primarily, or after loud noises. It is present within the first 3 weeks of life in 75% of infants born after 28 weeks' gestation. In contrast, eye pressing, or gouging, and light gazing are abnormal behavioral mannerisms in visually-impaired children. A paradoxical pupillary response is rare but when present, it is highly suggestive of congenital stationary night blindness, achromatopsia, or optic nerve hypoplasia. A paradoxic response refers to an immediate constriction during the first 20 seconds after room lights are turned off, followed by a slow dilation after 1 minute.

28. D)   Retinochoroiditis typically involves the retinal periphery and infrequently involves the macula.

Toxoplasmosis is one of several congenital infections that may cause damage to ocular structures. They are represented by the acronym TORCHS: *TO* = toxoplasmosis, *R* = rubella, *C* = cytomegalic inclusion disease, *H* = herpes simplex, and *S* = syphilis.

Toxoplasmosis is caused by a protozoan with a propensity to infect the retina and other CNS structures. It is highly prevalent in North America. Cats shed oocysts in their feces, which may remain infective for up to 1 year. Ingestion of food contaminated by oocysts or undercooked meat containing tissue oocysts may result in human infection.

Maternal infection early in pregnancy results in a greater risk of transmission to the fetus. The organism may produce a retinochoroiditis, which is usually bilateral and frequently involves the macula. Inactive lesions may re-activate later in life, producing whitish, elevated lesions and a severe vitreitis resulting in a "headlight through fog" appearance on ophthalmic examination.

29.   C)   4 to 6 weeks after birth

The American Academy of Pediatrics' guidelines suggest performing screening eye examinations on all infants born at less than 30 weeks of gestation or weighing less than 1300 g. Infants are not born with ROP; they develop it after birth. Therefore, initial screening examinations should be performed late enough so that there is a low incidence of false-negatives yet early enough so that early detection of disease is possible. Examination of infants at birth or even 1 to 2 weeks after birth would result in many false-negatives, that is, infants who do not manifest ROP at the time of examination but who go on to develop ROP at a later time. At 8 to 10 weeks of age, some infants who had ROP at 4 to 6 weeks of age will progress to more advanced stages, possibly resulting in irreversible damage to the retina.

30.   A)   5 contiguous clock hours of stage 3 plus

The degree of retinal vascular abnormality in ROP is divided into five stages (Table 5-2). *Stage 1* describes a demarcation line separating vascularized retina posteriorly from avascular retina anteriorly. *Stage 2* develops when the demarcation line of stage 1 becomes an elevated ridge. If ROP progresses and the ridge develops extraretinal fibrovascular extensions into the overlying vitreous, this is called *stage 3* (Fig. 5-31). *Stage 4* describes a subtotal retinal detachment, and *stage 5* describes a total retinal detachment. *Plus disease* is characterized by engorged veins and tortuous retinal arterioles. It may be associated with rapid progression of ROP.

The Cryotherapy for ROP Cooperative Group found that in very-low-birthweight (<1251 g) infants with *threshold ROP*—stage 3 ROP involving 5 or more contiguous clock hours of retina or 8 non-contiguous clock hours in zone 1 or zone 2 and plus disease—transscleral cryotherapy applied to avascular retina significantly reduces the final incidence of blindness.

TABLE 5-2. Classification of ROP

Location
    Zone I—circle centered on optic disc with radius of twice the disc-macula distance
    Zone II—from outside Zone I to a circle with radius of disc to nasal ora serrata
    Zone III—remaining crescent of temporal retina

Extent
    Number of clock hours of involvement

Staging
    Stage 1—demarcation line
    Stage 2—ridge
    Stage 3—ridge with extraretinal fibrovascular proliferation
    Stage 4—subtotal retinal detachment
        A. extrafoveal detachment
        B. foveal detachment
    Stage 5—total retinal detachment

Plus disease—venous engorgement and arterial tortuosity

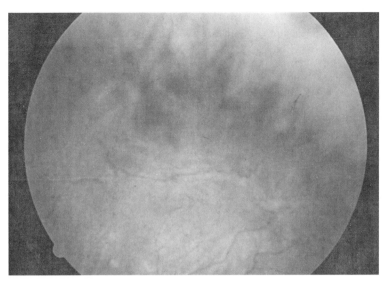

FIGURE 5-31

31. C) Twins

The major risk factors for developing ROP include hyperoxia, low gestational age, and low birth weight.

32. C) Males are affected more frequently than females.

Coats' disease is a retinal vascular disorder characterized by intraretinal and subretinal leakage of lipid from telangiectatic retinal vessels. It is usually diagnosed between 18 months and 10 years of age, and the most common presenting signs are leukocoria and strabismus. Boys are affected approximately three times more frequently than girls. Coats' disease is not hereditary and is unilateral in 90% of cases. Exudative retinal detachments (Fig. 5-32) occur in approximately two-thirds of eyes. Treatment is

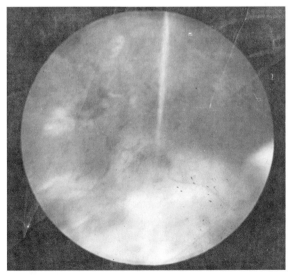

FIGURE 5-32

directed at obliterating leaking abnormal vessels by cryotherapy or photocoagulation. Scleral buckling may be performed on eyes with retinal detachments.

33. A)   Background diabetic retinopathy rarely occurs under the age of 20 years.

Whereas proliferative diabetic retinopathy rarely occurs under the age of 20 years, approximately 50% of patients with JODM for more than 7 years will have evidence of background retinopathy when examined by photography or angiography. In patients with JODM for more than 15 years, 90% will develop retinopathy.

Nonproliferative changes seen in the pediatric population include microaneurysms, cotton-wool spots, hard exudates, retinal hemorrhages, areas of nonperfusion, intraretinal microvascular abnormalities, and venous dilation.

Retinopathy rarely occurs fewer than 3 years after the onset of JODM. Because increased growth hormone levels during adolescence may be associated with progression of retinopathy, teenage diabetics should be examined for the presence of retinopathy within 5 years of diagnosis.

34. D)   Kearns-Sayre syndrome

Wagner vitreoretinal dystrophy is characterized by vitreoretinal degenerative changes, including an optically empty vitreous, high myopia, perivascular lattice degeneration, and retinal detachment. Cataract formation may also be associated with this disorder.

Stickler syndrome describes findings typical of Wagner dystrophy in association with the systemic features of Marfanoid habitus, Pierre-Robin anomaly, progressive joint degeneration, arthritis, deafness, and heart defects. It is an autosomal dominant disease with variable expressivity.

Characteristic findings in the autosomal recessively inherited Goldmann-Favre dystrophy include vitreous strands and veils, an optically empty vitreous, foveal and peripheral retinoschisis, attenuated retinal vessels, optic nerve pallor, and cataract formation. Both the ERG and EOG are abnormal, differentiating this condition from juvenile retinoschisis, in which the EOG is normal.

Although a characteristic of Kearns-Sayre syndrome is pigmentary degeneration of the retina, visual function is typically preserved. There is no significant vitreous involvement. Other features of this syndrome include progressive external ophthalmoplegia and, importantly, heart block, which may result in sudden death. Inheritance is via mitochondrial DNA, and onset is before the age of 20 years.

35. A)   The X-linked form is least common but most disabling.

The overall incidence of retinitis pigmentosa in the United States is approximately 1:3500. About half of these cases are sporadic, 22% are autosomal dominant, 16% are autosomal recessive, and 9% are X-linked recessive. The X-linked form is the most rapidly progressive and disabling, whereas the dominant form is least progressive and disabling.

ERG abnormalities precede ophthalmoscopically visible changes and subjective visual complaints. Early ERG evidence includes an increased rod threshold with a normal cone response and a decreased scotopic b-wave. Progression of the disease results in a nonrecordable ERG. The EOG is abnormal. The earliest visual field defect is characteristically an inferotemporal scotoma that enlarges to form a ring or annular scotoma.

The typical funduscopic findings include attenuation of the retinal vessels, mid-peripheral pigmentary changes, and optic disc pallor. Retinitis pigmentosa can occur without pigmentary changes in a form known as *retinitis pigmentosa sine pigmento*. Associated findings may include myopia, vitreous opacities, posterior subcapsular cataract, retinal pigment epithelial atrophy, cystoid macular edema, glaucoma, and keratoconus.

36. B) Night blindness and loss of peripheral vision frequently develop late in the course of the disease.

Characteristics of cone dystrophies include decreased central vision, color blindness, and photophobia, which develop within the first or second decade of life. The mode of inheritance is usually autosomal recessive; however, most familial cases are autosomal dominant.

Night blindness and loss of peripheral vision are uncommon even in advanced cases, distinguishing this disorder from retinitis pigmentosa. Subjective visual complaints typically precede macular changes on eye examination. The most common abnormality is the "bull's-eye" macular lesion, followed by the "salt-and-pepper" appearing macula with diffuse pigment stippling. The least common form is characterized by atrophy of the choriocapillaris, choroidal vessels, pigment epithelium, and photoreceptors. Some patients may develop a pattern of degeneration that mimics closely that of Stargardt's disease or fundus flavimaculatus. Optic atrophy, especially temporally, may occur as well.

ERG findings of decreased amplitude on the single-flash photopic and flicker responses along with reduced flicker fusion frequency confirm the diagnosis. Ultimately, visual acuity ranges from 20/60 to 20/400 with symmetric involvement of both eyes.

37. D) Fluorescein angiogram

This is a patient with Stargardt's disease, which is thought to be a result of lipofuscin accumulation within the retinal pigment epithelium; this in turn results in a characteristic "silent choroid" effect on fluorescein angiogram in which the lipofuscin blocks underlying choroidal fluorescence. The macula may exhibit a mottled hyperfluorescent appearance. The majority of patients have normal results on electrophysiologic tests, although ERG amplitudes are frequently in the low-normal range. When the peripheral retina is predominantly involved with the macula affected to a lesser degree, the term *fundus flavimaculatus* is used.

38. A) EOG

Best's vitelliform dystrophy is an autosomal dominant disorder characterized by an abnormal EOG in carriers, asymptomatic patients with normal-appearing fundi, as well as in affected individuals; and a normal ERG. Both ERG and EOG are needed to confirm this diagnosis.

In the early (pre-vitelliform) stage, the retina may appear normal, although the EOG is abnormal. In the vitelliform stage, a cyst-like yellow-orange lesion develops, typically in the macula, between the ages of 4 and 10 years. It is usually 1 to 5 disc-diameters in size and has a "sunny-side-up" egg yolk appearance. Central vision is usually good at this stage. With time, the vitelliform stage evolves into the "scrambled egg" stage, in which the material within the cystic structure becomes granular in appearance. The vision usually remains good at this stage. However, as the disease progresses, atrophy of the macula occurs. Subretinal neovascularization and hemorrhage and serous detachment of the retinal pigment epithelium may occur as well. Most patients see well for many years, but, ultimately, central vision decreases to 20/100 or worse.

39. A)   Figure 5-15

40. A)   Figure 5-16

41. C)   Figure 5-18

42. B)   Figure 5-17

43. C)   Figure 5-18

44. C)   Figure 5-19

Figure 5-15 = morning glory disc
        5-16 = optic nerve colobome
        5-17 = optic nerve pit

Figure 5-18 = optic nerve hypoplasia
        5-19 = hyaloid remnant
        5-20 = myelinated nerve fibers

Morning glory disc anomaly is characterized by an excavated nerve with overlying glial proliferation. The surrounding retina is often thrown into folds. There is an association of retinal detachment. Most cases are unilateral.

Optic nerve colobomas represent the same developmental problems as chorioretinal and uveal colobomas; specifically, a failure of the fetal fissure to close properly. They are most commonly located inferonasally. The coloboma can involve the macula and result in poor vision.

Optic pits may be considered a small coloboma. Pits usually occur inferotemporally but can be anywhere. They are associated with serous elevation of the macula, which tends to occur during the second or third decade of life.

Optic nerve hypoplasia can be profound with severe visual loss. The hypoplastic nerve often appears pale. When viewed, the surrounding scleral rim often deceivingly gives the impression of a normal nerve. A thin ring of pigment can be seen surrounding the nerve tissue, giving rise to the double ring sign. Strabismus, amblyopia, nystagmus, and an afferent pupillary defect can be associated findings. On occasion, vision in these eyes has been known to improve with amblyopia therapy. De Morsier's syndrome is associated with optic nerve hypoplasia, as well as hypothalamic and pituitary dysfunction. The latter can manifest as growth retardation, which can be treated with growth hormone supplementation. These children need to see a pediatric endocrinologist for work-up. Optic nerve hypoplasia has many important associations: fetal alcohol syndrome and maternal ingestion of LSD, quinine, and phenytoin. Both macular and optic nerve hypoplasia may be found with aniridia.

Usually, the myelination stops at the lamina cribrosa; however, myelination onto the surface of the retina appears as white, feathery radiating fibers. The myelin can obscure the view of retinal vessels and the macula.

Persistence of remnants of the hyaloid system is a common finding. There is a wide range of findings from a small Bergmeister's papilla (fibrous remnant of vasculature on the optic nerve head) to persistent blood-containing hyaloid vessels. The Mittendorf dot seen in Figure 5-21 is a remnant of the hyaloid vessel on the posterior lens capsule.

45. D)   The Reese-Ellsworth classification of retinoblastoma provides prognostic
information about patient survival.

Retinoblastoma is the most common ocular malignant tumor of childhood. It most
commonly presents as leukocoria, but it can present as strabismus, uveitis, cellulitis,
angle closure glaucoma, or hyphema. These atypical presentations are worrisome
because of the delay in diagnosis. The disease is caused by a mutation in the long
arm of chromosome 13 (13q14). Two mutations (Knudsen's 2-hit hypothesis) in this
region are necessary for the appearance of retinoblastoma. Approximately two-thirds
of the cases are unilateral and nonhereditary. All patients with familial disease, all
nonfamilial bilaterally affected patients, and about 15% of nonfamilial unilaterally
affected patients can transmit the disease in an autosomal dominant pattern with
high penetrance. The Reese-Ellsworth classification (Table 5-3) was developed in the
1950s as a guide for predicting visual prognosis in eyes treated by methods other
than enucleation. It has been used erroneously to predict patient prognosis for life.
Newer chemotherapeutic agents with better intraocular penetration are showing
promise as first line therapy. Patients with the hereditary form are predisposed to
developing secondary malignancies later in life, most commonly sarcomas. Tumors
occur in both the radiated and nonradiated patients, but they tend to appear 5 years
earlier in the radiated group.

Table 5-3. Reese-Ellsworth Classification

Group 1: Very favorable
   A. Solitary tumor less than 4 disc diameters (DD) in size, at or behind the equator
   B. Multiple tumors, none over 4 DD in size, all at or behind the equator

Group 2: Favorable
   A. Solitary tumor, 4 to 10 DD in size, at or behind the equator
   B. Multiple tumors, 4 to 10 DD in size, behind the equator

Group 3: Doubtful
   A. Any tumor anterior to the equator
   B. Solitary tumor, larger than 10 DD, behind the equator

Group 4: Unfavorable
   A. Multiple tumors, some larger than 10 DD in size
   B. Any lesion extending anteriorly to the ora serrata

Group 5: Very unfavorable
   A. Massive tumors involving over half the retina
   B. Vitreous seeding

46. A)   *craniosynostosis*—this patient would likely demonstrate midfacial hypoplasia,
V-pattern exotropia, proptosis, and telecanthus

This patient has the characteristic appearance of craniosynostosis, which is caused by
a premature closure of the cranial sutures by early childhood. Common findings
include midfacial hypoplasia, proptosis, telecanthus, V-pattern exotropia, oral and
dental problems, and respiratory problems. This child has Pfeiffer's syndrome, an
autosomal dominant condition that includes shallow orbits, syndactyly, and short
digits.

47.   D)   Toxoplasmosis

A ruptured dermoid cyst can incite a tremendous amount of inflammation. Rhabdomyosarcoma presents with rapid proptosis and reddish discoloration of the eyelids, mimicking orbital cellulitis. However, the redness is generally not accompanied by increased warmth. Other things to consider include pseudotumor, leukemia, eosinophilic granuloma, and infantile cortical hyperostosis. Toxoplasmosis is limited to intraocular inflammation and does not cause periocular inflammation.

48.   C)   Lymphoma

The hallmark of JXG is spontaneous hyphema from vascularized iris lesions. The lesions represent benign tumors found in the skin, iris, and orbit, which consist of lipid-filled histiocytes and Touton giant cells. Leukemic infiltration of the anterior segment may lead to heterochromia iridis and spontaneous hyphema. When there is deep corneal involvement, severe herpetic uveitis may be accompanied by hyphemas. Other causes of hyphemas in children include trauma, ROP, PHPV, Coats' disease, and retinoblastoma. Intraocular lymphoma is found in older patients and presents as a uveitis masquerade with primarily posterior segment inflammation.

49.   D)   dermoid cyst

Neuroblastoma is the most common source of orbital metastasis in children. Metastatic neuroblastoma produces proptosis with periorbital ecchymosis. Bilateral involvement is seen in half of the cases. Orbital infiltration by leukemia causes lid swelling, proptosis, and ecchymosis. Lymphangioma lesions consist of lymph-filled channels lined by endothelium and separated by thin, delicate walls with small blood vessels that are broken easily. Lymphangiomas infiltrate orbital tissues extensively, and intralesional bleeding is common. Dermoid cysts may rupture and spill their contents, inciting a significant amount of inflammation, but bleeding does not occur.

50.   C)   poor prognosis if diagnosed before 1 year of age

Neuroblastoma is the most frequent source of orbital metastasis in children. Metastases occur from the adrenals, mediastinum, and neck. Approximately 20% of all neuroblastoma patients exhibit ocular involvement, which can be the initial manifestation of the tumor. The mean age of presentation in orbital neuroblastoma metastasis is about 2 years. Their prognosis is very poor in general, but prognosis is considerably better in infants under 1 year of age. Spontaneous regression of this tumor may be seen in rare instances.

51.   A)   Sturge-Weber syndrome

Neurofibromatosis may be transmitted in an autosomal dominant fashion with complete penetrance and variable expressivity; however, half of all cases result from new mutations. Tuberous sclerosis may be inherited in an autosomal dominant fashion with irregular penetrance; up to 80% of cases result from new mutations. von Hippel-Lindau disease has a hereditary basis in 20% of cases and is transmitted in an autosomal dominant pattern with irregular penetrance and variable expressivity. The Sturge-Weber and Wyburn-Mason syndromes have no known mode of inheritance.

52. C)   Lisch nodules appear in over 90% of patients over the age of 6 years but are nondiagnostic because they may appear in normal patients as well.

Neurofibromatosis is a progressive disorder with a wide range of clinical manifestations. It occurs in 1 of 3000 births. Café-au-lait spots appear in over 99% of patients, and if five or more spots greater than 0.5 cm in diameter are observed, the diagnosis is established. Tumors of the CNS occur in 5% to 10% of patients. These patients are at increased risk for other malignancies as well, including neurofibrosarcomas, Wilms' tumor, rhabdomyosarcoma, pheochromocytomas, and leukemia.

Lisch nodules (melanocytic hamartomas) (Fig. 5-33) on the iris appear in over 90% of patients over the age of 6 years and are useful for establishing or excluding the diagnosis of neurofibromatosis. They are not found in the normal patient population. Plexiform neurofibroma involving the upper eyelid may produce ptosis and is associated with glaucoma in up to 50% of patients.

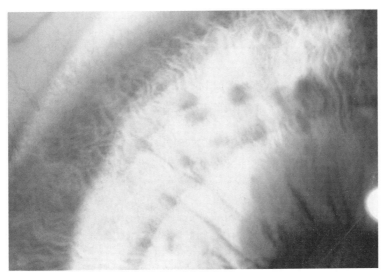

FIGURE 5-33. From Wright K. Textbook of ophthalmology. Baltimore: Williams & Wilkins, 1997.

53. B)   low flow lesion angiographically

The lesion pictured is a capillary hemangioma. Typically, these lesions appear within a short time after birth. They are composed of blood vessels that have an abnormal growth proliferation. These lesions can be located superficially or deep in the orbit. Some can present with both a superficial and a deep component. The capillary hemangiomas are characteristically high flow lesions, in contrast to cavernous hemangiomas, which are hemodynamically low flow. The majority of capillary hemangiomas will undergo spontaneous involution. Approximately 70% of these lesions will resolve before 7 years of age.

54. C)   Corticosteroids

The treatment of capillary hemangiomas depends on many factors, including vision, location, size, and systemic condition. Small lesions without visual compromise can be observed and vision can be monitored. Larger lesions can affect the patient's coagulation status by decreasing platelets. Thrombocytopenia secondary to sequestration of platelets in the tumor is termed the *Kassabach-Merritt syndrome.*

The lesion pictured demonstrates visual compromise, so observation alone is not possible. Corticosteroids can be administered topically, orally, or by intralesional injection. Complications of steroid injection include hypopigmentation and thinning of the skin, and very rarely central retinal artery occlusion. Surgical excision would also be an additional treatment option.

55. C)   Amblyopia

Lesions such as this can cause amblyopia in young children. Visual deprivation can occur if the lesion is so large that the lid obscures the visual axis. Even if the lesion does not block vision, it can cause astigmatism and a blurred image. These patients need to be observed closely with refractions to ensure that amblyopia does not develop.

56. B)   Inferior oblique

The inferior and superior obliques are abductors of the eye in synergy with the lateral rectus. The superior, inferior, and medial recti are all adductors.

57. D)   Inferior rectus

The primary action of the inferior rectus is depression of the globe. Its effect is greatest when the eye is abducted 23° from the midline.

58. D)   Temporal displacement of the corneal light reflex that does not shift during cover-uncover or alternate cover testing represents a positive angle kappa.

Positive angle kappa represents a slight temporal position of the fovea relative to the optical axis (Fig. 5-34). This causes a slight temporal rotation of the globe to keep the image on the fovea. This, in turn, causes the corneal light reflex to be displaced nasally. The deviated light reflex remains stable with cover testing as the fovea never spontaneously moves relative to the optical axis (Fig. 5-35). If simply covering and uncovering one eye reveals a re-fixation movement in the other eye, a tropia has been diagnosed. The alternate cover test dissociates the two eyes and allows measurement of the tropia plus the phoria. This patient's macula has been dragged temporally as a result of the scarring secondary to ROP (Fig. 5-36).

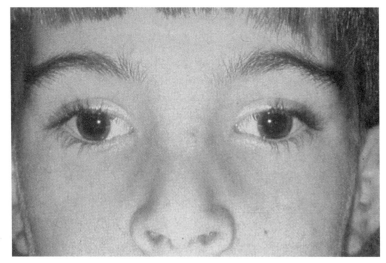

FIGURE 5-34. From Wright K, et al. Pediatric ophthalmology and strabismus. St. Louis: Mosby, 1995.

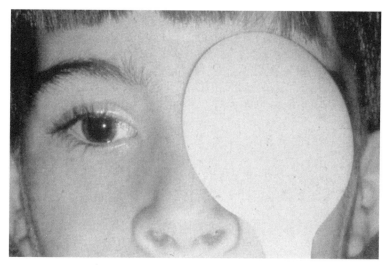

FIGURE 5-35. From Wright K, et al. Pediatric ophthalmology and strabismus. St. Louis: Mosby, 1995.

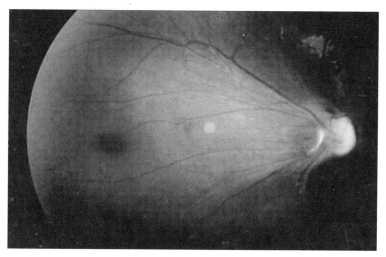

FIGURE 5-36. From Wright K, et al. Pediatric ophthalmology and strabismus. St. Louis: Mosby, 1995.

59. C) The Bruckner test uses the red reflex to determine the presence of strabismus. If strabismus is present, the fixing eye will have the brighter reflex.

The Bruckner test is a bilateral red reflex test, and if strabismus is present the brighter reflex is in the deviated eye. This is because the light reflects from peripheral retina in the deviated eye. Because there is less pigment in the peripheral retina than the macula, there is more reflection of light from the peripheral retina of the deviated eye.

60. A) The cover-uncover test will demonstrate a tropia; when the fixing eye is covered, the other eye will display an abduction movement.

This child has pseudo-strabismus. A broad nasal bridge with epicanthal folds can sometimes obscure the nasal sclera and simulate esotropia. As the child grows, the nasal bridge will not be as prominent and the folds may disappear. Cover testing will reveal orthophoria. DVD and inferior oblique overaction develop in association with congenital esotropia in up to 60% to 70% of cases.

61. B)   The frontal lobes control the slow pursuit movement.

OKN occurs in response to a repetitive visual stimulus moved across the visual field. The slow phase occurs in the direction of the moving stimulus; the fast phase occurs as a saccadic re-fixation movement in the opposite direction. The parieto-occipital lobe controls the slow pursuit component, whereas the frontal lobes control the saccadic component. In patients with congenital motor nystagmus, a reversal of the OKN response may occur. An OKN response elicited in an infant indicates that some visual input is present.

62. A)   Right superior oblique

The Parks' three step test, listed here, helps to identify a vertical muscle palsy:

1.   Determine which eye is hypertropic. This tells you that the involved muscle is one of the two depressors in the hypertropic eye, or one of the two elevators in the other eye. With this first step complete, choices are narrowed from eight muscles down to four muscles as shown in Figure 5-37.

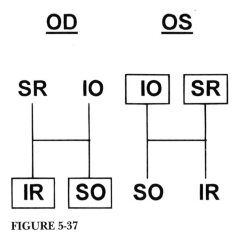

FIGURE 5-37

2.   Decide in which gaze the hypertropia is worse. By using the field of action of the four vertically acting muscles, the choices can always be narrowed down to two. In this example, the right hypertropia, which is worse on left gaze, indicates either the right superior oblique (the depressor of the right eye in left gaze) or the left superior rectus (the elevator of the left eye in left gaze) as shown in Figure 5-38.

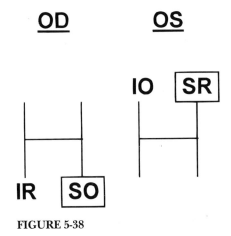

FIGURE 5-38

3. Determine if right or left head tilt worsens the hypertropia. This is the hardest step to understand, but it is really quite simple. When a normal patient tilts his head, one eye intorts and the other eye extorts. The intorters are the superior muscles (superior rectus and superior oblique) and the extortors are the inferior muscles (inferior rectus and inferior oblique). When the head tilts to the right, the right eye intorts and the left eye extorts. This means that both right superior muscles fire to cause the intorsion and both left inferior muscles fire to cause extorsion.

With this in mind, consider the previous example. Remember we have already determined that the palsy is either the right superior oblique or the left superior rectus. If the hyper gets worse with head tilt to the right, then the palsy is either in the right intorter or the left extorter. The right superior oblique is a right intorter, and if it is weakened, the unopposed action of the right superior rectus will cause the right eye to elevate further and worsen the right hyper (Fig. 5-39). In the left eye, the muscle in question is the left superior rectus, which is an intorter and should not be stimulated while extorting with right head tilt.

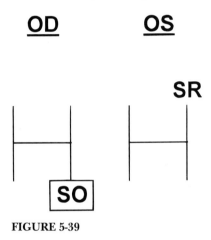

FIGURE 5-39

Two quick and easy patterns to memorize:

RIGHT(hyper) LEFT(gaze) RIGHT(tilt)—right superior oblique palsy
LEFT(hyper) RIGHT(gaze) LEFT(tilt)—left superior oblique palsy

63. D) Most applicable when a single muscle is involved

The Parks' three-step test is very useful in determining the specific pattern of deviations in single muscle palsies or overactions. The results are inconsistent or unreliable when more than one muscle is affected. The test is not able to distinguish between restrictive or paralytic palsies and congenital or acquired conditions. As with all tests, it is an adjunct to other clinical signs and symptoms in determining the involved muscle and whether it is palsied or overacting.

64. D) has its insertion near the macula

The following muscles correspond to each answer:

    A = superior oblique
    B = superior rectus
    C = inferior rectus
    D = inferior oblique

Congenital esotropia is a syndrome consisting of the following features:

1. Large angle esotropia, usually greater than 30 PD
2. Onset usually during the first few months of life, by definition by 6 months of age
3. Cross-fixation may be present
4. Latent nystagmus
5. Dissociated vertical deviation (in up to 60%–70%)
6. Inferior oblique overaction with V-pattern esotropia (in up to 60%–70%)
7. Mild hyperopia, + 1.00 to + 2.00 D

The above case is a classic case of congenital ET with inferior oblique overaction demonstrating both the V-pattern and the right hypertropia on left gaze and left hypertropia on right gaze.

65.   C)   dense amblyopia

Congenital esotropia, Möbius syndrome, and congenital fibrosis syndrome all can present with both eyes in the adducted position. Because the patient is cross-fixating, dense amblyopia is unlikely.

66.   D)   forced duction testing

By patching one eye, a patient with cross-fixation will have to abduct to see things in the temporal field. Doll's head movements generated by gentle, but rapid, turning of the baby's head can induce abduction past midline. The presence of a good saccadic abduction movement generated by an OKN drum can also indicate a well-functioning lateral rectus. If an eye in full adduction is secondary to a palsy, there most likely would not be enough lateral rectus function to generate a normal saccade. Forced duction testing identifies restriction not paresis.

67.   A)   always high AC/A ratio

Accommodative esotropia is acquired, developing as the child begins to accommodate around the age of 1 to 2 years, but can occur in infancy. Children with esodeviations usually suppress the deviated eye. Because the deviation is acquired, many patients spontaneously alternate fixation, so less than half will have amblyopia. Patients who constantly suppress one eye develop amblyopia. Patients are usually hyperopic with greater than 3.00 D of hyperopia. Approximately 20% have a high AC/A ratio and will benefit from bifocals.

**68.   B)   Dcc ortho wearing full distance correction of + 1.00 D OU
              Ncc ET15 wearing full distance correction of + 1.00 D OU**

The indication for prescribing bifocals to treat esotropia is specific. The patient must be able to fuse in the distance and be esotropic at near while wearing the full hyperopic correction. Giving a bifocal to a patient who has a deviation at distance despite full hyperopic correction will have no effect on the distance deviation. This patient needs surgery.

69.   B)   Acquired onset from infancy to 4 years of age

Accommodative esotropia occurs from infancy to 4 years of age with hypermetropia ranging from 2.00 to 7.00 D. Most neonates are not yet accommodating, so the esotropia is acquired when the infant starts to accommodate to bring vision in focus. As a result of the hyperopia, additional accommodative effort to bring images into focus is required, and an over-convergence response is seen. Accommodative esotropias are usually hyperopic but rarely more than + 7.00 D because if they are very hyperopic they develop bilateral amblyopia and do not even try to accommodate.

70. D)   amblyopia

Suppression occurs when the eyes are deviated or tropic, and there is excellent stereo acuity when the eyes are aligned with intermittent exotropia. During periods of visual concentration, these children often maintain straight eyes with bifoveal fusion and thus develop excellent stereopsis. Because both eyes are stimulated during times of fusion, amblyopia is rare. They do not have monofixation because monofixation is associated with a constant small-angle strabismus, and stereopsis is often worse than 70 seconds of arc.

71. B)   observe the child; tell the parents you are satisfied because this is the desired result postoperative day 1

An immediate overcorrection of 8 to 12 PD is a desirable result. Often, over the first or second postoperative week, the effect of the surgery will lessen and the eyes will straighten. At 8 years old, suppression is unlikely.

72. D)   Cannot determine from the information provided

This common pattern of exodeviation requires further evaluation. Exotropia that is farther rather than closer in the distance could represent either pseudo divergence excess or true divergence excess. One test that could be helpful is the 30-minute patch test. With this dissociating patch on for 30 minutes, the near deviation often increases and approximates the distance deviation. This deviation would then be classified as a pseudo-divergence excess.

A + 3.00 D lens may also prove helpful to look for high AC/A ratio patients. This classification is important both for determining how far to recess the recti muscles and for prognosis.

73. D)   A deviation of greater than 15 PD

The maintenance or preservation of good binocular function is the goal of surgery for intermittent exotropia. Warning signs that binocular function is becoming threatened are increasing deviation in the tropia phase, increasing ease of dissociation, and poor recovery of fusion. The size of the deviation is of little concern if the patients are able to fuse easily.

74. A)   orthoptic therapy with a base out prism or pencil push-up exercises

This patient demonstrates convergence insufficiency. This condition is best treated with orthoptic convergence training exercises. Base out prism therapy and pencil push-up exercises builds up convergence amplitudes. Reading glasses would help accommodative insufficiency but not convergence insufficiency. Very few physicians, if any, advocate surgery for this problem.

75. B)   Duane's type I

Sherrington's law states that when one extraocular muscle is stimulated, the ipsilateral antagonist is inhibited. In Duane's type I, the lateral rectus muscle is innervated by part of the medial rectus subdivision of the third nerve. This may be a result of a congenital agenesis of the abducens nucleus, which has been demonstrated pathologically. As a result of this aberrant innervation when the medial rectus is stimulated to contract, the lateral rectus also receives stimulatory impulses, thus violating Sherrington's law. Hering's law states that when an extraocular muscle receives stimulation, its yoke muscle (the prime mover in the contralateral eye in the same field of gaze) receives equal innervation. An exception to Hering's law is DVD. In DVD, one eye elevates, extorts, and abducts without any innervation to the contralateral eye.

76.   A)   Duane's retraction syndrome type I

77.   D)   Absence of electrical activity in the left lateral rectus muscle on abduction, with paradoxical activity on adduction

78.   D)   glaucoma

Duane's retraction syndrome (DRS) occurs in approximately 1% of all patients with strabismus. Its clinical features include a unilateral or bilateral abnormality of horizontal gaze, retraction of the globe on attempted adduction, and upshooting or downshooting of the globe on adduction. The left eye is affected more frequently than the right, and females are affected more frequently than males.

DRS may be divided into three types. *DRS type I* is characterized by marked limitation of abduction with normal or minimal restriction of adduction. Electromyography reveals an absence of electrical activity in the lateral rectus muscle on abduction with paradoxic activity on adduction. *DRS type II* is characterized by marked limitation of adduction with normal or minimal restriction of abduction. Electromyography reveals electrical activity of the lateral rectus muscle both on adduction and abduction. *DRS type III* is characterized by marked restriction of abduction as well as adduction. Electromyography reveals electrical activity of both the lateral and medial rectus muscles on both adduction and abduction.

Type I is the most common form of DRS, and type III is the least common. Although the majority of patients with DRS type I and type II will have straight eyes, some type I patients develop an esodeviation in primary position and some type II patients develop an exodeviation. Amblyopia may be present in 10% to 14% of patients with DRS.

Several ocular and systemic anomalies have been associated with DRS: cataracts, iris anomalies, Marcus Gunn jaw winking, microphthalmos, crocodile tears, Goldenhar's syndrome, maternal thalidomide use, and Klippel-Feil syndrome.

Brown's syndrome is characterized by the inability to actively or passively elevate the eye in the adducted position. It may be acquired or congenital. There is normal or nearly normal elevation of the eye in abduction.

79.   B)   A Faden procedure may reduce the upshoot of the affected eye on adduction.

The incidence of amblyopia in patients with Duane's retraction syndrome is only approximately 10%. The lid fissure narrowing is secondary to retraction of the globe with co-contraction of the medial and lateral rectus muscles. The strabismus is generally noncomitant. A *Faden procedure* (posterior fixation of the horizontal rectus muscles near the equator) may reduce the upshoot of the affected eye on adduction, as it stops vertical slippage of the lateral rectus muscle.

80. A) Esodeviation

Congenital third nerve palsy may result in complete or partial loss of superior, medial, and inferior rectus function, as well as inferior oblique and levator function. The eye is usually deviated down and out. Aberrant reinnervation may manifest as abnormal pupillary constriction with adduction.

81. D) recess-resect with supraplacement of the lateral rectus and infraplacement of the medial rectus

This patient exhibits a significant V-pattern without significantly overacting inferior obliques. In general, inferior oblique surgery is indicated for overaction of 2+ or more. Without significant oblique overaction, offsetting the horizontal muscles can correct as much as 30 PD of an A- or V-pattern. Horizontal muscle offset changes the vector of forces. The medial recti are moved toward the apex of the A- or V-pattern while the lateral recti are moved in the opposite direction. A recess-resect procedure is useful in cases in which surgery must be limited to one eye or when an incomitant deviation exists. Horizontal offset may be performed in conjunction with the recess-resect, but it may not correct large A- or V-patterns. In this case, the procedure of choice would be to recess the lateral recti for the appropriate deviation in primary position and offset the lateral recti superiorly.

82. C) The deviated eye extorts as it elevates.

DVD is present in 60% to 80% of patients with congenital esotropia. DVD is usually bilateral and asymmetric. The etiology is unknown but appears to be associated with an early disruption of binocular development. Thus, high-grade stereopsis and bifoveal fixation are not seen. During times of visual inattention, the nonfixating eye slowly drifts up, extorts, and abducts without a corresponding hypotropia of the fellow eye on alternate cover testing. This is the hallmark of this disorder—it does not obey Hering's law. DVD can simulate Inferior Oblique Overaction (IOOA) in side gaze when the nose acts as an occluder. The hyperdeviation in DVD is of the same amount in adduction, abduction, and primary position. This is in contrast to IOOA, in which the hyperdeviation is greatest in its field of action.

83. B) Occlude one eye for 30 minutes and remeasure the deviation.

This patient exhibits a difference of greater than 10 PD between near and distance. The patch test needs to be performed to differentiate a pseudo-divergence excess from a true divergence excess. This differentiation helps when deciding on the amount of surgery to perform and on the prognosis. The patient is monocularly occluded for 30 to 60 minutes and remeasured without letting him restore binocular fusion. The patch dissociates the eyes to suspend all tonic fusional convergence and to reveal the full latent deviation at near, eliminating the distance/near disparity.

84. B) Remeasure the deviation with a + 3.00 D add OU.

This child exhibits true divergence excess. He needs to be measured with a + 3.00 D add to determine if he has a high AC/A ratio. If the near deviation increases close to the distance deviation with a + 3.00 D add, he has a high AC/A. This factor is important because these patients are prone to overcorrection (75% overcorrection) if surgery for the full distance deviation is performed. Parents should be aware of the poor prognosis before surgery and of the possible need for bifocals to decrease the high AC/A ratio postoperatively.

85. A)   Observe and have the patient return in 2 weeks.

A small esotropia of 8 to 15 PD postoperatively is desirable, with 20 PD being the upper limit of normal. Postoperative diplopia associated with an initial overcorrection is normal and usually resolves by 1 to 2 weeks. In younger children (<4 years old), part-time alternate patching helps prevent the development of suppression. Patients with residual exotropia of more than 20 PD in the first postoperative week are unlikely to improve, and many will worsen.

86. C)   Prescribe enough base out prism to alleviate the diplopia but leave a small residual esophoria.

Prescribe just enough prism to alleviate the diplopia but leave a residual esophoria to encourage divergence. If the consecutive esotropia is present only at near, one can consider a bifocal add, miotics, or even base out prism. If the esotropia persists after 8 weeks, consider reoperation (usually a bilateral medial rectus recession). If the patient demonstrates lateral incomitance or significant limitation of abduction, a slipped muscle is a possibility.

87. B)   Lateral rectus recessions plus infraplace the lateral recti

This patient has high-grade stereoacuity and thus bifoveal fusion during his phoric phase. He also has a significant A-pattern from bilateral superior oblique overaction. Typically, one would operate on the superior obliques for significant overaction, but in patients with high-grade stereopsis, superior oblique tenotomies could cause consecutive superior oblique paresis with intractable torsional diplopia. In this case, vertical offsets of the horizontal muscles or the Wright superior oblique tendon expander should be done. The Wright silicone expander controls the amount of superior oblique weakening, is reversible, and alleviates the hyper inside gaze. The surgery of choice is lateral rectus recession with infraplacement to alleviate the A-pattern.

88. C)   superior oblique overaction with A-pattern is common

The picture exhibits a patient with limited elevation on adduction, which is consistent with Brown's syndrome. Brown's syndrome can be congenital or acquired, and it represents an inelastic superior oblique muscle tendon complex that leads to a restriction of passive or active elevation in adduction. There is often a downshoot of the eye on adduction and always limited elevation in adduction. This condition can be differentiated from inferior oblique palsy with exaggerated forced duction testing. Associated superior oblique overaction is uncommon.

89. A)   Patients with this condition have normal vertical fusion amplitudes.

This patient has congenital fourth nerve palsy. Longstanding fourth nerve palsy results in ocular torticollis with a compensatory head tilt to the side of the palsy that can lead to facial asymmetry of the dependent side. These patients have large vertical fusional amplitudes that help differentiate them from acquired fourth nerve palsies. The superior oblique tendon is rarely long or floppy or absent. When the child has fixation preference for the affected eye, the contralateral superior rectus muscle can appear to underact (inhibitional palsy of the contralateral antagonist) and the contralateral inferior rectus can undergo contracture, leading to a "double elevator palsy."

90. C)   Botox has been proven to be effective as the primary treatment of most types of strabismus.

Botox is a purified form of botulinum toxin type A, derived from the Hall strain of *Clostridium botulinum.* It blocks neuromuscular conduction by binding to receptor sites on motor nerve terminals interfering with the release of ACh into the synaptic cleft. When injected intramuscularly, Botox produces a localized chemical denervation muscle paralysis. The nerve ending atrophies but will resprout over time. Paralysis onset occurs in 2 days, increases in intensity over the next week, and lasts 3 months in extraocular muscles. Botox is indicated for blepharospasm associated with dystonia. The efficacy of Botox in strabismus is low and surgery remains the primary treatment for most types of strabismus. Multiple injections may be necessary but should not exceed 200 units in 1 month to decrease the incidence of antibody production. Reported side effects include ptosis, diplopia, and spatial disorientation. These are, fortunately, temporary. Perforation of the globe has been reported. Systemic effects of Botox are not seen because a dose over 100 times greater than the normal amount is required for toxicity.

91. C)   blepharospasm

Botox is the treatment of choice for most types of blepharospasm associated with dystonia.

92. D)   is often associated with intermittent exotropia

Latent nystagmus increases with monocular occlusion, when the fixing eye is in abduction (null point in adduction) and the fast phase is toward the fixing eye. It is associated with disruption of early binocular visual development (congenital ET, congenital monocular cataracts), not acquired strabismus (intermittent XT or accommodative ET).

93. C)   latent nystagmus with face turn to place the fixing eye in the null point

See answer for 92.

94. C)   prescribe full hyperopic correction + 3.00 OU

Reduce the latent nystagmus by correcting the residual esotropia and improving binocular fusion.

The best way to correct the small esotropia is by giving the hyperopic correction. Improving binocular fusion will reduce the latent nystagmus, thus reducing the face turn.

When one eye is occluded, the unoccluded eye remains in the adducted position and the patient may turn his and her face to the ipsilateral side to look straight ahead. The degree of esotropia increases when a base out prism is placed in front of the fixating eye, and the pupil constricts when the eye assumes its adducted position (indicating that this is an accommodative effort). Inferior oblique overaction and dissociated vertical deviation occur less frequently in patients with nystagmus blockage syndrome than in patients with essential infantile esotropia.

95. D)   optic atrophy

The classic triad of spasmus nutans includes monocular or dissociated small-amplitude nystagmus, head bobbing, and torticollis. The differential diagnosis for this disorder includes patients with chiasmatic gliomas and subacute necrotizing encephalomyopathy. Features of these two disorders may include optic atrophy, irritability, vomiting, and increased intracranial pressure. Spasmus nutans should be considered only after these two disorders are excluded. Spasmus nutans usually disappears within 2 years of onset.

96. A) oscillopsia is frequently present

Congenital motor nystagmus is a conjugate, jerk nystagmus that manifests in the perinatal period. It may be associated with a null point and a head turn to minimize the nystagmus. The visual acuity is relatively good—ranging from 20/20 to 20/70—and oscillopsia is typically absent. The nystagmus ceases when the patient is asleep.

97. D) Arnold-Chiari malformation

Congenital sensory nystagmus can result from a number of causes in which visual information does not reach the occipital cortex properly. Media opacities, such as congenital cataracts, foveal or optic nerve hypoplasia, and retinal degenerations, may all lead to sensory nystagmus. An Arnold-Chiari malformation causes a downbeat motor nystagmus.

98. B) Visual training, including muscle exercises, ocular pursuit, or tracking exercises, has been proven to improve academic abilities of dyslexic or learning disabled children.

Subnormal reading and learning may be a reason for an ophthalmologic evaluation. There is little evidence that reading abilities result from problems in the visual system; instead, the problem lies within the CNS and the interpretation of visual symbols. Eye defects do not cause reversal of letters, words, or numbers. Visual training has not been proven to be helpful in dyslexia. It is interesting to note that dyslexia is more common in languages in which certain letters or symbols have more than one sound. Boys are more likely to have dyslexia than girls.

99. D) MH can be triggered by succinylcholine, enflurane, and lidocaine

The incidence of MH is between 1:6000 and 1:30000, but it is thought to be higher in children. The mortality rate used to be as high as 70%, but it is less than 10% now. MH is triggered by succinylcholine, halothane, enflurane, and isoflurane. All local anesthetics may be used safely. Creatine phosphokinase is elevated in up to two-thirds of MH patients, but normal results have no predictive value and should not be relied upon. Frequently, the earliest sign is tachycardia or elevated end-tidal carbon dioxide. Other early signs include unstable blood pressure, tachypnea, sweating, muscle rigidity, cyanosis, and dark urine. A rise in temperature is a later sign.

100. A) Dantrolene

Dantrolene is a muscle relaxant that stabilizes cell membranes and prevents the release of calcium from the sarcoplasmic reticulum of the muscle cells. Adjunctive measures include discontinuation of the offending agent, cooling of the patient, hydration, hyperventilation, and bicarbonate for the acidosis.

Notes

Notes

6

Plastics

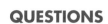

QUESTIONS

1. Which statement about the orbital septum is FALSE?

   A) During entropion repair, it is very important to recognize the orbital septum of the lower eyelid as being different from the aponeurosis or lower eyelid retractors.
   B) The orbital septum arises from a condensation of the periosteum of the orbital rim called the *arcus marginalis.*
   C) The orbital septum inserts on the superior border of the tarsus in the upper eyelid.
   D) The orbital septum serves as a barrier to the spread of infection from the superficial eyelids to the orbital tissues.

2. Which statement concerning the medial canthal area is TRUE?

   A) All of the attachments anchoring the tarsi to the medial orbital wall lie anterior to the lacrimal sac and attach to the maxillary portion of the frontal bone.
   B) The lacrimal sac lies posterior to the orbital septum.
   C) The muscle pump of the lacrimal pump mechanism is innervated by the fifth cranial nerve.
   D) Lockwood's ligament attaches posterior to the lacrimal sac.

3. Which statement regarding fat encountered during eyelid surgery is FALSE?

   A) Preaponeurotic fat is orbital fat.
   B) Extraconal orbital fat is an important landmark in identifying the levator aponeurosis.
   C) The removal of fat from the upper eyelid nasal, central, and lateral fat pads may be done with impunity.
   D) In the upper eyelid, the nasal fat pad is small, whereas the lateral fat pad is the small fat pad in the lower eyelid.

4. Which statement regarding Whitnall's ligament (superior transverse ligament) is FALSE?

   A) Whitnall's ligament attaches medially to the trochlea, laterally to the capsule of the lacrimal gland, and to the lateral orbital wall.
   B) This ligament is a condensation of the sheath of the levator muscle and serves as a check ligament to prevent excessive elevation of the eyelid.
   C) Whitnall's ligament acts to change the direction of pull of the levator muscle from horizontal to vertical.
   D) This ligament passes anterior to the lacrimal gland.

5. Which statement about eyelid anatomy is FALSE?

   A) The gray line is formed by the muscle of Riolan and represents the observable edge of the pretarsal orbicularis at the eyelid margin.
   B) The posterior lamella of the eyelid consists of the conjunctiva and tarsus.
   C) The mucocutaneous junction occurs where the eyelashes emerge from the eyelid.
   D) The peripheral and marginal arterial arcades allow for anastomosis between the internal and external carotid systems.

6. Features of the orbicularis muscle include:

A)   closure of the eyelid, depression of the eyebrow, and facilitation of tear drainage

B)   pretarsal orbicularis inserts temporally to become the lateral canthal tendon, contraction narrows the palpebral fissure, and the orbital portion of the muscle inserts medially on the posterior lacrimal crest

C)   the deep head of the medial pretarsal muscle is called *Horner's tensor tarsi* and innervation by cranial nerve III muscle is divided into three segments (pretarsal, preseptal, and orbital)

D)   the zygomaticofacial nerve innervates the upper lid orbicularis, the frontal branch of cranial nerve VII sends motor fibers to the upper lid orbicularis, and the preseptal orbicularis divides to encompass the lacrimal gland

7. Which one of the following muscle groups is paired INCORRECTLY?

A)   Tensor tarsi muscle—deep head of the pretarsal orbicularis

B)   Nasalis—preseptal orbicularis

C)   Superciliary corrugator muscle—orbital orbicularis

D)   Frontalis—procerus muscle

8. Which structure and its bony framework are paired INCORRECTLY?

A)   Lacrimal sac fossa—lacrimal and maxillary bones

B)   Optic canal—greater and lesser wings of the sphenoid bone

C)   Inferior orbital fissure—maxilla, zygomatic bone, palatine bone, and greater wing of the sphenoid bone

D)   Anterior and posterior ethmoidal foramen—ethmoid and frontal bones

9. The carbon dioxide laser has all of the following characteristics EXCEPT:

A)   wavelength in the infrared spectrum

B)   able to be seen by the human eye

C)   utilized for orbital tumor excision

D)   operates at 10.6 μm

10. The site of action of botulinum toxin type A (Botox), when used to treat facial movement disorders, is the:

A)   motor nerve terminal, inhibiting acetylcholine release

B)   motor nerve terminal, promoting cholinesterase release

C)   plasma membrane (sarcolemma) of the striated muscle, inhibiting acetylcholine release

D)   plasma membrane (sarcolemma) of the striated muscle, promoting cholinesterase release

11. Which one of the following is NOT a feature of basal cell carcinoma?

A)   Pearly elevated margins

B)   Spread to regional lymph nodes

C)   Ulcerated epithelium

D)   Telangiectatic vessels

12. The following factors are all associated with cutaneous cancers EXCEPT:

    A) increased sun exposure
    B) increased age
    C) red hair
    D) increased natural skin pigmentation

13. Features most consistent with a malignant eyelid lesion include:

    A) tenderness, erythema, alteration in pigmentary pattern
    B) disruption of tarsal architecture, raised pearly margins, pruritus
    C) lash loss, central ulceration, rapid growth
    D) ipsilateral lymph node metastasis, hyperkeratosis, dark pigmentation

14. A 40-year-old, red-haired, blue-eyed man of Irish descent living in Tucson, Arizona presents with a raised firm nodule with telangiectasia on his lower eyelid. This lesion most likely represents:

    A) nodular basal cell carcinoma
    B) morpheaform basal cell carcinoma
    C) squamous cell carcinoma
    D) sebaceous adenocarcinoma

15. Features of a keratoacanthoma include all of the following EXCEPT:

    A) spontaneous resolution
    B) loss of eyelashes
    C) ulcerated crater filled with lipids
    D) rapid growth

16. The 5-mm raised skin lesion with central ulceration is least likely to be which of the following?

    A) Keratoacanthoma
    B) Squamous cell carcinoma
    C) Basal cell carcinoma
    D) Malignant melanoma

17. The CT examination in Figure 6-1 is from a 55-year-old man. Which one of the following is LEAST likely in the differential diagnosis?

A)   Metastatic prostate carcinoma
B)   Sphenoid wing meningioma
C)   Fibrous dysplasia
D)   Metastatic melanoma

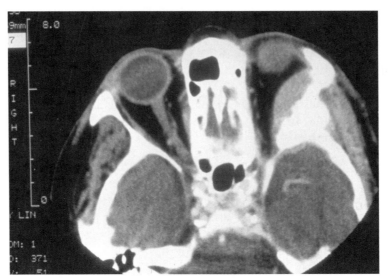

FIGURE 6-1

Questions 18–19

The defect of this eyelid (Fig. 6-2) of a 65-year-old woman resulted after a Mohs' surgical procedure.

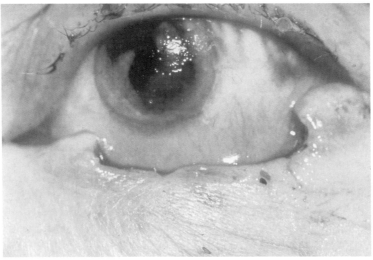

FIGURE 6-2

18. What surgical method would be the most appropriate for reconstruction?

    A) Cutler-Beard flap
    B) Bipedicle myocutaneous flap
    C) Full-thickness skin graft
    D) Hughes bridge flap

19. What is the LEAST likely cause that led to the eyelid defect pictured in Figure 6-2?

    A) Basal cell carcinoma
    B) Metastatic cancer
    C) Sebaceous cell carcinoma
    D) Squamous cell carcinoma

20. All of the following statements concerning lymphatic and venous drainage are true EXCEPT:

    A) lymphatic vessels of the orbit drain along the lateral portion of the cavernous sinus
    B) lymphatic vessels serving the medial portion of the upper eyelid drain into submandibular lymph nodes
    C) lymphatic vessels serving the lateral portions of the upper eyelid drain into preauricular nodes
    D) pretarsal venous drainage of the medial upper eyelid is into the angular vein and the lateral venous drainage is into the superficial temporal vein system

21. Xanthelasma eyelid lesions have all the following features EXCEPT:

    A) associated with systemic hyperlipidemic conditions in approximately 25% of patients
    B) located in the basal epithelial layer of the skin
    C) associated with the Erdheim-Chester disease
    D) microscopically contain foamy histiocytes

22. Which of the following glands are matched with their CORRECT types of secretions?

    A) Moll—apocrine, main lacrimal gland—eccrine, meibomian glands—apocrine
    B) Glands of Krause—holocrine, gland of Zeis—apocrine, goblet cells—holocrine
    C) Glands of Wolfring—eccrine, gland of Moll—apocrine, goblet cells—holocrine
    D) Main lacrimal gland—eccrine, meibomian glands—holocrine, gland of Zeis—apocrine

23. Which gland does NOT contribute to the aqueous layer of the tear film?

    A) Krause
    B) Main lacrimal
    C) Zeis
    D) Wolfring

24. Which statement about eyelid abnormalities is FALSE?

    A) Congenital coloboma of the eyelid always involves the lower eyelid and can vary from a small notch to a complete absence of the eyelid.
    B) Cryptophthalmos is a rare condition that is caused by a lack of differentiation of eyelid structures and is characterized by absence of a palpebral fissure with uninterrupted skin from the forehead over the eye to the skin of the cheek.
    C) Ankyloblepharon filiforme adnatum is a form of ankyloblepharon in which the eyelid margins are connected by thin strands of tissue.
    D) Distichiasis is a condition in which an accessory row of eyelashes grows from or are posterior to the meibomian orifices.

25. A patient calls to report pain, sudden swelling, and decreased vision the night after a blepharoplasty procedure. What should be done?

    A) Advise the patient to use ice packs to decrease the swelling.
    B) Set up an appointment for the patient to see you the next day.
    C) Make arrangements to see the patient as soon as possible.
    D) Reassure the patient that discomfort, swelling, and blurry vision are normal postoperative findings.

26. Which one of the following is found in the blepharophimosis syndrome?

    A) Euryblepharon
    B) Ankyloblepharon
    C) Epiblepharon
    D) Telecanthus

27. A 10-year-old girl has bulging and blepharoptosis of both upper eyelids and repeated episodes of eyelid inflammation and swelling. What is the most likely diagnosis?

    A) Blepharochalasis
    B) Dermatochalasis
    C) Steatoblepharon
    D) Blepharospasm

28. The proper surgical procedure for repair of a ptotic upper eyelid exhibiting a high eyelid crease, a margin to reflex distance (MRD) of 0 mm, and excellent levator function would be:

    A) resection of the superior tarsal muscle
    B) unilateral frontalis suspension using autogenous fascia lata
    C) reattachment of the dehisced levator aponeurosis
    D) plication of the levator muscle (16 mm)

29. The most common form of blepharoptosis is:

    A) involutional blepharoptosis (aponeurotic ptosis)
    B) neurogenic blepharoptosis
    C) myogenic blepharoptosis
    D) mechanical blepharoptosis

30. In myogenic congenital ptosis, the levator complex (in the ptotic eye) is:

    A) disinserted from the tarsus
    B) histologically different from normal levator complex with decreased muscle fibers and fatty infiltrates
    C) innervated by cranial nerve VII
    D) absent below Whitnall's ligament

31. In patients with ptosis, the 2.5% phenylephrine hydrochloride test:

    A) will activate the sympathetic receptors in Müller's muscle, resulting in elevation of the lid
    B) can be used to assess the approximate elevation of the lid with external levator advancement
    C) dilates the pupil so that the contralateral eyelid may drop
    D) does not affect blood pressure through systemic absorption of the phenylephrine

32. Which one of the following statements regarding blepharoplasty is FALSE?

    A) Repair of lower eyelid dermatochalasis and/or steatoblepharon may be followed by lower eyelid retraction.
    B) A retroblepharoplasty (transconjunctival blepharoplasty) is a procedure primarily used to perform upper eyelid surgery when trying to avoid an anterior incision.
    C) The advantage of eyelid crease fixation in conjunction with blepharoplasty is that it aligns the eyelid crease and the postoperative scar.
    D) Damage to the inferior oblique muscle is a potential complication of both anterior and posterior approaches to lower eyelid blepharoplasty.

33. Materials used for frontalis suspension of the eyelid include all of the following EXCEPT:

    A) silicone
    B) Gore-Tex
    C) supramid
    D) polyglactin 910 (Vicryl)

34. All of the following statements are true in describing the lacrimal gland EXCEPT:

    A) the lateral horn of the levator separates the orbital and palpebral lobes
    B) the orbital and palpebral lobes have separate excretory glands that empty into the conjunctival fornix approximately 5 mm above the superior margin of the tarsus
    C) the lacrimal glands are exocrine glands
    D) blood supply is provided by the lacrimal artery, a branch of the ophthalmic artery

35. The osteotomy site fashioned at the time of a dacryocystorhinostomy (DCR):

    A) is adjacent to the valve of Hasner
    B) enlarges the opening of the common duct
    C) is adjacent to the superior turbinate
    D) is within 10 mm of the cribriform plate

36. What is the most common reason for failure of a DCR?

    A) Obstruction at the level of the common caniculus or bony ostomy site
    B) Unsuspected lacrimal sac tumor
    C) Recurrent infection of the lacrimal sac
    D) Dacryoliths (lacrimal stones)

37. The Jones I test (Primary Dye Test):

    A) accurately defines the location of a nasolacrimal system obstruction
    B) involves irrigating the lacrimal sac with fluid
    C) has a high false-negative rate
    D) is a reliable indicator of nasolacrimal duct obstruction

38. What is the most frequently seen primary malignant tumor of the lacrimal sac?

    A) Fibrous histiocytoma
    B) Hemangiopericytoma
    C) Squamous cell carcinoma
    D) Lymphoma

39. Which one of the following is an indication for probing of the nasolacrimal system?

    A) Acute episode of acquired dacryocystitis
    B) Intermittent acquired inflammatory nasolacrimal system obstruction
    C) Congenital nasolacrimal duct obstruction unresponsive to massage
    D) Work-up of all patients with epiphora

40. Adult patients presenting with epiphora with an obstruction at the sac–duct junction would be expected to have:

    A) negative dye disappearance test/positive Jones III
    B) positive dye disappearance test/positive Jones I
    C) positive dye disappearance test/negative Jones I
    D) negative dye disappearance test/negative Jones II

41. Which one of the following statements regarding dacryocystograms is TRUE?

    A) They are a required part of the work-up in acquired nasolacrimal system obstruction.
    B) They are an excellent test of nasolacrimal function.
    C) They demonstrate canaliculi well.
    D) They demonstrate the nasolacrimal sac well.

42. All of the following statements regarding tumors of the nasolacrimal sac are true EXCEPT:

    A) They may produce painless irreducible swelling of the lacrimal sac.
    B) They may produce bleeding on attempted probing.
    C) They do not usually produce secondary dacryocystitis.
    D) They may produce epiphora.

43. In regard to canalicular trauma, all of the following are true EXCEPT:

    A) One may wait 24 to 48 hours after injury to allow soft tissue swelling to decrease.

    B) Upper canalicular trauma alone should never be surgically repaired so as not to risk damage to the remaining nasolacrimal system.

    C) Silicone stents should be left in place for 3 to 6 months.

    D) Surgical microanastomosis of the cut canalicular ends with silicone stent intubation offers the best possibility of successful repair.

44. Regarding the canalicular system, which statement is FALSE?

    A) The ampulla has the largest diameter of the canalicular system.

    B) A common canaliculus is present in approximately 30% of the population.

    C) The canaliculus has a diameter of approximately 1.0 mm.

    D) The average distance from the punctum to the nasolacrimal sac is approximately 10 mm.

45. Regarding irrigation of lacrimal outflow system, which statement is FALSE?

    A) Syringing saline into the lower canaliculus that irrigates into the nose indicates that no obstruction exists and that the system is functioning normally.

    B) Irrigation of the upper punctum with regurgitation through the upper punctum suggests an upper canalicular obstruction.

    C) Irrigation of the lower canaliculus into the sac with complete regurgitation through the upper punctum suggests obstruction of the nasolacrimal sac or duct.

    D) It may be helpful to recover fluid from the nose to examine for casts.

46. Chronic use of the following medications has been reported to cause canalicular stenosis EXCEPT:

    A) echothiophate

    B) idoxuridine

    C) epinephrine

    D) atropine

47. All of the following are indications for a conjunctivodacryocystorhinostomy (Jones tube procedure) EXCEPT:

    A) lacrimal canaliculi have been destroyed

    B) canalicular remnants cannot be anastomosed with the intranasal cavity

    C) common canalicular obstruction combined with nasolacrimal duct obstruction

    D) paralytic or scarred eyelids with absent canalicular pumping mechanism

48. In acute dacryocystitis:

    A) topical antibiotics without systemic antibiotics should be prescribed

    B) cool compresses are applied to the medial canthus

    C) diagnostic probing may be therapeutic in adults

    D) most adults will need a DCR for correction of outflow obstruction

Questions 49–52

A 12-year-old boy involved in a motor vehicle accident 3 months ago presents with a complaint of left-sided epiphora since the accident, along with a 1-week history of fever and progressive swelling, redness, and pain in the left medial canthal region with mucopurulent discharge from the medial canthus (Fig. 6-3).

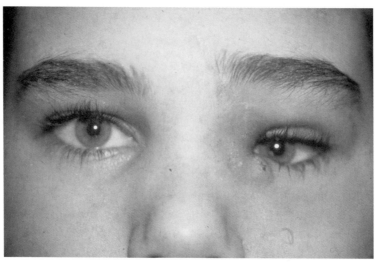

FIGURE 6-3

49. Appropriate initial work-up of this patient includes all of the following EXCEPT:

    A)   a complete ophthalmic exam
    B)   CT scan of the orbits and sinuses
    C)   probing and irrigation of the left nasolacrimal system
    D)   culture and Gram stain of the medial canthal discharge

50. Appropriate initial therapy of this patient would include all of the following EXCEPT:

    A)   DCR
    B)   IV antibiotics
    C)   topical antibiotic drops
    D)   incision and drainage of any pointing abscess

51. In acquired nasolacrimal system obstruction, where is the blockage most frequently located?

    A)   Canaliculi
    B)   Nasolacrimal sac
    C)   Nasolacrimal duct
    D)   Inferior turbinate

52. What is the most common bacterial etiology in acute dacryocystitis?

    A)   *Actinomyces israelii*
    B)   *Pseudomonas aeruginosa*
    C)   *Streptococcus pneumoniae*
    D)   *Staphylococcal* species

Questions 53–55

A mother brings her 12-month-old child to you because of chronic right-sided epiphora. She has been massaging the right nasolacrimal sac for the past 6 months; however, the epiphora has persisted (Fig. 6-4).

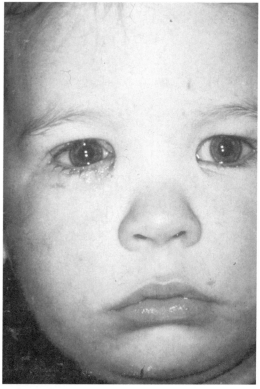

FIGURE 6-4

53. In congenital nasolacrimal system obstruction, where is the level of the obstruction?

A) Common canaliculus
B) Lacrimal sac
C) Valve of Rosenmüller
D) Valve of Hasner

54. The next therapeutic recommendation would include:

A) continuing massage
B) nasolacrimal system probing
C) DCR
D) observation, as most congenital obstructions resolve without therapy

55. Silicone stent intubation (with possible inferior turbinate infracture) is indicated in this patient when:

A) massage therapy has proven unsuccessful
B) dacryocystography (DCG) shows obstruction at the level of the nasolacrimal duct
C) nasolacrimal system probing has proven unsuccessful
D) the patient is older than 12 months

Questions 56–58

The 60-year-old woman pictured in Figure 6-5 reports a 3-month history of intermittent tearing and mattering in her right medial canthus. Additionally, she has noted focal swelling and tenderness near her lid margins.

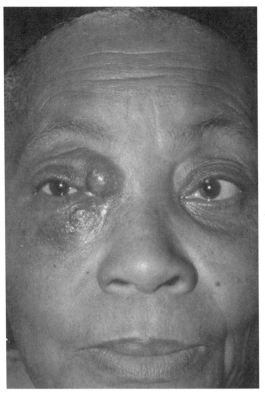

FIGURE 6-5

56. All of the following organisms are associated with canaliculitis EXCEPT:

  A) Actinomyces
  B) Candida
  C) Acanthamoeba
  D) Streptomyces

57. Which one of the following suggests a diagnosis of canaliculitis?

  A) Mucopurulent reflux from punctum with compression of the lacrimal sac
  B) Gritty sensation on probing with yellow-tinged concretions
  C) A palpable subcutaneous mass above the medial canthal tendon
  D) Palpable masses in the lacrimal sac

58. Treatment of canaliculitis includes all of the following EXCEPT:

  A) canalicular curettage
  B) canalicular incision and débridement
  C) canalicular irrigation
  D) oral penicillin

59. Trachoma can cause all of the following changes EXCEPT:

A) distichiasis
B) punctal stenosis
C) conjunctival scarring
D) entropion

60. All of the following pairs match mechanisms of involutional entropion with the surgical repair EXCEPT:

A) horizontal lower lid laxity—lateral tarsal strip
B) dehiscence of the lower lid retractors—retractor advancement
C) overriding of the pretarsal orbicularis by the preseptal orbicularis—excision of a strip of preseptal orbicularis
D) inward rotation of the lid by steatoblepharon—lower lid blepharoplasty

61. Clinical clues to the disinsertion of the lower lid retractors include all of the following EXCEPT:

A) white line below the tarsal border caused by the dehisced edge of the disinserted retractors
B) higher than normal lower eyelid position
C) decreased movement of the lower lid on downgaze
D) shrinking of the inferior conjunctival fornix

62. Which one of the following is the LEAST common form of ectropion?

A) Congenital
B) Paralytic
C) Mechanical
D) Cicatricial

63. Repair of lower eyelid involutional entropion would be BEST accomplished by:

A) suturing the orbicularis to the inferior fornix
B) suturing the retractors to the tarsus
C) suturing the orbital septum to the capsulopalpebral head
D) suturing the Lockwood's ligament to the conjunctiva and suspensory ligament of the fornix

64. The most common cause of upper eyelid retraction is:

A) recession of the superior rectus muscle
B) congenital eyelid retraction
C) surgical overcorrection of blepharoptosis
D) thyroid eye disease

Questions 65–68

65. An 11-year-old girl presents with acute, unilateral, left-sided periocular pain, proptosis, and double vision (Fig. 6-6). Which condition would NOT be included in the differential diagnosis?

A) Cavernous hemangioma
B) Sinusitis with orbital abscess
C) Traumatic retrobulbar hemorrhage
D) Orbital lymphangioma

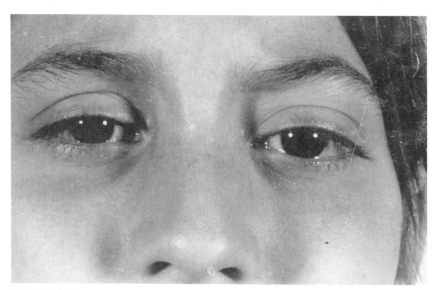

FIGURE 6-6

66. Twenty-four hours later (and without any treatment), the pain has resolved. Periocular ecchymosis has developed, and the double vision has stabilized (Fig. 6-7). The MRI results are also available (Fig. 6-8). The most likely diagnosis based on the clinical history and the MRI findings is:

A) rhabdomyosarcoma
B) capillary hemangioma
C) orbital abscess
D) lymphangioma

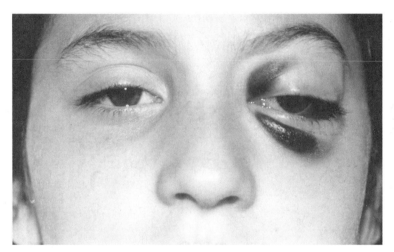

FIGURE 6-7

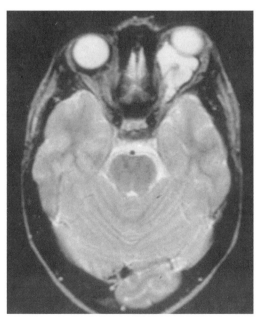

FIGURE 6-8

67. If the patient was losing vision because of this process, you would consider:

    A) open surgery to excise the lesion in its entirety
    B) CT-directed drainage of the encysted blood
    C) biopsy of the lesion to establish diagnosis and drain
    D) B and C

68. This disease process is an example of:

    A) the most common cause of proptosis in children
    B) the most common primary orbital malignancy in children
    C) a tumor that may enlarge with upper respiratory infections
    D) an orbital vascular lesion that will involute after intralesional corticosteroids

69. In orbital infectious disease:

    A) the presence of a subperiosteal collection of fluid is an indication for surgery
    B) the onset of decreased vision and an afferent pupillary defect in the presence of an orbital abscess is an indication for surgery
    C) proptosis and limitation of motility differentiate an orbital abscess from orbital cellulitis
    D) the maxillary sinus is the most common sinus involved when orbital cellulitis occurs as a result of sinusitis

70. An 8-year-old boy has a 2-week history of rapidly progressing superonasal mass that does not affect vision. Examination shows proptosis pushing the child's right eye down and out. The best management includes all of the following EXCEPT:

    A) CT scan
    B) anterior orbitotomy with biopsy
    C) MRI scan
    D) observation

Questions 71–74

71. The patient in Figures 6-9 and 6-10 has a history of increasing painless proptosis over the past 4 years. She is 48 years old and is otherwise healthy. Based on the history, the CT scan (Fig. 6-11), and the ultrasound (Fig. 6-12), what is the most likely diagnosis?

A) Optic nerve glioma
B) Cavernous hemangioma
C) Metastatic breast cancer
D) Benign mixed cell tumor of the lacrimal gland

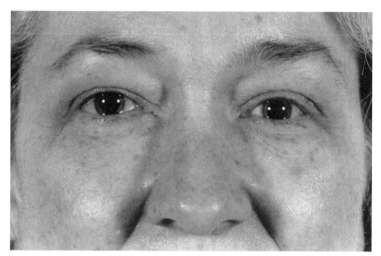

FIGURE 6-9

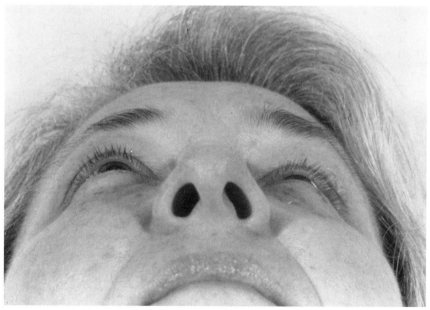

FIGURE 6-10

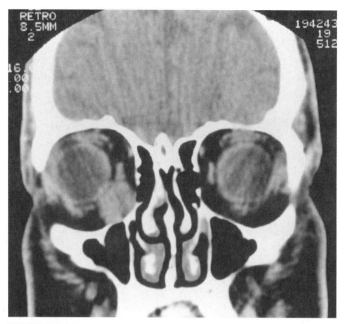

FIGURE 6-11

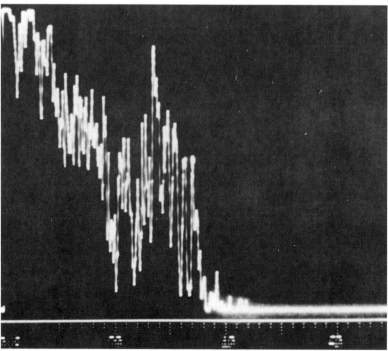

FIGURE 6-12

72. The orbital ultrasound shows:

    A) tissue of homogenous character
    B) high internal reflectivity
    C) B scan identifying tumor in the anterior inferior orbit
    D) low amplitude internal echoes

73. If the lesion in Figure 6-11 is NOT surgically removed, the patient can expect:

    A) slow growth over several years
    B) erosion of surrounding bony structure
    C) displacement of the globe downward and medially
    D) potential for malignant conversion of the presently benign lesion

74. Surgical removal of the lesion in Figure 6-11 would best be approached by:

    A) a lateral orbitotomy with en bloc removal of the mass
    B) incisional biopsy followed by radiation or chemotherapy
    C) an anterior approach through the inferior fornix
    D) a medial orbitotomy with reflection of the medial rectus muscle

75. Where do orbital floor fractures most commonly occur?

    A) Along the infraorbital canal
    B) Within the zygoma medial to the infraorbital canal
    C) Within the zygoma medial to the inferior orbital fissure
    D) Within the maxilla medial to the infraorbital canal

76. A 7-year-old white boy presents with a sudden onset of rapid evolution of unilateral ptosis for approximately 1 week. Examination shows significant edema in the periorbital area with a palpable mass in the superior nasal quadrant of the eyelid. Biopsy is performed immediately and the diagnosis of rhabdomyosarcoma is made. How is rhabdomyosarcoma best treated?

    A) Radiation with or without additional chemotherapy
    B) Total surgical excision
    C) Exenteration
    D) Chemotherapy alone

77. Which one of the following is the most common primary malignancy of the orbit in children?

    A) Neuroblastoma
    B) Rhabdomyosarcoma
    C) Ewing's sarcoma
    D) None of the above

Questions 78–79

The CT scan in Figure 6-13 is from a 60-year-old woman who presented with painless swelling of the lacrimal gland and anterior orbit for approximately 2 months. There was no significant past or current ophthalmic history. The patient's medical history was noncontributory.

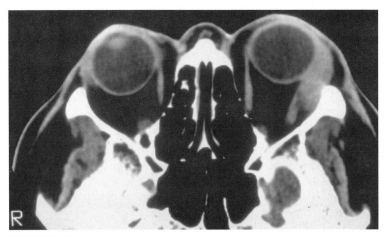

FIGURE 6-13

78. What is the most likely diagnosis?

A) Primary lacrimal gland lymphoma
B) Pleomorphic adenoma
C) Adenoid cystic carcinoma
D) Malignant pleomorphic adenoma

79. What is the most accurate description of the pathology specimen taken from this lesion?

A) Spindle cells with both ductal epithelium and a mixed stromal pattern
B) "Swiss cheese" pattern—hyperchromatic small cells proliferating around nerves
C) Ductal epithelium in a tubular formation with malignant degeneration
D) Mixture of both B and T cells, with predominance of B cells

80. Enophthalmos in one eye without previous injury is suspicious for:

A) cavernous hemangioma
B) metastatic breast carcinoma in a woman
C) orbital cellulitis
D) all of the above

81. The most common cause of bilateral exophthalmos in adults is:

A) cavernous hemangioma
B) pseudotumor
C) thyroid-related orbitopathy
D) metastatic disease

82. What is the most common cause of unilateral childhood exophthalmos?

    A) Capillary hemangioma
    B) Thyroid-related orbitopathy
    C) Orbital hemorrhage
    D) Orbital cellulitis

83. Predisposing conditions for mucormycosis include:

    A) diabetes
    B) renal disease
    C) dehydration
    D) all of the above

84. Proper treatment of orbital mucormycosis includes all of the following EXCEPT:

    A) stabilizing the underlying disease process
    B) débridement of all devitalized tissue, including exenteration if necessary
    C) amphotericin B for 6 weeks
    D) radiation to the orbit

Questions 85–87

85. A 55-year-old white man presents with bilateral proptosis, double vision, and chemosis. Figure 6-14 is an external photograph. What is the most likely diagnosis?

    A) Thyroid-related orbitopathy
    B) Orbital cellulitis
    C) Lymphangioma
    D) Meningioma

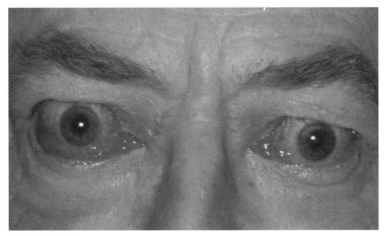

FIGURE 6-14

86. Concerning thyroid-related orbitopathy, the most common recommended surgical order of therapy is:

A)   orbital decompression, strabismus surgery, and eyelid retraction surgical repair
B)   eyelid retraction surgery, orbital decompression, and strabismus surgery
C)   orbital decompression and eyelid retraction surgery repair
D)   eyelid retraction surgery, strabismus surgery, and orbital decompression

87. A CT is performed on this patient with thyroid orbitopathy. Which feature, as demonstrated by CT, helps to clarify that this process is more likely thyroid-related orbitopathy than orbital inflammatory syndrome?

A)   Enlarged extraocular muscle
B)   Absence of a thickened tendon of the extraocular muscle insertion
C)   Enlarged lacrimal glands
D)   Periorbital soft tissue edema of the lids

88. A histopathologic slide of an orbital tumor is shown in Figure 6-15. This tumor is best treated by:

A)   exenteration and removal of involved bone
B)   radiation therapy
C)   chemotherapy
D)   all of the above

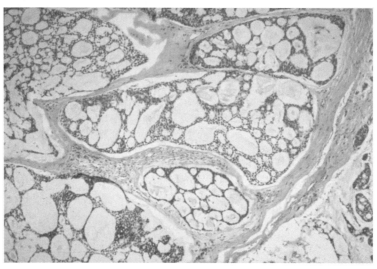

FIGURE 6-15

Questions 89–97 (Fig. 6-16 to 6-22)

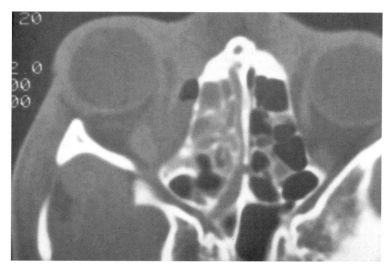

FIGURE 6-16

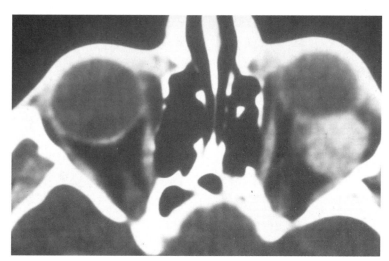

FIGURE 6-17

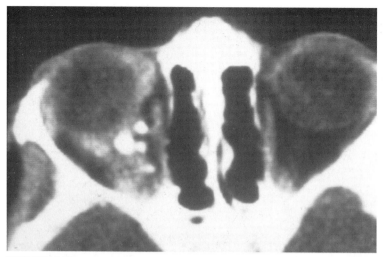

FIGURE 6-18

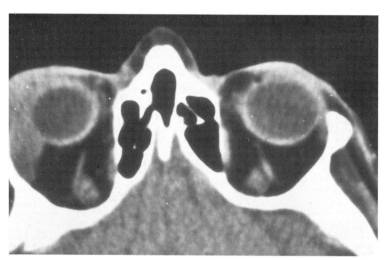

FIGURE 6-19

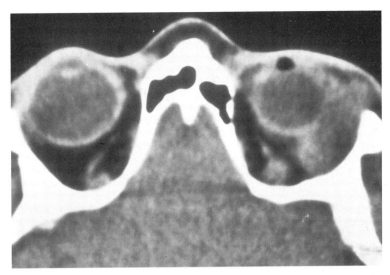

FIGURE 6-20

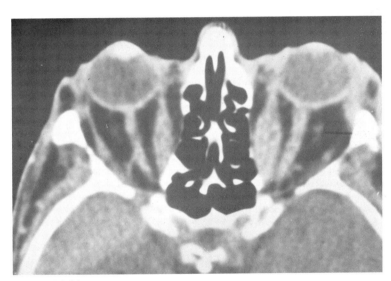

FIGURE 6-21

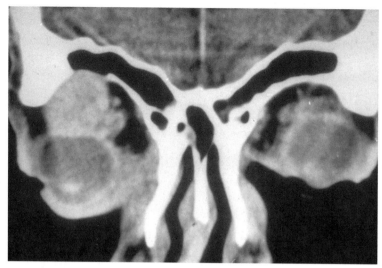

FIGURE 6-22

89. *Staphylococcus aureus* is the most common pathogen in patients who have the process as demonstrated in:

A) Figure 6-16
B) Figure 6-18
C) Figure 6-19
D) None of the above

90. Which two CTs best demonstrate orbital processes with a vascular origin?

A) Figures 6-17 and 6-19
B) Figures 6-17 and 6-18
C) Figures 6-16 and 6-17
D) Figure 6-17 only

91. The lesion shown in Figure 6-17 was found in a 30-year-old woman who noticed mild proptosis that accelerated during her pregnancy. This lesion caused retinal striae and hyperopia. Which etiology is most likely?

A) Metastatic breast carcinoma
B) Cavernous hemangioma
C) Dermoid cyst
D) Hemangiopericytoma

92. Histologic examination of a biopsy specimen from the lesion shows Dutcher body formations that are intranuclear periodic acid-Schiff (PAS)-positive inclusions of immunoglobulin. Which CT demonstrates a characteristic lesion consistent with this finding?

A) Figure 6-18
B) Figure 6-19
C) Figure 6-20
D) Figure 6-22

93. A 45-year-old white man presents with gradual painless proptosis in the right eye that has displaced the globe inferiorly and medially. A firm lobular mass is palpated near the superior lateral orbital rim. Vision is not affected. CT is obtained and the lesion is demonstrated in Figure 6-20. The next step in therapy should be:

A) a 2-week course of systemic corticosteroids
B) incisional biopsy
C) excisional biopsy
D) metastatic work-up

94. A 70-year-old patient presents with severe pain in the left orbit over the past month. Limitation of upgaze and lateral gaze is present. Vision is not affected. CT is obtained and demonstrated in Figure 6-22. Microscopic pathologic review is most likely to show:

A) tubules—solid nests of cells in a cribriform Swiss cheese pattern with perineural invasion
B) Flexner-Wintersteiner rosettes
C) psammoma bodies
D) Antoni A and Antoni B cells with nuclear palisades

95. Orbital decompression is performed in this condition for extreme proptosis, and development of compressive optic neuropathy occurs as demonstrated on which CT?

A) Figure 6-17
B) Figure 6-20
C) Figure 6-21
D) Figure 6-16

96. The etiology of the process defined on CT in Figure 6-16 can be from:

A) paranasal sinusitis
B) previous trauma
C) dacryocystitis
D) all of the above

97. Which CT demonstrates a condition in which proptosis increases with the Valsalva maneuver?

A) Figure 6-17
B) Figure 6-18
C) Figure 6-20
D) Figure 6-22

98. All of the following are considered a part of a syndrome of craniofacial synostosis EXCEPT:

A) Crouzon's
B) Treacher-Collins
C) Apert's
D) plagiocephaly

99. All of the following clinical findings can be associated with Goldenhar's syndrome EXCEPT:

A) eyelid colobomas
B) lipodermoids
C) Duane's syndrome
D) proptosis

100. Which systemic condition is incorrectly paired with a skin lesion?

A) Sturge-Weber syndrome (encephalo-trigeminal angiomatosis)—nevus flammeus (port wine stain)
B) Ataxia telangiectasia—café-au-lait spots
C) Incontinentia pigmenti—hyperpigmented macules ("splashed paint")
D) Tuberous sclerosis—facial angiofibromas (adenoma sebaceum)

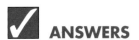 **ANSWERS**

1. C) The orbital septum inserts on the superior border of the tarsus in the upper eyelid.

   The orbital septum is a fibrous sheet that arises from the arcus marginalis, which lies at the junction of the periorbital periosteum (periorbita) and the pericranium. The septum extends toward the eyelid margins to fuse with the levator aponeurosis in the upper eyelid and the lower eyelid retractors (aponeurosis) of the lower eyelid. The septum is immediately deep to the orbicularis oculi muscle and superficial to the preaponeurotic orbital fat. During blepharoptosis surgery and other procedures, such as entropion repair of the lower eyelid, it is important to realize that the aponeurosis and lower eyelid retractors are located deep to the orbital septum and deep to the preaponeurotic fat. Therefore, in an anterior approach during blepharoptosis or entropion repair, the orbital septum must be incised to reach the eyelid retractors.

2. D) Lockwood's ligament attaches posterior to the lacrimal sac.

   The medial canthal area is complex in its anatomic structures. The medial canthal tendon has anterior and posterior portions. The anterior portion attaches to the frontal process of the maxillary bone and serves as the origin of the superficial head of the pretarsal orbicularis. The posterior portion inserts on the posterior lacrimal crest and fossa. The posterior limb of the medial canthal tendon, the deep head of the pretarsal orbicularis, and the deep head of the preseptal orbicularis muscles are important in maintaining apposition of the eyelids to the globe. The lacrimal sac is positioned anterior to the orbital septum and, therefore, does not lie within the orbit.

   During contraction of the orbicularis, the preseptal portion of the orbicularis exerts traction on the fascia lateral to the lacrimal sac (lacrimal diaphragm) as part of the lacrimal pump process. The orbicularis oculi is innervated by cranial nerve VII, not cranial nerve V.

   Lockwood's ligament (Lockwood's suspensory ligament) acts as a suspensory system for the globe. It is the lower eyelid retractor system with contributions from intermuscular septae and Tenon's capsule. Posteriorly, it arises from fibrous attachments to the inferior side of the inferior rectus muscle and continues anteriorly as the capsulopalpebral fascia (lower eyelid retractors). Medial and lateral horns extend to attach to the retinacula. The medial retinaculum attaches to the posterior lacrimal crest, and the lateral retinaculum attaches to the lateral orbital tubercle of Whitnall. These tissues form a suspensory hammock for the globe.

3. C) The removal of fat from the upper eyelid nasal, central, and lateral fat pads may be done with impunity.

   Orbital fat is located posterior to the orbital septum and is commonly encountered during eyelid surgery. The orbital fat is divided into intraconal fat (central) that is located inside of the muscle cone, and extraconal fat (peripheral) that is located outside of the muscle cone.

   The removal of extraconal orbital fat is commonly done during upper and lower eyelid blepharoplasty. Numerous fine connective tissue septae course through the orbital fat and condense in several areas to form compartments. The upper eyelid has a small medial fat pad and a larger preaponeurotic fat pad (located between the orbital septum and levator aponeurosis), which primarily is located centrally. The orbital lobe of the lacrimal gland is located laterally and should not be removed.

The color of the medial or nasal upper eyelid fat is typically whiter or paler when compared with the yellow color of the preaponeurotic, centrally and laterally located fat. The upper eyelid medial fat pad often moves anteriorly with aging more than the preaponeurotic fat, which results in a bulge that is located inferior to the trochlea area of the upper medial orbit.

The lower eyelid has a small lateral fat pad and a larger medial fat pad. The small fat pad is located inferiorly to the lateral canthus and is separated from the large fat pad by fibrous tissue connecting the capsulopalpebral fascia and the orbital septum. Posteriorly, the main fat pad of the lower eyelid is divided into two fat pads by the inferior oblique muscle. Therefore, some references will state that the lower eyelid has three fat pads instead of two.

It is important to realize that this is normal fat that occupies the orbit and is bulging from a weakening of the orbital septum. This fat may serve a role in protection of the globe and facilitate its movement. Removal of too much fat may result in restriction of the extraocular muscles or a cicatricial blepharoptosis. In addition, aggressive removal of fat without careful attention to hemostasis can also result in an orbital hemorrhage and blindness.

4. D) This structure passes anterior to the lacrimal gland.

The superior transverse ligament, or *Whitnall's ligament,* arises from the compaction of the sheath of the anterior portion of the levator muscle. Medially, it arises from the connective tissue of the trochlea. Laterally, it attaches to the capsule of the orbital lobe of the lacrimal gland and to the lateral orbital wall above the lateral orbital tubercle. There are extensions to the medial and lateral retinacula. This structure acts to change the direction of pull of the levator muscle from horizontal to vertical and serves to limit the elevation of the eyelid. Although Whitnall's ligament attaches to the fascia on the superior and medial surfaces of the lacrimal gland; it does not pass anteriorly to the lacrimal gland. The lacrimal gland is divided into orbital and palpebral lobes by the lateral horn of the levator aponeurosis.

5. C) The mucocutaneous junction occurs where the eyelashes emerge from the eyelid.

The eyelid is divided by some references into the anterior and posterior lamella. The anterior lamella consists of the skin and the orbicularis oculi (eyelid protractor) muscle. The posterior lamella consists of the conjunctiva, tarsus, and retractors. The eyelid may be subdivided further to include a middle lamella composed of the eyelid retractors. The mucocutaneous junction occurs posterior to the eyelashes near the opening of the meibomian glands. The gray line represents the marginal edge of the pretarsal orbicularis and would be considered part of the anterior lamella.

The ophthalmic (orbital) artery branches from the internal carotid system and contributes to the palpebral arterial arcades. The angular artery and the malar branch of the transverse facial artery, as branches of the facial artery, also contribute to the arcades. The facial artery branches from the external carotid system.

6.   A)   closure of the eyelid, depression of the eyebrow, and facilitation of tear drainage

The orbital portion of the orbicularis muscle runs from the anterior limb of the medial canthal tendon, the orbicularis muscle is innervated by cranial nerve VII (not III), and the origins of the preseptal orbicularis wrap around the lacrimal sac, not the lacrimal gland.

   The orbicularis muscle is divided into pretarsal, preseptal, and orbital parts. The orbital portion is involved in forced eyelid closure. The pretarsal portion arises from the posterior lacrimal crest and anterior limb of the medial canthal tendon. The lateral portion of the pretarsal muscle becomes the lateral canthal tendon. The deep head of the pretarsal muscle (*tensor tarsi muscle of Horner*) encircles the canaliculi to facilitate tear drainage. The corrugator draws the head of the brow to the nose, and the procerus depresses the eyebrow. The preseptal orbicularis originates from the fascia around the lacrimal sac and posterior lacrimal crest. Superficial origins arise from anterior fibers of the medial canthal tendon. Laterally, it forms the lateral palpebral raphe overlying the lateral orbital rim. The orbital portions of the orbicularis originate from the anterior medial canthal tendon and periosteum.

7.   B)   Nasalis—preseptal orbicularis

The pretarsal portion of the orbicularis lies anterior to the tarsus. Medially, the pretarsal muscle divides into two heads. The superficial head becomes the medial canthal (palpebral) tendon, and the deeper head passes posteriorly to insert on the posterior lacrimal crest and is also referred to as the *tensor tarsi muscle of Horner.* Laterally, the lateral palpebral tendon arises from the pretarsal orbicularis muscles and attaches to the lateral retinaculum, which attaches to the lateral orbital tubercle of Whitnall.

   The superciliary corrugator muscle arises from the periosteum of the frontal bone and inserts laterally into the subcutaneous tissue. The superciliary corrugator muscle is responsible for the vertically oriented glabellar skin creases (rhytids). Its inferior fibers are continuous with the orbicularis muscle. The procerus muscle interdigitates with the inferior edge of the frontalis muscle and is responsible for the horizontal lines seen at the nasion and the dorsum of the nose. The nasalis muscle is located on the lateral aspect of the nose and is a separate muscle from the preseptal orbicularis.

8.   B)   Optic canal—greater and lesser wings of the sphenoid bone

The lacrimal sac fossa consists of the maxillary bone anteriorly and the lacrimal bone posteriorly. The lacrimal gland fossa is located in the frontal bone in the anterior lateral orbit. The optic canal passes through the lesser wing of the sphenoid, NOT between the greater and lesser wings of the sphenoid bone.

   The inferior orbital fissure is bordered medially by the maxillary bone, anteriorly by the zygomatic bone, and laterally by the greater wing of the sphenoid and is also bounded by the palatine bone. The anterior and posterior ethmoidal foramina are located at the junction of the ethmoid and frontal bones.

9.   B)   able to be seen by the human eye

The carbon dioxide laser operates at a wavelength in the infrared portion of the electromagnetic spectrum. At 10.6 μm or 10600 nm, the carbon dioxide laser is not within the visible spectrum, which means that it is not visible to the human eye. The laser may be visibly guided with a helium-neon (HeNe) laser-aiming beam. The carbon dioxide laser is absorbed by water. The increase in temperature ultimately causes cell destruction. The carbon dioxide laser has a high absorption coefficient with water that is inversely proportional to the absorption length, which is very small. Therefore, carbon dioxide has the ability to remove tissue in small increments. The laser has wide application for orbital tumor removal (Fig. 6-23).

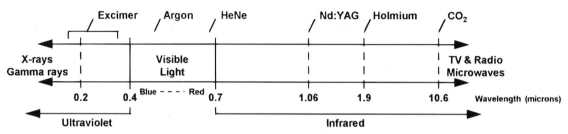

FIGURE 6-23. Modified from Trost D, Zacherl A, Smith MFW. Surgical laser properties and their tissue interactions. St. Louis: Mosby, 1992:133.

10. A)   motor nerve terminal, inhibiting acetylcholine release

Botulinum toxin type A inhibits acetylcholine release by binding to receptors of the motor nerve terminals. The denervation that results usually lasts several months. Some patients develop antibodies to the medication, resulting in a decreased efficacy of the botulinum toxin. Botulinum toxin does not affect the function but may actually increase the level of acetylcholinesterase. In addition, there is no direct effect of botulinum toxin type A on the striated muscle. The introduction of botulinum toxin type A in medicine has a variety of applications. Examples include benign essential blepharospasm, hemifacial spasm, paralytic strabismus, spasmodic dysphonia, and torticollis. Although botulinum toxin is a potent paralytic agent, the doses used for an adult are well below the amount necessary for systemic toxicity.

11. B)   Spread to regional lymph nodes

Basal cell carcinoma is the most common primary eyelid malignancy and is located most frequently on the lower eyelid. Nodular basal cell carcinoma has the classic appearance of a pearly raised nodule with centrally ulcerated epithelium. Basal cell carcinoma may recur locally, but basal cell carcinoma is unlikely to metastasize to regional lymph nodes.

12. D)   increased natural skin pigmentation

Sun exposure, fair skin, family history of skin cancer, previous patient history of skin cancer, and red hair are all associated with increased risk of skin cancers. Having more darkly pigmented natural skin pigmentation is not associated with increased risk for cutaneous cancer.

13. C)   lash loss, central ulceration, rapid growth

Erythema, pruritus, and dark pigmentation are not associated with malignancy. Although most cancers have slow, progressive growth, rapid growth does not rule out a malignancy.

14. A) nodular basal cell carcinoma

Basal cell carcinoma is the most common eyelid malignancy. Basal cell carcinoma accounts for over 90% of eyelid malignancies and is 40 times more common than squamous cell carcinoma. Basal carcinoma occurs most commonly on the lower eyelid (50% to 60%), near the medial canthus (25% to 30%), the upper eyelid (10% to 15%), and in the lateral canthus (5%). Nodular basal cell carcinoma occurs most commonly.

Clinically, telangiectasia and smoothing of the skin texture are early findings. These early changes may be followed by elevation and rolling of the edges of the lesion and central ulceration.

Histopathologically, nodular basal cell carcinoma consists of basal cell nests, and peripheral palisading may be present. Ulceration may be observed both clinically and histologically. Although morpheaform or fibrosing basal cell carcinoma is much more aggressive, it is less common. Histopathologically, morpheaform tumors occur in peripheral radiating cords without peripheral palisading.

Squamous cell carcinoma is less common but is more aggressive than basal cell carcinoma. Squamous cell carcinoma can arise from actinic (solar) keratosis and has been associated with human papilloma virus lesions. Sebaceous adenocarcinoma arises from the tarsal plate of meibomian glands or from other sebaceous glands or periocular tissues. Sebaceous adenocarcinoma is a very aggressive and malignant tumor.

15. C) ulcerated crater filled with lipids

Keratoacanthoma is a form of pseudoepitheliomatous hyperplasia. The lesion is typically a rapidly growing circular lesion that has a central ulceration filled with keratin. The lesion may cause disruption of the architecture of the lid margin or the cilia. Left untreated, the lesion may resolve spontaneously. Because of the possibility of an underlying malignancy and because the pathologist will need to examine the whole lesion, an excisional biopsy is recommended.

16. D) Malignant melanoma

Many skin lesions develop central ulceration. Some ulcerated lesions, such as the papillomatous lesion with central ulceration seen in molluscum contagiosum, are considered benign. A keratoacanthoma arises quickly and often has central ulceration. Keratoacanthomas typically are less apt to be malignant but can develop into squamous cell carcinoma. Both squamous cell carcinomas and basal cell carcinomas can have central ulcerations. A small melanoma would be least likely to have central ulceration.

17. D) Metastatic melanoma

The CT demonstrates a hyperostotic lesion of the left lateral orbital wall. Choices A, B, and C typically are associated with hyperostosis. In this patient, choices A and B are the most likely possibilities. Fibrous dysplasia can present with hyperostosis, although it normally presents in a somewhat younger patient population. Melanoma, in contrast, will metastasize to the extraocular muscles without hyperostosis.

18. D) Hughes bridge flap

Before selecting an appropriate reconstructive technique, it is necessary to assess the defect. There are numerous methods of reconstructing a defect. In Figure 6-2, there is an approximately 75% full-thickness defect of the lower eyelid, including both the anterior and posterior lamellae. Neither a bipedicle myocutaneous flap nor a full-thickness skin graft adequately replaces the posterior lamella (tarsal plate). The Hughes flap transposes a bridge flap of tarsus and conjunctiva into the defect. In addition, a full-thickness skin graft or advancement flap is used to replace the anterior lamella. A Cutler-Beard flap is a reconstructive technique that replaces full-thickness defects of the upper eyelid with a full-thickness tissue flap from the lower eyelid on the same side. Composite grafting, lateral cantholysis and direct closure, and a tarso-conjunctival flap with a myocutaneous flap (Hews' procedure) are additional reconstructive options.

19. B) Metastatic cancer

Basal cell carcinoma, metastatic cancer, sebaceous cell carcinoma, and squamous cell carcinoma are all malignant. In the malignant category of eyelid lesions, basal cell carcinoma is the most commonly encountered lesion. It is followed in decreasing frequency by squamous cell carcinoma, sebaceous cell carcinoma, and metastatic eyelid lesions.

20. A) lymphatic vessels of the orbit drain along the lateral portion of the cavernous sinus

No lymphatic vessels or nodes are typically present within the orbit. The conjunctiva does have lymphatic vessels. The statements regarding lymphatic and venous drainage of the upper eyelid are correct.

21. B) located in the basal epithelial layer of the skin

Xanthelasma are typically flat, yellow skin lesions, located in the dermis. Histologically, these lesions consist of foamy histiocytes. The majority of patients do not have an associated hyperlipidemic condition. *Erdheim-Chester* disease is a multisystem disease with lipogranuloma formation in the liver, heart, kidneys, and bones. Histologically, these lipogranulomas contain histiocytes, Touton giant cells, lymphocytes, and plasma cells. Ophthalmic manifestations of this disease can include proptosis and xanthelasma-like skin lesions (Fig. 6-24).

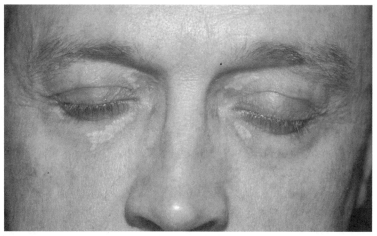

FIGURE 6-24

22. C)   Glands of Wolfring—eccrine, gland of Moll—apocrine, goblet cells—holocrine

23. C)   Zeis

GLANDS	LOCATION	SECRETION	CONTENT
Lacrimal	orbital lobe	eccrine	aqueous
	palpebral lobe	eccrine	aqueous
Accessory lacrimal	plica, caruncle	eccrine	aqueous
Krause	lid	eccrine	aqueous
Wolfring	lid	eccrine	aqueous
Meibomian	tarsus	holocrine	oil
Zeis	follicles of cilia	holocrine	oil
	lid, caruncle	holocrine	oil
Moll	lid	apocrine	mucous
Goblet cell	conjunctiva	holocrine	mucous
	plica, caruncle	holocrine	

24. A)   Congenital coloboma of the eyelid always involves the lower eyelid and can vary from a small notch to a complete absence of the eyelid.

Colobomas are more common in the upper eyelid, but that they can occur in either or both. When the coloboma is in the medial upper lid, it is usually an isolated finding, whereas in the lower lid, it is often associated with other congenital anomalies such as clefting problems. Not only is surgical repair indicated but also the eye must be protected with lubrication before surgery to prevent drying of the cornea and conjunctiva.

Cryptophthalmos is a condition that results from a failure of the eyelids to develop and separate. This condition is usually associated with a malformed eye. *Ankyloblepharon* is a term used to describe fusion of all or part of the eyelids. *Distichiasis* refers to an extra row of eyelashes arising posterior to the normal row of eyelashes. This term should not be confused with *trichiasis*, which is used to describe misdirected eyelashes rather than an extra row.

25. C)   Make arrangements to see the patient as soon as possible.

Pain, proptosis, periorbital ecchymosis, and decreased vision are the hallmarks of a postoperative orbital hemorrhage and possible compressive optic neuropathy. This patient requires immediate attention and evaluation. In the postoperative patient with a vision-threatening hemorrhage, the incision may be opened, the hematoma drained, and the tissue evaluated for control of active bleeding.

26. D)   Telecanthus

Blepharophimosis means horizontal palpebral fissure narrowing. The *blepharophimosis syndrome* (congenital eyelid syndrome) is typically congenital and consists of a widened intercanthal distance (*telecanthus*), blepharoptosis, blepharophimosis, and epicanthus inversus. It has autosomal dominant inheritance. Lower eyelid ectropion is also commonly seen in this condition. Other associated findings include poor development of the orbital rims and nasal bones as well as hypertelorism.

Euryblepharon is a horizontal widening of the palpebral fissure. *Ankyloblepharon* is a partial or complete fusion of the eyelids. *Epiblepharon* is commonly seen in Asian children and is caused by altered lower eyelid retractor (*aponeurosis*) attachments, which allow overriding of the pretarsal orbicularis above the eyelid margin. The result is posterior misdirection of the lower eyelashes and potential keratopathy.

27. A) Blepharochalasis

Blepharochalasis is a rare inherited condition that occurs more commonly in young females than in males and consists of repeated bouts of eyelid inflammation and edema. Recurrent idiopathic eyelid swelling eventually leads to blepharoptosis secondary to dehiscence or attenuation of the levator aponeurosis. Anterior bulging of the lacrimal gland or orbital fat may also occur.

Dermatochalasis refers to the excess eyelid skin that occurs with aging. *Steatoblepharon* refers to the bulging of orbital fat that also commonly occurs with aging or attenuation of the orbital septum. Blepharospasm may be associated with blepharoptosis and entropion caused by aponeurotic dehiscence. Dermatochalasis, steatoblepharon, and blepharospasm typically are not associated with repeated bouts of eyelid edema and inflammation.

28. C) reattachment of the dehisced levator aponeurosis

This patient has the classic signs of a blepharoptosis secondary to an acquired dehiscence of the levator aponeurosis. The patient exhibits a high eyelid crease or high eyelid pull, excellent levator function, and thinning of the eyelid superior to the upper tarsal plate. Therefore, surgery to reanastomose the dehisced end of the levator to the superior aspect of the tarsus would correct the blepharoptosis in the most anatomically proper fashion. Repair of the dehisced aponeurosis alone does not give as long lasting a result as suturing the aponeurosis to the edge of the tarsus.

29. A) involutional blepharoptosis (aponeurotic ptosis)

Ptosis (blepharoptosis) describes drooping of the upper eyelid and can have many different causes. Attempts to classify blepharoptosis can be confusing because there may be overlap of the categories. The term *congenital* means the blepharoptosis was present at birth, whereas *acquired* blepharoptosis describes blepharoptosis occurring after birth. Neither of these terms addresses the etiology of the observed blepharoptosis.

Acquired blepharoptosis is the most common ptosis. There are many different types of acquired blepharoptosis, which are often categorized by their etiology. The most common type of acquired blepharoptosis is involutional or aponeurotic blepharoptosis, which is caused by dehiscence of the levator aponeurosis.

Acquired neurogenic blepharoptosis occurs when there is a disruption of the normal innervation to the upper eyelid retractors. A traumatic blepharoptosis caused by a cranial nerve III injury is one example. Another example is acquired Horner's syndrome, in which there is interruption of sympathetic innervation to the superior tarsal muscle, resulting in miosis, anhydrosis, and a subtle upper eyelid blepharoptosis. Marcus Gunn jaw winking is an example of congenital neurogenic blepharoptosis and is also referred to as *synkinetic blepharoptosis*. This condition is characterized by an aberrant connection of the levator muscle innervation and the motor supply to the ipsilateral lateral pterygoid muscle.

Aberrant regeneration of cranial nerve III after trauma can result in a ptotic upper eyelid that exhibits synkinetic or abnormal movements. Abnormal regeneration and growth of the motor fibers from the inferior division of cranial nerve III into the superior division of this nerve may result in an eyelid that is ptotic in primary gaze but exhibits retraction in medial or inferior gaze as a result of stimulation of the levator muscle. Myasthenia gravis is caused by a defect at the neuromuscular junction and could be classified as a neurogenic blepharoptosis.

Mechanical blepharoptosis can be acquired or congenital. A tumor or hematoma involving the levator muscle, for example, could be a cause of an acquired or congenital blepharoptosis. Traumatic blepharoptosis can result from injury to the levator muscle, the aponeurosis, or the superior tarsal muscle, or innervation of any of these structures. Acquired myogenic blepharoptosis is rare. Some examples include oculopharyngeal dystrophy, chronic progressive external ophthalmoplegia, and other muscular diseases such as muscular dystrophy.

The most common type of congenital blepharoptosis is myogenic blepharoptosis due to poor development of the levator muscle. These terms are often used interchangeably. Myogenic blepharoptosis is due to dysgenesis of the levator muscle. Striated muscle fibers are diminished, and fibrosis as well as occasional fat may be present in the muscle. This abnormality decreases the ability of the muscle to contract and relax.

30. B)   histologically different from normal levator complex with decreased muscle fibers and fatty infiltrates

Myogenic congenital ptosis is the result of dysgenesis of the levator muscle complex. Both histopathologically and clinically, the complex is atrophic with replacement of muscle fibers by fibrous or adipose tissue. In myogenic ptosis, the levator aponeurosis will insert on the tarsus. Congenital dehiscence of the levator aponeurosis has been described but would not fall into the category of myogenic ptosis. Although the levator complex may be abnormal, the complex is still present below Whitnall's ligament. The levator is still innervated by cranial nerve III, but patients may use cranial nerve VII to elevate the brow and thus the lids.

31. A)   will activate the sympathetic receptors in Müller's muscle, resulting in an elevation of the lid

The 2.5% phenylephrine hydrochloride test will activate the sympathetic fibers of Müller's muscle. The resultant elevation of the lid simulates the position of the lid after conjunctivomüllerectomy. The alteration of the lid position also helps the surgeon evaluate the effect of Hering's law on the contralateral eyelid. Lid position, not pupillary dilation, is responsible for this effect. Phenylephrine can elevate systemic blood pressure. Digital punctal occlusion can be used to help prevent this side effect.

32. B)   A retroblepharoplasty (transconjunctival blepharoplasty) is a procedure primarily used to perform upper eyelid surgery when trying to avoid an anterior incision.

Dermatochalasis is a term used to describe redundant eyelid skin of the upper or lower eyelids. *Steatoblepharon* describes bulging orbital fat that commonly occurs with aging and is often removed during blepharoplasty. This fat tends to bulge forward with the aging process and may be related to a weakening or stretching of the orbital septum.

A retroblepharoplasty (transconjunctival blepharoplasty) or blepharoplasty via the transconjunctival approach is used in lower eyelid blepharoplasty, NOT upper eyelid blepharoplasty. The advantage of this approach is to avoid a visible scar on the skin of the eyelid. One disadvantage of this approach is that it does not allow for skin removal and is best used in patients with significant lower eyelid steatoblepharon without coexisting significant dermatochalasis.

Blepharoplasty of the upper eyelid is typically done using an eyelid crease incision. When the skin is reapproximated, the suture needle should be passed into the fascia located posterior to the orbicularis. This step accentuates the crease fixation and allows the healed incision to be hidden in the upper eyelid crease.

The inferior oblique muscle originates at the lacrimal spine located on the medial inferior orbital rim. The origin or muscle belly of the inferior oblique can be injured easily during lower eyelid blepharoplasty when the eyelid fat pad is removed.

Lower eyelid retraction is a common complication of lower eyelid blepharoplasty. Although the mechanism is unknown, the retraction may be related to scarring of the lower eyelid retractors and/or excessive removal of skin or muscle proportional to the eyelid's horizontal laxity.

33. D)   polyglactin 910 (Vicryl)

Numerous materials have been described for use in frontalis suspension. These materials include donor fascia lata, autogenous fascia lata, temporalis fascia, supramid, silicone, and Gore-Tex. An absorbable suture such as Vicryl would not be effective in suspending the eyelid for the long term.

34. B)   the orbital and palpebral lobes have separate excretory glands that empty into the conjunctival fornix approximately 5 mm above the superior margin of the tarsus.

The excretory ducts from the orbital lobe of the lacrimal gland pass into the palpebral lacrimal gland. The ducts continue, then empty into the conjunctival fornix.

35. D)   is within 10 mm of the cribriform plate

The osteotomy site created at the time of a DCR or CDCR is at the level of the middle turbinate. This site is most often within 10 mm of the cribriform plate. Typically, the lacrimal sac is divided and secured to the nasal mucosa. This division allows an open outlet from the common opening into the nasal cavity. The valve of Hasner is clinically significant more often in patients with a congenital tearing problem. This valve is located at the distal end of the nasolacrimal duct under the inferior turbinate.

36. A)   Obstruction at the common canaliculus or bony ostomy site

The two most common causes of DCR failure are obstruction at the common canaliculus and obstruction at the bony ostomy site. Recurrent obstruction can result in recurrent infection and dacryolith formation. Unsuspected tumors may also cause recurrent obstruction but are not the major cause of DCR failure.

37. C)   has a high false-negative rate

The Primary Dye Test (Jones I test) determines whether the tears are passing into the nose under normal physiologic pumping conditions. In this test, 2% fluorescein is instilled in the precorneal tear film. Topical anesthetics and decongestants are sprayed in the ipsilateral inferior turbinate, and a rolled cotton fluff is inserted in the inferior meatus. After 5 minutes, the cotton is removed and examined for fluorescein. If no dye is present, a functional block is possible. However, in 20% to 30% of normal patients, no dye is noted, thus decreasing the reliability of this test when accomplished alone. This test does not indicate where an obstruction exists within the nasolacrimal system. Irrigation of the nasolacrimal system is accomplished on the Secondary Dye Test (Jones II test).

38.   C)   Squamous cell carcinoma

Although rare, primary malignancies most frequently are of the papillary carcinoma group and are divided into three histologic subgroups: squamous cell, transitional cell, and mixed cell. They are treated by local excision and have a favorable prognosis.

The second most common primary lacrimal sac malignancies are lymphomas. These are treated by radiotherapy after biopsy and systemic evaluation have been completed. Complete excision is not usually necessary.

39.   C)   Congenital nasolacrimal duct obstruction unresponsive to massage

Probing of the nasolacrimal duct is not indicated in acute dacryocystitis. It is also rarely effective in acquired nasolacrimal duct obstruction. Probing of the duct is not indicated in the routine work-up of patients with epiphora.

The majority (80% to 90%) of congenital nasolacrimal duct obstructions resolve by 12 months of age. Thereafter, spontaneous resolution becomes less likely and probing is encouraged. In the face of chronic mucopurulent discharge, probing may be considered at 6 to 12 months or sooner, given the clinical situation. After 18 to 24 months of age or after multiple failed probings, consideration may be given to silicone stent intubation of the nasolacrimal system.

40.   C)   positive dye disappearance test/negative Jones I

The dye disappearance test, Jones I, Jones II, and canalicular probing and irrigation all provide information that leads to a proper diagnosis in a patient with a tearing problem. The dye disappearance test is performed by placing fluorescein in the cul-de-sac and observing the degree of clearing after 5 minutes. A positive test is interpreted as significant retention of dye after 5 minutes. It does not localize an abnormality within the system but assesses the overall clinical functioning of the lacrimal system. Jones I is positive if dye can be visualized within the nasal cavity. Jones II is a method for determining if dye has entered the lacrimal sac. A positive Jones II indicates dye is in the nasal cavity after lacrimal irrigation. Jones III is useful when assessing the functioning of a surgical osteotomy site. A positive Jones III means dye is found in the nasal cavity of a post DCR or CDCR patient.

In this question, the site of blockage is known. Therefore, a Jones II test is unnecessary because this test determines the functioning of the lacrimal pump and canalicular system. In this case, there is no indication of lacrimal surgery, so a Jones III also does not apply. Table 6-1 diagrams the various situations and the dye pattern that generally apply.

TABLE 6-1. Functional Lacrimal System Tests

Test	Method	Interpretation	Comments
Dye disappearance test (DDT)	2% fluorescein placed in conjunctival cul-de-sac OU and amount of dye present at 5 minutes is observed	Pooling of dye on side with more nasolacrimal system obstruction	Relative information compared to other eye. Nonlocalizing.
Jones I	Fluorescein placed in conjunctival cul-de-sac and cotton swab used to recover dye from nose	Fluorescein on cotton swab indicates functioning nasolacrimal system	High false negative rate (no dye recovered, but patent NLD system). May be positive in mild obstruction of NLD.
Jones II	After DDT or Jones I, lacrimal sac cannulated and irrigated with saline. Fluid from nose recovered.	Dye recovered = lower lacrimal system obstruction. Clear fluid recovered = obstruction before lacrimal sac	Does not indicate funtional status of NLD system

41. D)   They demonstrate the nasolacrimal sac well.

DCG involves forcibly injecting radiopaque dye into the lower canaliculus, with radiographs being taken thereafter. Because force is used, it is not a test of lacrimal function. Because the lacrimal cannula is inserted into the canaliculus, a DCG usually does not demonstrate the canalicular system well. A DCG can show the size and filling defects within the sac (diverticula, fistulas, lacrimal tumors, stricture locations). In most situations, diagnosis of a nasolacrimal system obstruction can be made without the use of a DCG.

42. C)   They do not usually produce secondary dacryocystitis.

Clinical signs of lacrimal sac tumors include epiphora, irreducible swelling of the lacrimal sac, bleeding on attempted probing and irrigation, and secondary dacryocystitis.

43. B)   Upper canalicular trauma alone should never be surgically repaired so as not to risk damage to the remaining nasolacrimal system.

Studies have demonstrated that in up to 50% of patients tested, creation of a monocanalicular state resulted in symptomatic epiphora. Canalicular trauma affects a generally younger patient population. In Figure 6-25, the probe is within the upper canaliculus. Leaving open the possibility of future trauma and disease to the remaining canaliculus, and considering present surgical techniques with a high success rate of repair, many recommend attempted repair of all recent canalicular lacerations. Additionally, acute trauma is generally easier to repair before scarring. One may wait a few days to allow acute soft tissue swelling to decrease before attempted repair. The longer the silicone stents remain in place, the better the likelihood of patency for the system (after all surrounding scarring has occurred). Many doctors prefer silicone stent intubation with microanastomosis of the lacerated canalicular system to maximize the success of canalicular patency.

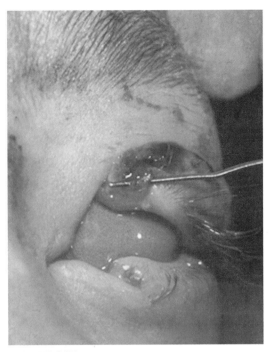

FIGURE 6-25

44. B)   A common canaliculus is present in approximately 30% of the population.

The punctum is perpendicular to the lid margin and approximately 2 mm from the ampulla. The canaliculus then turns horizontally and travels approximately 8 mm to the nasolacrimal sac. The ampulla has the largest diameter of the canalicular system (approximately 2 mm). The canaliculus has an average diameter of 1 mm. These relationships are important to keep in mind when probing the canalicular system.

45. A)   Syringing saline into the lower punctum that irrigates into the nose indicates that no obstruction exists and that the system is functioning normally.

The Jones II test alone is a nonphysiologic evaluation of absolute nasolacrimal system patency. Therefore, it gives no information on the adequacy of nasolacrimal drainage function. In a canalicular obstruction, irrigation would be expected to regurgitate from the punctum being tested. Reflux of fluid from the opposite punctum when the sac is irrigated indicates obstruction at the level of the sac or duct. Recovery of fluid in the nose after irrigation may be helpful in looking for casts or other debris. Additionally, when accomplished after a negative Jones I testing (no dye recovered from the inferior meatus after instillation of dye in the eye), retrieval of fluorescein-colored irrigant suggests dye-tinged fluid entered the sac, and a partial or functional block may exist.

46. D)   atropine

Canalicular stenosis may follow infections (herpetic, trachoma, infectious mononucleosis), inflammations (Stevens-Johnson syndrome, ocular pemphigoid), trauma (lacerations, chemical or thermal injuries, repeated probings), allergy, irradiation, tumors (rarely), canaliculitis, and use of eye drops. Eye drops, including antivirals, strong miotics, and epinephrine-containing compounds, have been implicated most frequently.

47. C)   common canalicular obstruction combined with nasolacrimal duct obstruction

A Jones tube (Fig. 6-26) is indicated in cases in which the canalicular system is disrupted and is inadequate to allow tear flow into the nose. In certain situations, even a patent canalicular system may require a Jones bypass conduit if the lacrimal pump mechanism is disrupted (scarred or paralytic lids). A canaliculodacryocystorhinostomy is indicated for a focal distal canalicular obstruction combined with nasolacrimal duct obstruction.

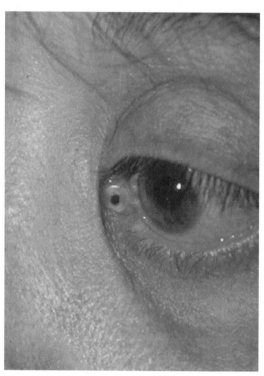

FIGURE 6-26

48. D)   most adults will need a DCR for correction of outflow obstruction

Acute dacryocystitis is treated with systemic antibiotics and warm compresses. Probing the system does not successfully treat the problem in adults. DCR is usually necessary to re-establish lacrimal outflow in adults.

49. C)   probing and irrigation of the left nasolacrimal system

In acute dacryocystitis, probing of the nasolacrimal system is not indicated. Complete ophthalmic evaluation is necessary to determine whether a surrounding orbital cellulitis is present. Culture and Gram stain may help direct antibiotic therapy. In situations of previous trauma, radiographic imaging will help evaluate any anatomic changes.

50. A) DCR

After a complete evaluation, the patient should be started on systemic (IV or oral) and topical antibiotics, warm compresses, and pain control. Additionally, if a pointing abscess is present, incision and drainage of the abscess may result in more rapid healing and patient comfort. A DCR is not indicated for an acute dacryocystitis.

51. C) Nasolacrimal duct

Although obstruction may be found anywhere in the lacrimal drainage system, acquired nasolacrimal system obstruction is seen most frequently at the level of the mid or lower duct. Obstruction results from chronic low-grade inflammation with ultimate fibrosis of the duct walls.

52. C) *Streptococcus pneumoniae*

Dacryocystitis results from tear stasis. Pneumococci are the most common organism in dacryocystitis. Other organisms include streptococci, diphtheroids, *Klebsiella pneumonia, Haemophilus influenzae, Pseudomonas aeruginosa,* and mixed organisms. Actinomyces and fungi, such as Candida, are also frequently seen.

53. D) Valve of Hasner

This is a relatively common cause of epiphora and is seen in 2% to 4% of newborn infants. In 80% to 90% of patients, the membranous valve of Hasner opens spontaneously or with gentle massage of the nasolacrimal sac within the first 6 to 12 months of life. The valve of Rosenmüller is located between the common canaliculus (sinus of Maier) and the lacrimal sac and prevents reflux back into the canalicular system. The valve of Krause (and sinus of Arlt) is located at the junction of the nasolacrimal sac and duct. The spiral valve of Hyrtle and the valve of Taillefer are located within the nasolacrimal duct (Fig. 6-27).

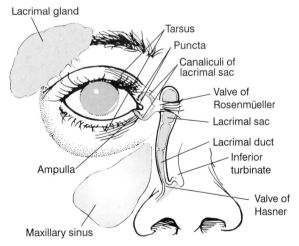

FIGURE 6-27. From Wright K. Textbook of ophthalmology. Baltimore: Williams & Wilkins, 1997.

54. B)   nasolacrimal system probing

55. C)   Nasolacrimal system probing has proven unsuccessful.

As mentioned in the previous answer, 80% to 90% of cases of congenital nasolacrimal duct obstruction resolve spontaneously by the first year of life. Thereafter, spontaneous resolution decreases significantly. The next appropriate step would be nasolacrimal system probing under general anesthesia. If the probing is unsuccessful, consideration may be given to silicone stent intubation of the nasolacrimal system (this may be combined with infracture of the inferior turbinate). Only after multiple failed probings and silicone stent intubations would a DCR be considered for a child.

56. C)   Acanthamoeba

Although *Actinomyces israelii* is associated most frequently with canaliculitis, multiple organisms have been shown to cause this disorder. Streptomyces, *Arachnia propionica* (previously Streptothrix), Nocardia, and fungi, such as *Candida albicans* and *Aspergillus niger,* have been documented to cause canaliculitis.

57. B)   Gritty sensation on probing with yellow-tinged concretions

Canaliculitis affects the inferior canaliculus most frequently. A diagnosis is suspected when focal swelling of the canaliculus is noted. Probing of the affected canaliculus gives gritty resistance, and frequently, yellow-tinged concretions are noted. Mucopurulent reflux on palpation of the lacrimal sac is seen more frequently in dacryocystitis. Palpable subcutaneous masses above the level of the medial canthal tendon would arouse suspicion of a lacrimal sac tumor, and palpable masses in the lacrimal sac would be more suspicious for dacryoliths.

58. D)   oral penicillin

Canaliculitis may be treated by external pressure and curettage of the concretions with irrigation of a penicillin solution. Topical penicillin may also be necessary. Occasionally, incision of the canaliculus may be indicated to débride the tissue. Oral antibiotics are not a method of treatment.

59. A)   distichiasis

The sequelae of trachoma are a result of the severe inflammatory reaction to the Chlamydial antigens in the conjunctiva. Shortening of the posterior lamella resulting in entropion, keratoconjunctivitis sicca, and trichiasis (misdirected lashes) occur, contributing to the high incidence of corneal ulcers and blindness in developing nations. *Distichiasis,* in contradistinction, is the growth of aberrant lashes in the meibomian gland orifices. These lashes are usually shorter and softer than the usual lid margin cilia. Distichiasis can be congenital or acquired secondary to conditions such as Stevens-Johnson syndrome or ocular cicatricial pemphigoid.

60. D)   inward rotation of the lid by steatoblepharon—lower lid blepharoplasty

Lower lid steatoblepharon is not a cause of lower lid entropion.

61. D)   shrinking of the inferior conjunctival fornix

With retraction of the lower lid retractors, the inferior cul-de-sac may be deeper rather than shallower.

62. A)   Congenital

Involutional is the most common form of ectropion. It is most commonly attributable to laxity of the eyelid that occurs with aging. Gravity is also a contributing factor. It is very rare to see ectropion at birth (congenital).

Paralytic ectropion occurs when there is interruption of the innervation to the orbicularis oculi as found in cranial nerve VII palsy or Bell's palsy. Mechanical ectropion may occur due to a lower eyelid tumor, severe edema, or any other condition that causes the lower eyelid to pull away from the globe.

Cicatricial ectropion arises from a relative shortening of the anterior lamella. Some etiologies that occur are scarring of the skin, chemical or thermal burns, chronic solar damage or inflammatory diseases of the skin, or skin tumors. Treatment of cicatricial ectropion often requires skin grafting.

63. B)   suturing the retractors to the tarsus

The cause of involutional entropion is a dehiscence of the lower eyelid aponeurosis (capsulopalpebral fascia). One way to repair an entropion is to repair the dehisced tissue by suturing the aponeurosis of the lower eyelid retractors to the inferior border of the tarsus. An entropion, therefore, is in many ways analogous to involutional blepharoptosis of the upper eyelid. Repair should be directed at reattaching the lower eyelid retractors and may be combined with other procedures, such as horizontal eyelid tightening procedures. The normal lower eyelid retractors consist of the capsulopalpebral fascia, the suspensory ligaments of the lower fornix, and the inferior tarsal muscle.

The distal portion of the capsulopalpebral fascia, known as the *aponeurosis,* is analogous to the levator aponeurosis of the upper eyelid. Some investigators think that the aponeurosis attaches to the inferior edge of the tarsus. We believe that the posterior portion of the aponeurosis inserts on the anterior border of the lower eyelid tarsus posteriorly and extends anteriorly into the subcutaneous tissue in a fashion similar to the anatomy of the upper eyelid. Inferior to the tarsus, the orbital septum fuses with the capsulopalpebral fascia just as the septum of the upper eyelid fuses with the levator aponeurosis. Reanastomosis of the dehisced lower eyelid aponeurosis does not provide an adequate anchoring of the tarsus for long-term repair of the entropion. However, suturing of the capsulopalpebral fascia (lower eyelid retractors) to the inferior border of the tarsus provides a strong anchor and may be used alone or in conjunction with other techniques for correction of the entropion.

Factors frequently mentioned in literature as causes of involutional entropion include increased horizontal eyelid laxity, the overriding of the preseptal orbicularis, and enophthalmos with fat atrophy. Although we agree that these findings are commonly associated with entropion, we suggest that these findings are incidental to aging (increased laxity and possible fat atrophy) and are not primary causes of the involutional entropic phenomenon. Common surgical procedures for correction of entropion are directed at stabilization of the anatomic abnormalities. Some examples include dehiscence repair with horizontal eyelid shortening, the Quickert four-snip procedure, the Bick procedure, the Wies procedure, the use of Quickert-Rathbun rotational sutures, and the use of a tarsal strip with dehiscence repair.

64.   D)   thyroid eye disease

Recession of the superior rectus muscle, congenital eyelid retraction, surgical overcorrection of blepharoptosis, and thyroid eye disease are all causes of upper lid retraction, but the most common cause is thyroid eye disease.

65.   A)   Cavernous hemangioma

Infection and hemorrhage can both present with rapidly developing proptosis. Orbital lymphangioma may produce acute proptosis when there is a hemorrhage from interstitial capillaries. The cavernous hemangioma is a slow-growing lesion that creates proptosis over years or months.

66.   D)   lymphangioma

The MRI scan shows a layered hemorrhage in the lobular and cystic mass behind the eye. The sinuses are clear of infection, making an orbital abscess unlikely. Acute bleeding would not be typical of a capillary hemangioma. The hemorrhage and ecchymosis would be more characteristic of lymphangioma than rhabdomyosarcoma.

67.   D)   B and C

The hemorrhage from an orbital lymphangioma can cause compressive optic neuropathy. In a patient with visual loss from optic nerve compression, drainage of the cyst with CT guidance or open surgery may be considered. Because the lymphangioma in this patient interdigitates with extraocular muscles and the optic nerve, it would be impractical to attempt total surgical excision of the lesion. Sometimes a lymphangioma will be more localized and amenable to surgical excision with preservation of normal structures. IV corticosteroids may also be beneficial.

68.   C)   a tumor that may enlarge with upper respiratory infections

Lymphangiomas may increase in size during viral infection, presumably caused by the lymphocytic components of the tumor. Orbital cellulitis is the most common cause of proptosis in children; lymphangioma is not a malignant tumor; and capillary hemangioma (not lymphangioma) responds to intralesional corticosteroids.

69.   B)   the onset of decreased vision and an afferent pupillary defect in the presence of an orbital abscess is an indication for surgery

Orbital infectious disease occurs most commonly as a result of spread from surrounding sinusitis, most commonly the ethmoid sinuses. Whether the presence of a subperiosteal fluid collection on CT (in the presence of stable vision and clinical signs) is an absolute indication for surgery is controversial. Most ophthalmologists would agree that medical management and careful observation may be employed when the patient's clinical signs are stable and the vision is normal. Proptosis and motility limitation help to differentiate orbital cellulitis from preseptal cellulitis. Indications for surgical intervention in orbital cellulitis include decreasing vision and afferent pupillary defect, failure to respond to IV antibiotics, and progression of clinical signs such as motility changes and proptosis.

70. D)   observation

Rapid evolution of unilateral proptosis in a child should be considered rhabdomyosarcoma until proven otherwise. This finding necessitates a biopsy and then radiation and chemotherapy. Other causes of superonasal masses include myocele, mucopyocele, encephalocoele, and neurofibroma.

71. B)   Cavernous hemangioma

72. B)   high internal reflectivity

73. A)   slow growth over several years

74. C)   an anterior approach through the inferior fornix

The patient is a middle-aged woman with very gradual onset of proptosis and no other symptoms. The CT scan shows a well-circumscribed, rounded mass inferonasal and anterior to the globe that displaces, but does not invade, surrounding tissue. The A-scan ultrasound shows high internal reflectivity consistent with nonhomogeneous tissue. These findings make the most likely diagnosis cavernous hemangioma. Typically, the cavernous hemangioma is a slow- growing mass that becomes symptomatic with proptosis or diplopia as the mass displaces the globe. The location of this lesion is surgically approached through the inferior conjunctival fornix.

75. D)   Within the maxilla medial to the infraorbital canal

With impact to the anterior orbit, forces are transmitted posteriorly. The weakest point along the floor is posterior and medial to the infraorbital canal. The convexity in the posterior orbital floor measures approximately 0.5 mm in thickness.

76. A)   Radiation with or without additional chemotherapy

Before 1965, the standard treatment for orbital rhabdomyosarcoma involved exenteration, and it had a poor survival rate. Since 1965, this mutilating procedure has been abandoned as primary management. Radiation and systemic chemotherapy are the mainstays of treatment based on the guidelines set forth by the Intergroup Rhabdomyosarcoma Study. The total dose of local radiation varies from 4500 to 6000 rad given over a period of 6 weeks. Chemotherapy is used to eliminate microscopic cellular metastasis. The survival rate using these modalities has improved significantly.

77. B)   Rhabdomyosarcoma

The most common primary malignancy in children is rhabdomyosarcoma. The most common metastatic tumor is neuroblastoma, and it may be bilateral. Neuroblastoma typically produces an abrupt ecchymotic proptosis that may be bilateral. Metastasis from neuroblastoma in children most frequently goes to the orbit, whereas metastasis from neuroblastoma in adults usually is found in the uveal tract. In children, the most common benign tumor is capillary hemangioma.

78. A)   Primary lacrimal gland lymphoma

Differentiating the variety of lacrimal gland lesions is often very challenging. The short history and the CT examination provided do allow for separating the lesions listed. The choices provided are all considered intrinsic lesions of the lacrimal gland. These lesions have typically been divided into lymphoproliferative lesions and epithelial tumors. Primary lacrimal gland lymphoma, pleomorphic adenoma, and adenoid cystic carcinoma are in the epithelial category. Adenoid cystic carcinoma and malignant pleomorphic adenoma are characteristically painful, with CT findings indicative of bone destruction. Pleomorphic adenoma, also referred to as a benign mixed cell neoplasm, usually has a 9-month or longer history of lacrimal gland enlargement. CT changes of bony erosion and expansion are also commonly seen. Lymphoma characteristically demonstrates "molding or putty-like" qualities on the CT. Lymphomas can present with both a short- and long-standing history of lacrimal gland swelling. In this case, when both history and CT examinations are analyzed, primary lacrimal gland lymphoma is the most appropriate answer.

79. D)   Mixture of both B and T cells, with predominance of B cells

Lymphomas have proliferation of lymphocytes, mostly of the B-cell variety. A pleomorphic adenoma or benign mixed cell lacrimal gland neoplasm can be found to have spindle cells with both ductal epithelium and a mixed stromal pattern. *Swiss cheese pattern* is a classic term for describing an adenoid cystic carcinoma. Ductal epithelium in a tubular formation with malignant degeneration describes a malignant pleomorphic adenoma.

80. B)   metastatic breast carcinoma in a woman

Metastatic breast cancer is by far the most likely to present with enophthalmos, but gastrointestinal and lung are among other tumors, including prostate, that occasionally present with enophthalmos. Cavernous hemangioma and orbital cellulitis are characterized by proptosis, not enophthalmos.

81. C)   thyroid-related orbitopathy

The most common cause of bilateral exophthalmos in adults is most often thyroid-related orbitopathy and less often pseudotumor, Wegener's granulomatosis, or neoplasm.

82. D)   Orbital cellulitis

The most common cause of unilateral childhood exophthalmos is most often orbital cellulitis, secondary to ethmoid sinusitis or respiratory tract infections.

83. D)   all of the above

Of patients with mucormycosis, 70% have diabetes mellitus, 5% have renal disease, 18% have other immunosuppressed states, 3% have leukemia, and only 4% have no systemic illness.

84. D)   radiation to the orbit

It is postulated that patients with diabetes do better than other patients with mucormycosis because they have a disease process that has the potential for control.

It is also necessary to treat concurrent bacterial infections. Débridement of all devitalized tissue until free bleeding tissue is encountered is extremely important; it may include external ethmoidectomy, Caldwell-Luc operations, intranasal ethmoidectomy, sphenoid sinusectomy, palate resection, and exenteration. Exenteration is reserved for potentially lethal disease that is progressing unresponsive to other forms of treatment or as a palliative treatment for severe pain. It has been demonstrated that the more extensive the débridement, the better the prognosis. Since the addition of treatment with amphotericin B, survival rates have jumped from 6% to 73%. Early diagnosis with local excision, systemic stabilization, and IV amphotericin give mucormycosis patients the best chance for survival.

85. A)   Thyroid-related orbitopathy

The clinical signs of thyroid-related orbitopathy can be generally grouped into two independent manifestations: type 1 and type 2 orbitopathy. Type 1 orbitopathy comprises symmetric proptosis with symmetric eyelid retraction, minimal orbital inflammation, and minimal extraocular muscle inflammation or restrictive myopathy. Type 2 orbitopathy comprises extraocular muscle myositis, restrictive myopathy, orbital inflammation, and chemosis. Compressive optic neuropathy is more commonly a feature of type 2 orbitopathy.

86. A)   orbital decompression, strabismus surgery, and eyelid retraction surgical repair

This order of therapy allows strabismus surgery to be performed after rather than before orbital decompression because decompression may alter ocular motility alignment. Furthermore, treatment of lower eyelid retraction must be performed after strabismus because recessing the inferior rectus can also cause an increase in lower eyelid retraction because of the connection of the inferior rectus to the lower lid retractors.

87. B)   Absence of a thickened tendon of the extraocular muscle insertion

It is possible to see enlarged extraocular muscles in both orbital inflammatory syndrome and thyroid-related orbitopathy. However, the tendon is almost never involved in thyroid orbitopathy, whereas the extraocular muscle tendon can be thickened in orbital inflammatory syndrome. The most commonly involved muscles in thyroid-related orbitopathy are the inferior rectus and the medial rectus. Lacrimal gland enlargement can occur in both entities.

88. D)   all of the above

The histopathologic slide of adenoid cystic carcinoma or cylindroma (Fig. 6-15) shows the most common malignant tumor of the lacrimal gland. These tumor cells grow in tubules, solid nests, or in a cribriform Swiss cheese pattern. Perineural invasion is frequently observed in microscopic sections. Exenteration is almost always performed. Radiation and chemotherapy may be useful in extensive tumors.

89. A)   Figure 6-16

Figure 6-16 shows a post-septal orbital cellulitis with a subperiosteal abscess demonstrated on axial CT scans. *Staphylococcus aureus* is the most common pathogen in children with orbital cellulitis. This infection responds quickly to penicillinase-resistant penicillin such as oxacillin.

90.   B)   Figures 6-17 and 6-18

Figure 6-17 demonstrates a cavernous hemangioma on an axial CT scan, which is the most common, well-circumscribed orbital lesion in adults. Figure 6-18 shows an orbital varix, which is an irregular mass with a phlebolith. Treatment for orbital varices is usually conservative. Because of the risks of optic nerve or globe damage, surgery is reserved for instances in which the varix is threatening vision. Complete surgical excision is difficult.

91.   B)   Cavernous hemangioma

Cavernous hemangioma is the most common benign neoplasm in adults. Proptosis is slowly progressive and growth may accelerate during pregnancy. Retinal striae, hyperopia and optic nerve compression, increased IOP, and strabismus may develop. Dermoid cysts occur less frequently but are found in the posterior orbit, usually in the superior and temporal portions. Metastatic breast carcinoma often causes enophthalmos. Hemangiopericytoma are encapsulated; however, they are quite rare.

92.   B)   Figure 6-19

The CT demonstrates a solid infiltrating tumor that has the characteristic putty-like molding of the tumor to preexisting orbital structures. Bone changes are usually not seen, and these lesions are usually not well-circumscribed. Lymphoplasmacytoid proliferation with Dutcher bodies should bring to mind the possibility of Waldenström macroglobulinemia or a systemic lymphoma with immunoglobulin production.

93.   C)   excisional biopsy

Figure 6-20 presents an axial CT showing a lacrimal gland mass with no bony erosion. The patient presents with painless proptosis. This mass is most likely benign mixed pleomorphic adenoma of the lacrimal gland as this is the most common epithelial tumor of the lacrimal gland. It is impossible to tell whether this lacrimal gland tumor is benign or malignant without a biopsy. Excisional biopsy is indicated because complete removal of the tumor within its pseudocapsule is necessary. Performing an incisional biopsy may allow the tumor cells to spill into the orbit. Such cells can lead to a proliferation of an infiltrative recurrent tumor requiring extensive surgery at a later date. Furthermore, incompletely excised benign mixed tumors may later develop into malignant mixed tumors of the lacrimal gland.

94.   A)   tubules—solid nests of cells in a cribriform Swiss cheese pattern with perineural invasion

Figure 6-22 shows a mass in the superolateral quadrant that is pressing the globe downward and is most likely of lacrimal gland origin. Bony erosion is present in the superior orbital roof, suggesting a malignant process. A painful orbital mass with rapid progression is most characteristic of adenoid cystic carcinoma, which is the most common malignant tumor of the lacrimal gland. The pain is caused by the perineural invasion and bony destruction. The course is rapid. Treatment consists of exenteration of the orbit with removal of any bone that is involved. Radiation and chemotherapy may be used in the treatment of extensive tumors. Psammoma bodies are composed of monotonous whorls of meningothelial cells interspersed with round calcified material found in meningiomas. Flexner-Wintersteiner rosettes are nearly pathognomonic for retinoblastoma. Antoni A and Antoni B are patterns of proliferation of Schwann cells that occur in Schwannomas.

95. C) Figure 6-21

Figure 6-21 demonstrates enlarged extraocular muscles in thyroid-related orbitopathy on an axial CT scan. Orbital decompression is indicated when there is severe proptosis that causes severe corneal exposure or, more commonly, when compressive optic neuropathy is demonstrated by visual field loss.

96. D) all of the above

Figure 6-16 shows a post-septal cellulitis demonstrated on axial CT scan. Causes of orbital cellulitis include: 1) extension of infection from periorbital structures (paranasal sinuses, face and eyelids, dacryocystitis, dental infection, and intracranial infections); 2) exogenous causes, including previous trauma or surgery; 3) endogenous causes, such as bacteremia with septic embolization; and 4) intraorbital causes, such as endophthalmitis and dacryoadenitis.

97. B) Figure 6-18

Figure 6-18 shows an axial CT scan that demonstrates an orbital varix with phleboliths present. Orbital varices occur primarily as dilations of preexisting venous channels. Because dilated veins are present, proptosis can increase after Valsalva or when the head is in a dependent position. Surgery to remove varices is reserved for instances in which the varix is threatening vision because of optic nerve or globe damage. Complete surgical excision is difficult because the varix is often intertwined with other normal orbital structures. Orbital hemorrhages may result from trauma or may occur spontaneously.

98. B) Treacher-Collins

Crouzon's and Apert's are both categorized as craniofacial synostosis. These conditions are the result of premature closure of one or more cranial sutures. Plagiocephaly does not describe a syndrome, but simply indicates the premature closure of one cranial suture. Treacher-Collins syndrome is in the general category of clefting syndromes. These patients typically have hypoplasia of the mid-face, pseudocolobomas of the eyelids, downward angle to the lateral canthi, and dental and ear anomalies.

99. D) proptosis

Goldenhar's syndrome involves abnormalities of the first and second branchial arches. Eyelid colobomas, lipodermoids, and Duane's syndrome are all part of a large list of clinical findings associated with Goldenhar's. Additional findings include microphthalmia, anophthalmia, optic nerve hypoplasia, ocular colobomas, preauricular fistulas and skin tags, and palatal and facial clefts. Proptosis is seen more often with the synostosis, which includes both Crouzon's and Apert's syndromes.

100. B)   Ataxia telangiectasia—café-au-lait spots

Sturge-Weber syndrome consists of facial cutaneous angioma, which is called *nevus flammeus* or *port-wine stain*. Ipsilateral vascular malformations of the leptomeninges are typically present and lead to seizures, calcifications of the brain, and mental deficiency. Sturge-Weber syndrome is not hereditary.

Ataxia-telangiectasia is autosomal recessive and affects the skin, eye, immune system, and brain. The conjunctival and skin lesions consist of telangiectatic changes, usually in sun-exposed areas. These patients typically have involvement of their cerebellum resulting in ataxia as well as difficulty in initiating saccades. Decreased T-cell function and thymus hypoplasia lead to recurrent infections. Café-au-lait spots are found in neurofibromatosis, not ataxia-telangiectasia.

Incontinentia pigmenti is a syndrome displaying X-linked dominant transmission and occurs almost exclusively in females. This condition affects the skin, the eye, and the brain. The skin appears normal at birth, but it gradually develops erythema, bullae, and verrucous lesions. Small, hyperpigmented macules described as "splashed paint" typically occur on the trunk. Associated findings may include seizures; mental deficiency; skull, dental, and palate deformities; microcephaly; hydrocephalus; and dwarfism. The eyes may develop peripheral retinal vascular pathology.

Tuberous sclerosis often occurs as a new mutation, or it may be transmitted as a dominant trait. The "ash leaf" or hypopigmented macule represents an early skin finding in this condition. Angiofibromas of the face (adenoma sebaceum) occur late in childhood and are progressive. Tuberous sclerosis is often associated with calcifications of the basal ganglion and periventricular areas of the brain, mental retardation, seizures, and retinal phakomas.

Notes

Notes

7

Pathology

QUESTIONS

1. Histologic examination of a corneal button received from penetrating keratoplasty showed two Bowman's layers. One was localized in its normal position and the other one was found in the superficial stroma. What is a possible reason for these findings?

    A) Status post photorefractive keratectomy with an excimer laser (PRK)
    B) Status post epikeratoplasty (epikeratophakia)
    C) Trauma
    D) Status post intrastromal keratomileusis (LASIK)

Questions 2–3

2. Which statement about rhabdomyosarcoma of the orbit is INCORRECT?

    A) It is the most common primary malignant orbital tumor in children.
    B) The embryonal type is the most common type.
    C) It originates from the extraocular muscles.
    D) Patients present usually with very rapid onset of unilateral proptosis that can simulate an orbital inflammation.

3. What cell type has the poorest prognosis?

    A) Mixed
    B) Pleomorphic
    C) Embryonal
    D) Alveolar

4. Examination of an eye enucleated for malignant melanoma of the choroid shows a glistening white irregular tumor arising from a ciliary crest measuring 3 mm × 2 mm × 2 mm. A histologic section is shown in Figure 7-1. Which statement is true?

A) This is an intraocular metastatic lesion from the uveal melanoma.
B) This is a rare tumor of the nonpigmented epithelium of the ciliary body.
C) This lesion can be found in approximately 25% of older patients.
D) This lesion leads to secondary angle closure if untreated.

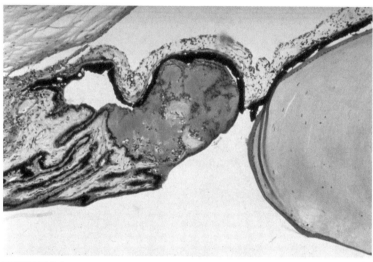

FIGURE 7-1

Questions 5–9 (Fig. 7-2 to 7-7)

A 42-year-old patient presents with a progressive decrease of visual acuity over 2 months in his right eye. Ophthalmologic examination (Fig. 7-2) shows an orange lesion temporal to the macula with associated retinal detachment in the inferior two quadrants. Fluorescein angiography (Fig. 7-3) displays a hyperfluorescent lesion with a hypofluorescent circular ring around the peripheral border of the lesion. Ultrasonography is shown in Figure 7-4. The patient was lost to follow-up, but returned 2 months later with a blind, painful eye, and the eye was enucleated. Histologic examination is shown in Figure 7-5. Figures 7-6 and 7-7 show higher magnifications of the area temporal to the macula, that is, the area of the clinically visible lesion.

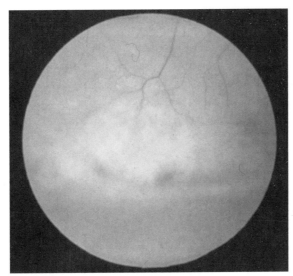

FIGURE 7-2

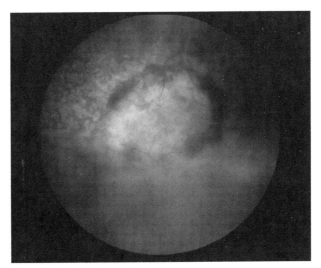

FIGURE 7-3

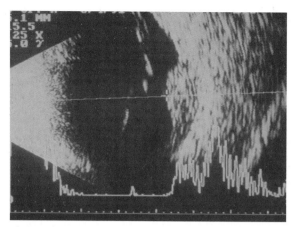

FIGURE 7-4

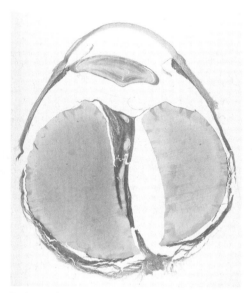

FIGURE 7-5

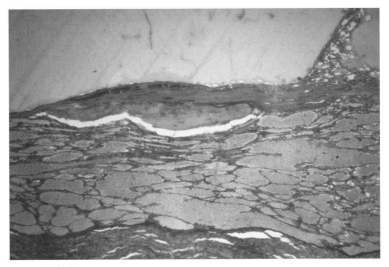

FIGURE 7-6

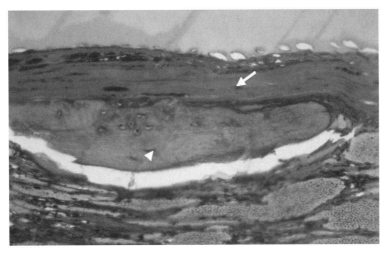

FIGURE 7-7

5. Figures 7-6 and 7-7 show an area of dense fibrous tissue (*arrow*) overlying an area of calcified tissue (*arrowhead*) in the plane of the retinal pigment epithelium and Bruch's membrane. Which statement is TRUE?

   A) These lesions developed from choroidal melanocytes (melanocytes of neural crest origin).
   B) The cells of origin for these lesions are the retinal pigment epithelial cells (cells of neuroectodermal origin).
   C) These lesions can undergo malignant transformation.
   D) The cell of origin of these lesions is unknown.

6. The histologic section of the enucleated eye is shown in Figure 7-5. What type of retinal detachment is present?

   A) Rhegmatogenous
   B) Tractional
   C) Exudative
   D) Artifactitious

7. The histologic section through the choroidal lesion is shown in Figure 7-6. Which statement isTRUE?

   A) This is a malignant lesion.
   B) Lakes of proteinaceous material are separated by fibrovascular septa.
   C) This lesion is consistent with a capillary hemangioma.
   D) Cavernous spaces filled with erythrocytes are present.

8. Which statement regarding the choroidal lesion in this patient is TRUE?

   A) Two clinical growth patterns, that is, a localized and a diffuse form, are observed.
   B) The reason for the retinal detachment is a choristoma in the choroid.
   C) This is a bilateral disease in most cases.
   D) This lesion may be found in association with similar lesions of the cerebellum.

9. A 5-year-old girl has a facial nevus flammeus and seizures. A choroidal biopsy shows a choroidal lesion similar to the histologic picture of Figure 7-6. Which statement is most likely TRUE?

   A) This is a condition with a high probability of spontaneous regression.
   B) Glaucoma is not a common feature of this disease.
   C) This disease is inherited in an autosomal recessive manner.
   D) Ipsilateral hemangiomas of the meninges are common.

10. Histologic examination of an eye bank eye shows peripheral retinal changes as shown in Figure 7-8. Which statement is TRUE?

    A) This is an infrequently observed change of the peripheral retina in older eyes.
    B) The cystic spaces typically develop first in the inner nuclear layer of the retina.
    C) A common late sequel is a rhegmatogenous retinal detachment.
    D) The lesion appears clinically as grayish bubbles posterior to the ora serrata.

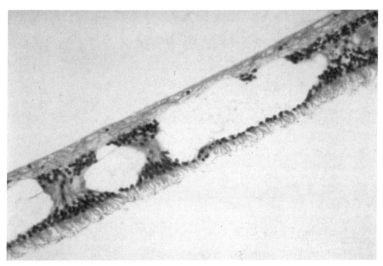

FIGURE 7-8

Questions 11–12 (Fig. 7-9 and 7-10)

A 72-year-old female had intracapsular cataract extraction 6 months ago. Recently she developed increased IOP that was unresponsive to topical treatment. Histologic sections through the anterior segment are shown in Figures 7-9 and 7-10. Figure 7-10 is a magnification of an area of Figure 7-9.

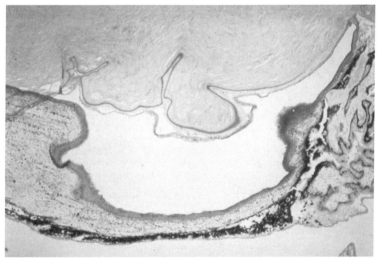

FIGURE 7-9

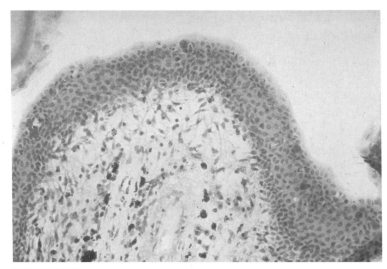

FIGURE 7-10

11. Which statement is CORRECT?

  A) This condition is a variant of the iridocorneal endothelial (ICE) syndrome.
  B) Surface epithelium is found in the anterior chamber.
  C) This is a congenital condition that manifests only in adults.
  D) This is a self-limited disorder in most cases.

12. Which stain highlights the characteristic features of the epithelium and allows identification of its origin in Figures 7-9 and 7-10?

  A) Hematoxylin-eosin
  B) Oil Red O
  C) Periodic acid-Schiff (PAS)
  D) Congo Red

13. During processing of tissue for histologic examination, water is removed and replaced by paraffin. Which statement is INCORRECT?

  A) IOLs made of PMMA are dissolved completely.
  B) Immunohistochemical stains of paraffin sections can be used for differentiation of tissue.
  C) Special stains, such as Oil Red O, can be used to identify lipids.
  D) The paraffin has to be removed before applying different stains.

Questions 14–15

A 16-year-old young man presented with a blind, painful eye. Ophthalmologic examination showed band keratopathy, and the anterior chamber and pupil were covered by a pigmented membrane. Ultrasonographic examination showed a microphthalmic eye with an irregular structure behind the lens extending to the optic disc. The eye was enucleated; gross examination is shown in Figure 7-11. The lens was replaced by a yellowish tissue and tractional membranes were extended to the ciliary body processes. A whitish strand-like structure extended through the vitreous cavity to the optic disc. Histologic examination is shown in Figures 7-12 and 7-13.

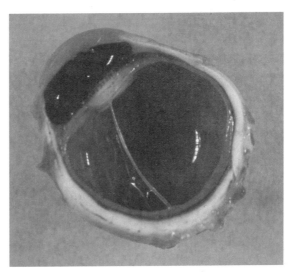

FIGURE 7-11

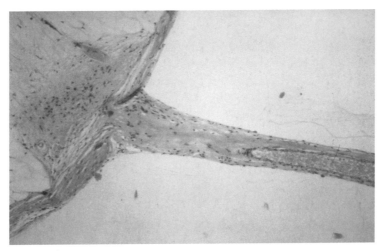

FIGURE 7-12

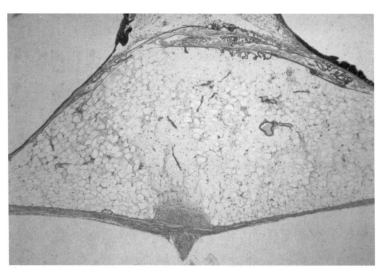

FIGURE 7-13

14. Which statement is INCORRECT?

    A) A microphthalmic eye is typical for this disease.
    B) This is a unilateral disease.
    C) Lipomatosis lentis can be a feature of this condition.
    D) The diagnosis is confirmed with CT and serologic studies.

15. What is the etiology of this condition?

    A) Developmental abnormality
    B) Intraocular infection
    C) Trauma
    D) Neoplasm

16. A 6-month-old child has an iris lesion and recurrent anterior chamber bleeding. A biopsy of this mass was performed. The histology is shown in Figure 7-14. Which statement is correct?

A) The lesion shows pleomorphic cells with a multinucleated tumor cell.

B) This is a benign cutaneous disorder rarely involving the eye.

C) Immunohistochemical stains for macrophages (histiocytes) are negative.

D) Most ocular lesions occur after 1 year of age in this disease entity.

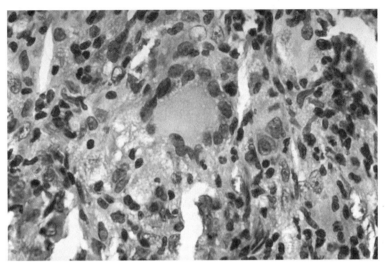

FIGURE 7-14

Questions 17–18 (Fig. 7-15 and 7-16)

A 72-year-old woman presents with a lesion in her right eye (Fig. 7-15) that had developed over the course of 2 years. The cherry red lesion is located in the bulbar conjunctiva in the area of the plica semilunaris next to the caruncle. Ophthalmologic examination is otherwise normal. Histologic examination is shown in Figure 7-16.

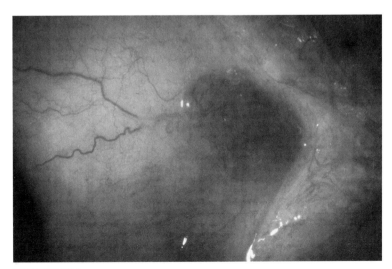

FIGURE 7-15

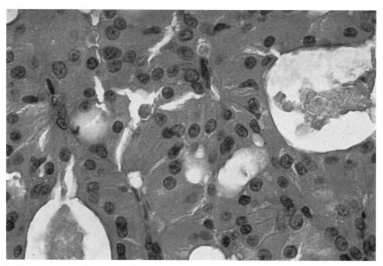

FIGURE 7-16

17. What is the disease process?

    A) Adenoid cystic carcinoma
    B) Oncocytoma
    C) Pyogenic granuloma
    D) Papilloma

18. The granular appearance of the cytoplasm of the cells in Figure 7-16 is caused by:

    A) rough endoplasmic reticulum
    B) multiple partially atypical mitochondria
    C) smooth endoplasmic reticulum
    D) polyribosomes

Questions 19–20 (Fig. 7-17 and 7-18)

A 23-year-old man presents with a hard, painless lump within the left lower eyelid for over 6 weeks. Histologic examination is shown in Figures 7-17 and 7-18.

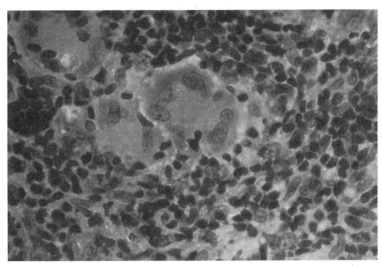

FIGURE 7-17

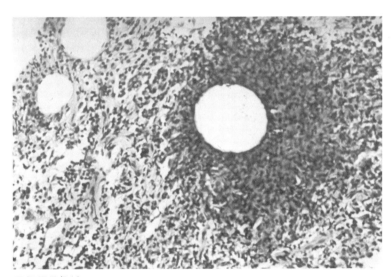

FIGURE 7-18

19. Which statement is CORRECT?

    A)   This can be a chronic inflammation of the Zeis sebaceous glands.
    B)   Excision with frozen section control of margins is the treatment of choice.
    C)   Histologic examination is not necessary because it is always a benign lesion.
    D)   Moll's glands can be the etiologic agent for this inflammation.

20. The clear spaces in Figure 7-18:

    A)   are features of xanthomas
    B)   are also visible on a frozen section
    C)   are consistent with a zonal lipogranuloma
    D)   are vascular channels

21. A 35-year-old woman has a history of recurrent "corneal inflammation." A large scar developed and a penetrating keratoplasty was performed. Histologic examination (Fig. 7-19) shows a granulomatous reaction to Descemet's membrane and the presence of retrocorneal tissue. What is the most likely etiologic agent for the keratitis?

    A)   Acanthamoeba
    B)   Herpes simplex
    C)   Pseudomonas
    D)   *Candida albicans*

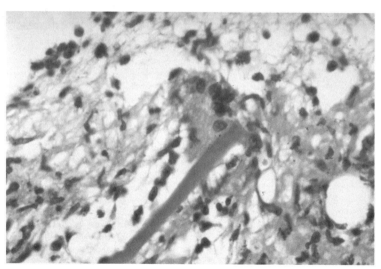

FIGURE 7-19

22. A 72-year-old woman has a history of cataract extraction with implantation of an anterior chamber IOL 5 months ago. She reports that the surgeon had "lost some lens material" during surgery. The eye was never "quiet" after surgery. Gross photos (Fig. 7-20) and a histologic section through the lens (Fig. 7-21) are shown. Which statement is INCORRECT?

A) The eye has a chronic choroidal detachment.
B) The lens nucleus was lost into the vitreous during cataract surgery.
C) The eye is hypotonous.
D) The disease is phacolytic glaucoma.

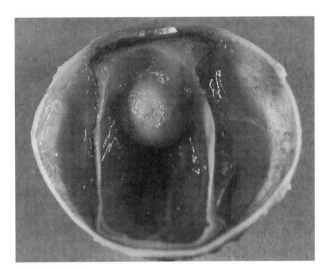

FIGURE 7-20

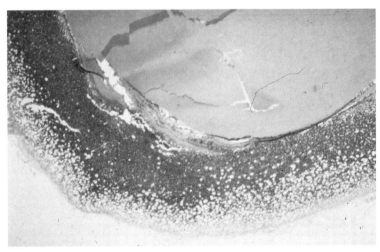

FIGURE 7-21

23. A lens capsule removed during cataract surgery is shown in Figure 7-22. Which statement is true?

A)   This condition can be caused by exposure to infrared radiation.
B)   Radial transillumination defects are found in the iris.
C)   The incidence of zonular dialysis during cataract surgery is higher in these patients.
D)   This condition is much more common in African Americans.

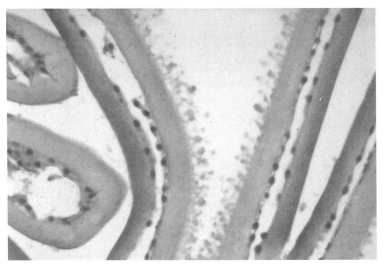

FIGURE 7-22

24. What is the abnormal condition in this histologic specimen (Fig. 7-23)?

A)   Basal laminar deposits
B)   Soft drusen
C)   Nodular drusen
D)   Basal linear deposits

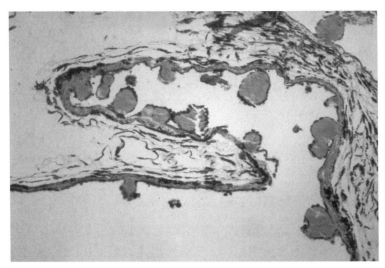

FIGURE 7-23

Questions 25–26 (Fig. 7-24 and 7-25)

A 72-year-old woman presents with a lesion on her eyelid. Histologic examination is shown in Figures 7-24 and 7-25.

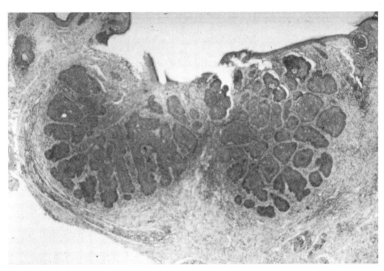

FIGURE 7-24

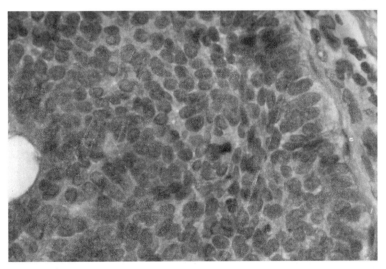

FIGURE 7-25

25. What is the most accurate diagnosis for this lesion?

A) Basal cell carcinoma, morphea type
B) Basal cell carcinoma, nodular type
C) Basal cell carcinoma, superficial type
D) Basal cell carcinoma, ulcerated type

26. What is the order of probability (from highest to lowest) of the location of this lesion?

A) Upper eyelid—lower eyelid—inner canthus—lateral canthus
B) Lower eyelid—inner canthus—upper eyelid—lateral canthus
C) Inner canthus—upper eyelid—lower eyelid—lateral canthus
D) Lower eyelid—upper eyelid—lateral canthus—inner canthus

27. Histologic examination of an optic nerve head is shown in Figure 7-26. Which statement is correct?

A) This histologic feature developed quickly over a few days.
B) A special stain for acid mucopolysaccharides (e.g., colloidal iron) can be positive within the optic nerve.
C) A central retinal artery occlusion is a possible cause.
D) In adults, the condition is reversible with appropriate treatment.

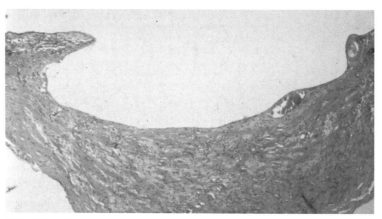

FIGURE 7-26

28. Histology of a conjunctival lesion is shown in Figures 7-27, 7-28, and 7-29. Which statement is true?

A) This is an inflammatory lesion with pseudoglands of Henle.
B) This neoplastic lesion contains epithelial embryonic rests.
C) This malignant lesion has glandular differentiation.
D) This lesion is always nonpigmented.

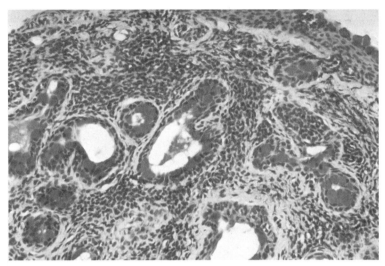

FIGURE 7-27

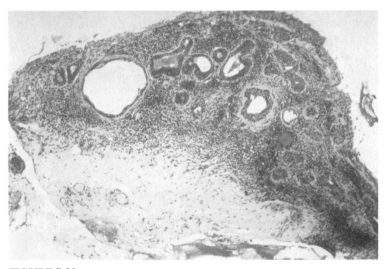

FIGURE 7-28

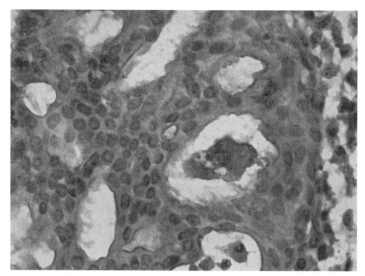

FIGURE 7-29

29. Figure 7-30 shows a histologic section through scleral tissue. Figure 7-31 is a higher magnification of the superior portion of Figure 7-30. What is the most likely scenario in this case?

   A)   Status postrepair of a scleral rupture
   B)   Status postrepair of retinal detachment
   C)   Status postpenetrating ocular trauma
   D)   Scleral staphyloma

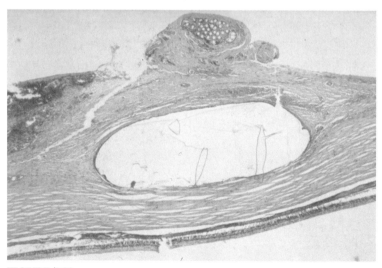

FIGURE 7-30

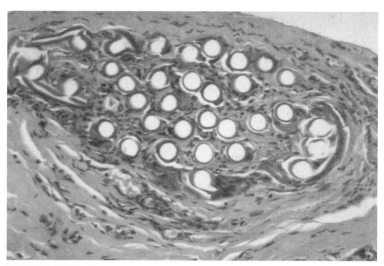

FIGURE 7-31

30. Homer-Wright rosettes are NOT found in which of these conditions?

A) Medulloblastoma
B) Retinoblastoma
C) Neuroblastoma
D) Rhabdomyosarcoma

31. Which condition is most likely associated with formation of intraocular cartilage?

A) Phthisis bulbi
B) Posterior persistent hyperplastic primary vitreous
C) Medulloepithelioma
D) Retinoblastoma

Questions 32–36 (Fig 7-32 to 7-38)

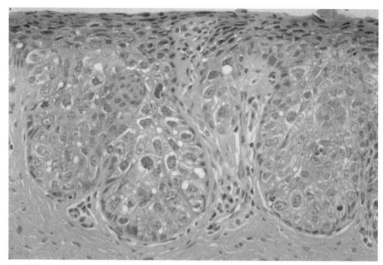

FIGURE 7-32

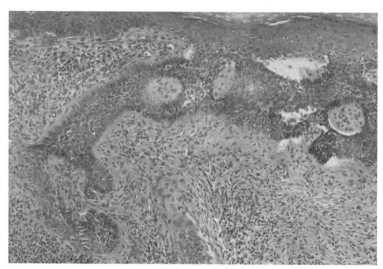

FIGURE 7-33

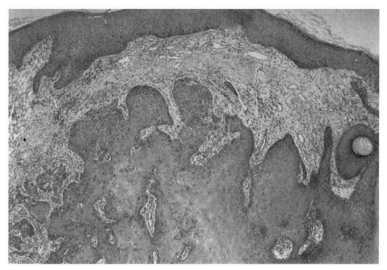

FIGURE 7-34

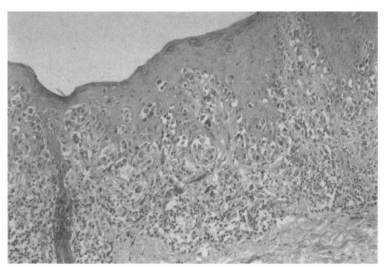

FIGURE 7-35

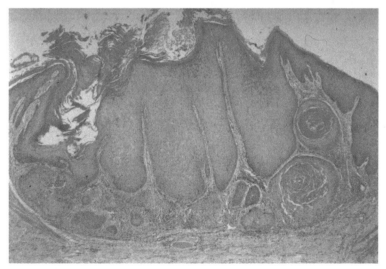

FIGURE 7-36

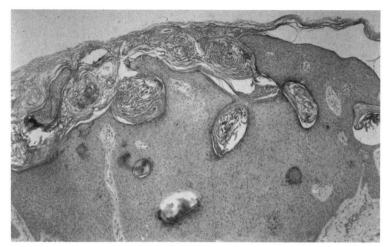

FIGURE 7-37

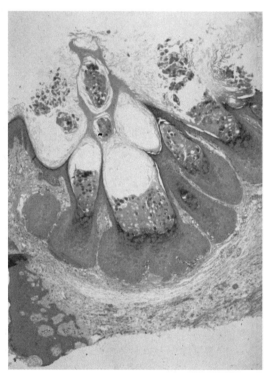

FIGURE 7-38

32. Which lesion may spontaneously disappear?

    A)   Figure 7-36

    B)   Figure 7-37

    C)   Figure 7-35

    D)   Figure 7-34

33. Which lesion is thought to be caused by sun exposure?

    A) Figure 7-36
    B) Figure 7-38
    C) Figure 7-37
    D) Figure 7-34

34. Which lesion is locally invasive with little potential for metastasis?

    A) Figure 7-35
    B) Figure 7-34
    C) Figure 7-32
    D) Figure 7-33

35. Which lesion can be found in association with the conjunctival reaction pictured in Figure 7-39?

    A) Figure 7-38
    B) Figure 7-32
    C) Figure 7-36
    D) Figure 7-33

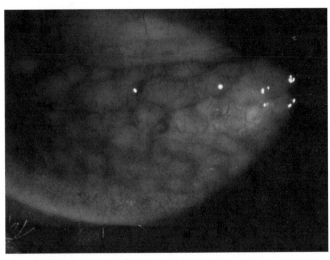

FIGURE 7-39

36. Which stain would be helpful in the diagnosis of Figure 7-32?

    A) Masson trichrome
    B) Gomori methenamine silver
    C) Oil Red O
    D) Gram stain

Questions 37–43

37. A 3-year-old patient presents with bilateral leukocoria. What is the LEAST likely diagnosis?

    A) Congenital cataracts
    B) Retinoblastoma
    C) Retinopathy of prematurity
    D) Metastasis

38. A CT scan was obtained and is shown in Figure 7-40. The right eye was subsequently enucleated. Which treatment would be LEAST effective for the left eye?

    A) Enucleation
    B) Radiation
    C) Chemotherapy
    D) Cryotherapy

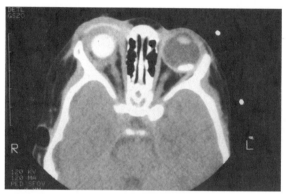

FIGURE 7-40

39. The ultrasound of the lesion in the left eye is shown in Figure 7-41. What is the source of the calcification?

    A) Metaplasia of cells with bone formation
    B) Calcium precipitation from the exudative fluid
    C) Localized abnormality of calcium metabolism
    D) Necrosis of tissue with calcification

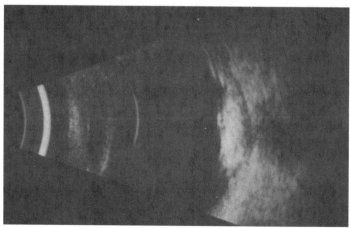

FIGURE 7-41

40. The histologic specimen is shown in Figure 7-42. Which cell is thought to be the most closely related to these cells?

A) Ganglion cell
B) Photoreceptor
C) Retinal pigment epithelium
D) Müller cell

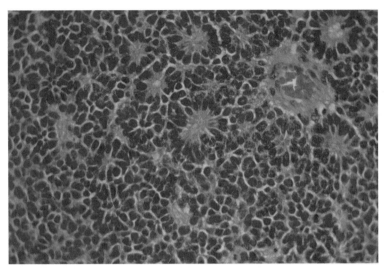

FIGURE 7-42

41. Which one of the following is NOT an indicator of a poorer prognosis?

A) Extrascleral extension
B) Tumor cells through the lamina cribrosa of optic nerve
C) Bilateral involvement
D) Tumor diameter greater than 10 DD

42. What type of secondary tumors are these patients at highest risk for?

A) Osteogenic sarcoma
B) Pheochromocytoma
C) Lymphoma
D) Neuroblastoma

43. What is the probability that this child will have an affected child?

A) 40%
B) 6%
C) 1%
D) 80%

44. The central portion of a corneal button (Fig. 7-43) was obtained at time of penetrating keratoplasty. What is the most likely cause for the transplantation?

    A) Pseudophakic bullous keratopathy
    B) Keratoconus
    C) Fuchs' dystrophy
    D) Congenital hereditary endothelial dystrophy

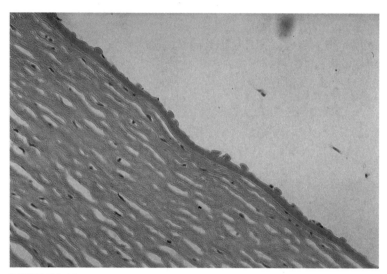

FIGURE 7-43

45. The nuclei of which cell type is NOT found in the layer of the retina indicated by the arrow in Figure 7-44?

    A) Bipolar cell
    B) Amacrine cell
    C) Ganglion cell
    D) Horizontal cell

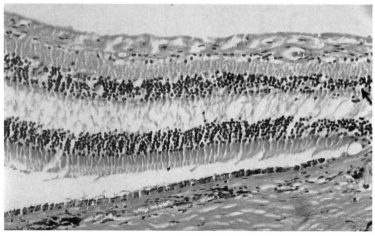

FIGURE 7-44

46. A patient is diagnosed with a malignant melanoma localized to the iris. Which statement is FALSE?

A) This melanoma may produce ipsilateral hyperchromia of the iris.
B) Metastases to liver and bone commonly occur.
C) Treatment is by iridectomy.
D) These lesions may be pigmented or amelanotic.

47. Which tumor is found in association with tuberous sclerosis?

A) Choroidal osteoma
B) Melanocytoma
C) Astrocytic hamartoma
D) Capillary hemangioma

48. Which one of the following retinal layers is most severely affected after a central retinal artery occlusion?

A) Inner plexiform layer
B) Retinal pigment epithelium
C) Outer nuclear layer
D) Inner nuclear layer

49. What do ghost cells represent?

A) Hemosiderin-laden macrophages
B) Denatured lens proteins
C) Spherical red blood cells
D) Inflammatory cells

50. Which disease entity does NOT belong to the group of histiocytosis X?

A) Eosinophilic granuloma of the bone
B) Juvenile xanthogranuloma
C) Hand-Schüller-Christian disease
D) Letterer-Siwe disease

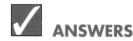 **ANSWERS**

---

1. B) Status postepikeratoplasty (epikeratophakia)

During epikeratoplasty, the epithelium of the recipient cornea is removed with Bowman's layer left in place. An epikeratoplasty lenticle is fashioned from a donor corneal button in the shape that gives the desired refractive power. This is done in such a way that the epithelium with its basement membrane, Bowman's layer, and anterior stoma are left intact and only Descemet's membrane and the deep stroma are removed. This tissue is transplanted onto the denuded Bowman's layer of the recipient. This condition is the only one in which two Bowman's layers are found in one corneal button. PRK ablates superficial layers and part or full thickness Bowman's layer in the center of the cornea. Intrastromal keratomileusis leaves Bowman's layer intact. Trauma can cause rupture of Bowman's layer but not complete duplication.

2. C) It originates from the extraocular muscles.

3. D) Alveolar

Children with rhabdomyosarcoma present with rapidly progressive unilateral, painless proptosis. Swelling and ecchymosis may resemble orbital cellulitis. The cell of origin is presumably an undifferentiated, pluripotent cell of the soft tissue. These cells have the capacity to differentiate toward muscle with production of myosin and actin and to show cross-striations. Immunohistochemistry shows positivity for vimentin, myosin, myoglobin, muscle-specific actin, and desmin. The embryonal type is the most common type, followed by the alveolar type. The prognosis is poorest for the alveolar type. The pleomorphic or well-differentiated type occurs in older patients and has the best prognosis.

4. C) This lesion can be found in approximately 25% of older patients.

Figure 7-1 shows a typical Fuchs' adenoma (Fuchs' reactive hyperplasia, coronal adenoma, Fuchs' epithelioma, benign ciliary epithelioma). This lesion is considered to be proliferative rather than neoplastic. The lesion is composed of basement membrane material (type IV collagen and laminin), acid mucopolysaccharides, glycoproteins, and proliferating cells of the nonpigmented ciliary body epithelium. It rarely may cause localized occlusion of the chamber angle. A metastatic lesion from a malignant melanoma would display mostly pleomorphic, pigmented cells with malignant features (high nuclear-cytoplasmic ratio, nucleoli, and mitotic figures).

5. B) The cells of origin for these lesions are the retinal pigment epithelial cells (cells of neuroectodermal origin).

The retinal pigment epithelium has the capability for fibrous and osseous metaplasia. This is a nonspecific reaction and is observed most often in phthisical eyes. This metaplasia can lead to intraocular ossification, even with intraocular hematopoiesis. The lesion is benign.

6. C) Exudative

The histologic section (Fig. 7-5) displays a complete retinal detachment with amorphous eosinophilic material under the retina. This material is not serous as it is in a rhegmatogenous retinal detachment, but contains an abundance of protein. The subretinal fluid in a retinal detachment caused by traction is mostly serous, and the histologic section would show fibrous preretinal membranes in the vitreous. Artifactitious detachments do not have subretinal fluid.

7. D) Cavernous spaces filled with erythrocytes are present.

Histologic section through this choroidal lesion shows a typical cavernous hemangioma, which is characterized by lakes of erythrocytes separated by thin fibrous septa. The lesion is histologically benign. A capillary hemangioma consists of multiple capillaries surrounded by epithelial cells and pericytes.

8. A) Two clinical growth patterns, that is, a localized and a diffuse form, are observed.

The patient has a choroidal hemangioma, mostly a unilateral lesion. This is an uncommon hamartoma that has been reported to exhibit two clinical growth patterns: 1) circumscribed tumors without systemic disease, and 2) diffuse tumors often associated with the Sturge-Weber syndrome. The lesion is histologically benign; however, the lesion can lead to an exudative retinal detachment if untreated. Therapeutic options are photocoagulation and cryotherapy. The solitary type is histologically characterized by a cavernous hemangioma with sharply demarcated pushing borders, often compressing surrounding melanocytes and choroidal lamellae. This is visible clinically as a ring of hyperpigmentation in the periphery of the lesion (Fig. 7-2) and on fluorescein angiography as a ring of blockage of the underlying choroidal fluorescence (Fig. 7-3). von Hippel-Lindau disease has vascular lesions of the retina and cerebellum; however, these are capillary hemangioblastomas.

9. D) Ipsilateral hemangiomas of the meninges are common.

The girl has meningocutaneous angiomatosis (Sturge-Weber syndrome, encephalotrigeminal angiomatosis). The syndrome consists of mostly unilateral meningeal calcifications, facial nevus flammeus (port-wine stain) frequently along the distribution of the trigeminal nerve, and congenital glaucoma (30%). Heredity does not seem to be an important factor. Histologically, the syndrome is characterized by cavernous hemangiomas of the skin, lids, choroid, and meninges. The disease has no tendency for spontaneous regression as observed with capillary hemangiomas of the child.

10. D) The lesion appears clinically as grayish bubbles posterior to the ora serrata.

The condition is called typical peripheral cystoid degeneration (TPCD) and is inevitable in adult eyes. The cystoid spaces develop first at the outer plexiform layer. If these spaces coalesce, typical degenerative retinoschisis results. In most cases, this is without clinical consequence. Very rarely, a retinal detachment can develop in the presence of holes in the inner *and* outer layers of the schisis cavity. In contrast, reticular cystoid degeneration is less common and develops in the nerve fiber layer.

11.   B)   Surface epithelium is found in the anterior chamber.

This condition is known as epithelial ingrowth (downgrowth) and occurs when surface epithelium of the eye gains access to the internal structure of the globe. This is generally seen after accidental or surgical penetration of the eye. The multilayered nonkeratinized squamous epithelium grows over any available surface and can cause an obstruction of the trabecular meshwork, thus causing a secondary glaucoma. In most advanced cases, the eye is lost. The ICE syndrome is characterized by a unilateral disease in young to middle-aged adults. Abnormal corneal endothelium grows over the trabecular meshwork and over the anterior iris surface. Secondary open-angle glaucoma may develop. Three different clinical phenotypes are known: Chandler's syndrome, Cogan-Reese (iris nevus), and essential iris atrophy.

12.   C)   Periodic acid-Schiff (PAS)

The epithelium in the anterior chamber covering the trabecular meshwork and growing over the iris is a nonkeratinized stratified squamous epithelium. To differentiate this epithelium according to conjunctival or corneal origin, the identification of goblet cells may help. Goblet cells are found in the conjunctival epithelium and are highlighted with a PAS stain (Fig. 7-10). Hematoxylin-eosin is the standard stain for most tissues. Oil Red O is an excellent stain for lipid; however, this must be done on fresh tissue. Congo Red is used to look for amyloid material. With a polarized microscope, amyloid stained with Congo Red demonstrates birefringence and dichroism.

13.   C)   Special stains such as Oil Red O can be used to identify lipids.

During the embedding process in paraffin, different organic solvents (alcohol, xylene) that dissolve and leach out the lipids are used. Therefore, fresh tissue or frozen section has to be used to preserve the lipids and apply a lipid stain such as Oil Red O or Sudan Red. Lipid stains are helpful when looking for sebaceous cell carcinoma.

14.   D)   The diagnosis is confirmed with CT and serologic studies.

15.   A)   Developmental abnormality

The patient has the anterior form of persistent hyperplastic primary vitreous. The embryonic primary vitreous and hyaloid vasculature system persist. This condition is mostly unilateral and is characterized clinically by leukocoria (the most common lesion simulating retinoblastoma). However, contrary to retinoblastoma, persistent hyperplastic primary vitreous is associated with a microphthalmic eye. Histologically, it is characterized by elongated ciliary processes, persistent hyaloid vessel (Fig. 7-12), retrolental fibrovascular tissue (with posterior lens capsule dehiscence) sometimes containing adipose tissue ("lipomatosis lentis") (Fig. 7-13), cartilage, and smooth muscle. The diagnosis is made clinically, and adjunctive tests are unrevealing.

16.   B)   This is a benign cutaneous disorder rarely involving the eye.

The child has juvenile xanthogranuloma (nevoxanthoendothelioma) of the iris. This is a benign cutaneous disorder of infants with typical raised orange skin lesions occurring singly or in crops and regressing spontaneously. Ocular involvement is rather rare and occurs mostly under 6 months of age. Children may present with spontaneous anterior chamber hemorrhage and secondary glaucoma. Histologically, the lesion is characterized by a diffuse granulomatous inflammatory reaction with many histiocytes and Touton giant cells, as seen in Figure 7-14. The histiocytes are positive for antibodies binding to macrophages (e.g., CD 68).

17.   B)   Oncocytoma

Ocular *oncocytomas* (adenolymphomatous tumor, apocrine cystadenoma, oxyphilic cell adenoma) are rare, mostly benign neoplasms and are mostly found on the caruncle. This tumor arises from accessory lacrimal glands in the caruncle, especially in elderly women. It also can arise from accessory lacrimal glands. Histologic examination reveals solid nests and cords of polyhedral cells exhibiting abundant, finely granular acidophilic cytoplasm and round to oval paracentral nuclei, usually containing a single prominent nucleolus. Cystic cavities are identified within the tumor. Adenoid cystic carcinoma (malignant cylindroma) occurs in the lacrimal gland in young adults. The tumor causes pain (infiltration of perineural lymphatics) and is histologically characterized by a "Swiss cheese" pattern. A *pyogenic granuloma* is a type of granulation tissue composed of inflammatory cells and budding capillaries that form a radial pattern. A *papilloma* is characterized by fronds or fingerlike projections of acanthotic epithelium overlying a fibrovascular stroma.

18.   B)   multiple partially atypical mitochondria

Electron microscopic examination shows a cytoplasm densely packed with mitochondria. The mitochondria are sometimes atypical. This is characteristic of oncocytomas.

19.   A)   This can be a chronic inflammation of the Zeis sebaceous glands.

This lesion is a chalazion. A chronic inflammation of the meibomian glands (deep chalazion) or Zeis sebaceous glands (superficial chalazion) results in a hard, painless nodule. Histologically, it is characterized by zonal granulomatous inflammation, including multinucleated giant cells, around clear spaces previously filled with lipid that is dissolved in the processing (Fig. 7-17). It is important to do a biopsy to exclude a sebaceous gland carcinoma in patients with recurrent chalazion. This type of carcinoma can mimic a recurrent chalazion or a chronic blepharitis. Moll's glands are apocrine sweat glands in the eyelid and are not associated with chalazion formation.

20.   C)   are consistent with a zonal lipogranuloma

The clear spaces in this chalazion were previously filled with lipid that dissolved out during tissue processing. The pathogenic principle of a chalazion is a lipogranulomatous inflammatory process. In contrast to xanthomas, the lipid is located in the extracellular space. In a frozen section without paraffin embedding, the lipid is preserved and visible. A vascular channel should at least show endothelial cells.

21.   B)   Herpes simplex

A granulomatous reaction to Descemet's membrane (including multinucleated giant cells) (Fig. 7-19) is most frequently seen with disciform keratitis with a history of herpes simplex or herpes zoster keratitis. This peculiar reaction to Descemet's membrane may be related to an altered antigenicity of the membrane and subsequent development of an autosensitivity reaction. This reaction is very uncommon with other etiologic agents.

22. D)   The disease is phacolytic glaucoma.

The patient has a phacoanaphylactic (phacoimmune) endophthalmitis. This disease develops after exposure of large amounts of lens antigen to the immune system and abrogation of tolerance to lens protein. It is clinically characterized by signs of chronic uveitis, choroidal detachment, and hypotonia bulbi. Normally, lens protein is recognized as "self." In the case of a breakdown of the T-cell tolerance, antibodies against the lens proteins may be produced, initiating a chronic inflammation. In this case, the lens nucleus was lost during cataract surgery (Fig. 7-20) and a phacoanaphylactic endophthalmitis developed. Histologically, it is characterized by activated neutrophils surrounding and "eating away" lens material (Fig. 7-21). These in turn are surrounded by epithelioid cells and occasionally multinucleated giant cells and granulation tissue (zonal granuloma). In contrast, phacolytic glaucoma is characterized by the leakage of denatured lens proteins through an intact capsule (e.g., hypermature cataract). This initiates a mild foreign body reaction, and macrophages get swollen and engulf denatured lens material. These macrophages can block the trabecular outflow and can cause a secondary open angle glaucoma (phacolytic glaucoma).

23. C)   The incidence of zonular dialysis during cataract surgery is higher in these patients.

The patient has pseudoexfoliation syndrome (basement membrane exfoliation syndrome). This is characterized by a deposition of a peculiar white, fluffy material on the lens capsule, the zonules, the ciliary epithelium, the iris pigment epithelium, and the trabecular meshwork. It is more common in Scandinavians and is quite rare in African Americans. The amorphous eosinophilic material lines up perpendicular to the lens (like iron filings lining up on a magnet). The iris pigment epithelium displays a sawtooth posterior configuration. The incidence of zonular dialysis during cataract surgery is higher in these patients. The iris may have peripapillary transillumination defects in this condition in contrast to the radial defects seen with pigment dispersion syndrome. Infrared radiation may cause "true exfoliation" of the lens capsule in glass blowers or welders.

24. C)   Nodular drusen

Nodular (hard) *drusen* consist of a focal thickening of the basement membrane of the retinal pigment epithelium. Clinically, they appear as small yellow or yellow-white spots measuring 50 μm in diameter. *Soft* (exudative, fluffy) *drusen* are bigger and appear less dense and more fluffy. *Basal laminar deposits* consist of banded basement membrane material (wide-spaced collagen) located between the basal plasmalemma of the retinal pigment epithelium and its basement membrane. *Basal linear deposits* refer to material located external to the basement membrane of the retinal pigment epithelium.

25. B)   Basal cell carcinoma, nodular type

Basal cell carcinoma is characterized histologically by a proliferation of basophilic cells. It is by far the most common malignant tumor of the eyelid. The tumor can be grouped into three types: nodular, superficial, and morpheaform. Ulceration and pigmentation may or may not occur. Typical features of the nodular type are peripheral palisading of the tumor cells. The superficial type shows irregular buds of basaloid cells arising from multiple foci of the epidermal undersurface. The morpheaform type is characterized by tumor cells growing in thin, elongated strands or cords, often only one cell layer thick ("Indian file" pattern).

26. B) Lower eyelid—inner canthus—upper eyelid—lateral canthus

The reason for this order is probably the amount of ultraviolet light exposure during life.

27. B) A special stain for acid mucopolysaccharides (e.g., colloidal iron) can be positive within the optic nerve.

Figure 7-26 shows an excavated, deeply cupped optic disc. The most likely cause is an elevated IOP over the course of many years. In the case of a cavernous optic atrophy (Schnabel's), cystic spaces generally posterior to the lamina cribrosa are found. The cystic spaces are filled with hyaluronic acid that stains positive with a stain for acid mucopolysaccharides (e.g., colloidal iron). A central retinal occlusion leads to an atrophic optic nerve; however, the disc is not excavated. Reduction and normalization of IOP can result in reversal of optic disc cupping, which is common in children and less frequent in adults.

28. B) This neoplastic lesion contains epithelial embryonic rests.

The histologic lesion shown in Figures 7-27, 7-28, and 7-29 consists of a proliferation of cells with bland nuclei in the epithelium and subepithelial layer. The subepithelial component contains cysts with a nonkeratinized squamous epithelium with goblet cells. The lesion represents a typical compound nevus of the conjunctiva. The subepithelial hamartomatous component, in addition to the nevus cells, frequently contains epithelial embryonic rests that may develop into epithelial cysts, as this case shows. The lesion can be pigmented or nonpigmented. In chronic conjunctivitis, a chronic inflammatory cell infiltrate is seen. Infoldings of the proliferated epithelium and goblet cells may resemble glandular structures in tissue sections and are called *pseudoglands* (Henle).

29. B) Status postrepair of retinal detachment

The histologic picture (Figs. 7-30 and 7-31) shows an empty cystic space in the sclera with an overlying polyfilamentous suture associated with a foreign body giant cell reaction. The empty scleral space represents a dissolved encircling band from prior surgery for retinal detachment. The polyfilamentous suture was used to fix the band to the sclera. A ruptured sclera should be associated with full thickness scleral scars. A scleral staphyloma is ectatic and thinned sclera lined by choroid with or without retina.

30. D) Rhabdomyosarcoma

Homer-Wright rosettes are characterized by cells that line up around an area containing cobweb-like material, but no acid mucopolysaccharides are present. These rosettes are not specific for retinoblastoma and are found also in neuroblastoma and medulloepithelioma. Rhabdomyosarcoma displays no rosette formation. In contrast, Flexner-Wintersteiner rosettes are the characteristic rosettes of retinoblastoma but are not always present. The presence of Flexner Wintersteiner rosettes makes the diagnosis of a well-differentiated retinoblastoma. In Flexner-Wintersteiner rosettes, the cells line up around an apparently empty central lumen. However, special stains show hyaluronidase-resistant acid mucopolysaccharides in the lumen.

31. C)   Medulloepithelioma

The medulloepithelioma (diktyoma) arises from the ciliary epithelium. Nonteratoid and teratoid varieties (presence of heteroplastic elements) are known. Both can be benign or malignant. The teratoid type may contain cartilage and/or rhabdomyoblasts. Phthisis bulbi can result in metaplasia of the retinal pigment epithelium with bone formation. Cartilage formation is virtually unknown. Posterior persistent hyperplastic primary vitreous is characterized by vitreous membranes extending from the disc usually toward the equatorial zone, posterior radial retinal folds, disturbance of macular function, and retinal detachment. Cartilage formation is not a feature of posterior persistent hyperplastic primary vitreous, contrasting with the anterior form in which it has been described in rare cases. Retinoblastoma displays calcification secondary to rapid proliferation and necrosis of cells, but no cartilage formation occurs.

32. A)   Figure 7-36

33. D)   Figure 7-34

34. D)   Figure 7-33

35. A)   Figure 7-38

36. C)   Oil Red O

The lesions pictured are enumerated:

> Figure 7-32 = sebaceous cell carcinoma
> Figure 7-33 = basal cell carcinoma, nodular
> Figure 7-34 = squamous cell carcinoma
> Figure 7-35 = malignant melanoma
> Figure 7-36 = keratoacanthoma
> Figure 7-37 = seborrheic keratosis
> Figure 7-38 = molluscum contagiosum

Sebaceous cell carcinomas may present insidiously as chronic, recurrent chalazia or blepharitis. If they are suspected, fresh tissue should be processed for lipid stains such as Oil Red O. They are notorious for skip lesions and require wide excision. Metastasis to regional lymph nodes is possible.

Basal cell carcinoma is the most frequently occurring eyelid lesion, often in sun-exposed areas. These may present as raised lesions with pearly borders, telangiectatic vessels, and an ulcerated crater (rodent ulcer). Histopathologically, there are palisading rests of basophilic cells with scanty cytoplasm and hyperchromatic nuclei. Basal cell carcinoma is locally invasive and rarely metastasizes.

Squamous cell carcinoma is also related to sun exposure. Proliferation of eosinophilic epithelium with rests of keratin pearls traverse the basement membrane into the underlying dermis. Surgical excision using the Mohs' technique is recommended. Metastasis occurs to regional nodes.

The keratoacanthoma may be confused with the squamous cell carcinoma; however, it presents much more rapidly. The central crater contains keratin. These may resolve spontaneously over several months.

Seborrheic keratoses are benign lesions that have a greasy, "stuck on" appearance. Pathologic examination shows hyperkeratosis and papillomatosis with keratin pseudo-horn cysts.

Molluscum contagiosum is caused by a pox virus and appears as raised, umbilicated lesions on the eyelid, face, and genital regions. Epithelium thickened by intracytoplasmic molluscum bodies are present in the central crater. These may be shed into the tear film from eyelid margin lesions, causing a chronic follicular conjunctivitis. Treatment is by cryotherapy, curettage, or excision.

37. D) Metastasis

Congenital cataracts, retinoblastoma, and retinopathy of prematurity, among others, are in the differential of bilateral leukocoria. Intraocular metastatic disease to the eyes is extremely rare in children.

38. D) Cryotherapy

The CT scan shows bilateral high density lesions consistent with calcification within the tumors. In this case of retinoblastoma, the right eye was enucleated. Treatment for the left eye includes enucleation, radiation, and chemotherapy. Cryotherapy may be effective for small lesions. For posterior lesions, as pictured, effective placement of cryotherapy would be difficult to achieve. Moreover, it would be ineffective for multicentric tumors. Chemotherapy or radiation is preferable to try to preserve vision in the left eye.

39. D) Necrosis of tissue with calcification

Retinoblastoma is a rapidly growing tumor that can outgrow its vascular supply. This rapid growth leads to necrosis of tissue and secondary calcification. Whitish flecks of calcification can be seen in the whitish substance of the tumor (Fig. 7-45).

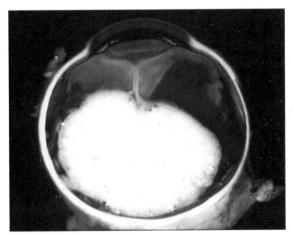

FIGURE 7-45

40.   B)   Photoreceptor

Figure 7-42 shows a Flexner-Wintersteiner rosette, characteristic of retinoblastoma. These rosettes represent abnormal photoreceptor differentiation. Homer-Wright rosettes and fleurettes are also along the spectrum of photoreceptor differentiation.

41.   D)   Tumor diameter greater than 10 DD

Extraocular spread of retinoblastoma indicates a poor prognosis. Patients with bilateral involvement may be at higher risk of trilateral retinoblastoma. The size of the tumor, per se, does not affect prognosis. Figure 7-46 shows tumor cells within the substance of the optic nerve.

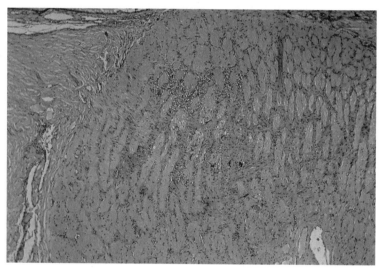

FIGURE 7-46

42.   A)   Osteogenic sarcoma

Secondary tumors are more common in these children and include osteogenic sarcoma, malignant melanoma, lymphoma and leukemia, rhabdomyosarcoma, and medulloblastoma. The most common malignancies are sarcomas, particularly osteogenic sarcoma.

43.   A)   40%

In this bilateral case, there is a high likelihood that a somatic, heritable mutation exists. Half of this child's offspring will receive the abnormal chromosome. With 80% penetrance, 40% of his children will be affected.

44.   C)   Fuchs' dystrophy

The cornea has multiple excrescences at the level of Descemet's membrane consistent with Fuchs' dystrophy. Keratoconus would have breaks in Bowman's layer and epithelium along with thinning and scarring of the cornea, but with a normal Descemet's membrane. Pseudophakic bullous keratopathy and congenital hereditary endothelial dystrophy have thickening of the corneal stroma and loss of endothelial cells.

45. C)   Ganglion cell

The ganglion cell nuclei are found in the innermost layer of nuclei. The inner nuclear layer contains cell bodies of the bipolar, amacrine, horizontal, and Müller cells. The outer nuclear layer has the cell bodies of the photoreceptors (Fig. 7-47).

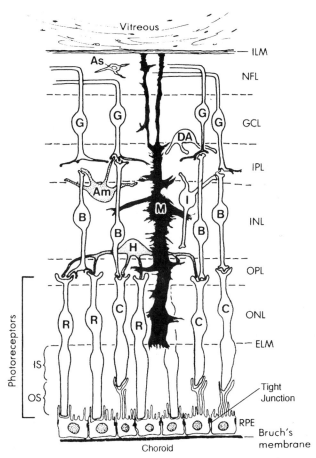

FIGURE 7-47. From Wright K. Textbook of ophthalmology. Baltimore: Williams & Wilkins, 1997:37.

46. B)   Metastases to liver and bone commonly occur.

If isolated to the iris, malignant melanoma behaves in a more benign fashion than does melanoma of the choroid. Involvement of the ciliary body or choroid portends a poorer prognosis. Metastases are rare, and localized iridectomy may remove the tumor entirely. These lesions may be pigmented or amelanotic. Ipsilateral hyperchromia may be present.

47. C)   Astrocytic hamartoma

Findings associated with tuberous sclerosis include astrocytic hamartomas, intracerebral calcification, seizures, mental retardation, adenoma sebaceum, and ash leaf spots. Capillary hemangiomas may be found in von Hippel-Lindau disease.

48. A)   Inner plexiform layer

The retinal arteries supply oxygen to the superficial layers of the retina, including the nerve fiber layer, ganglion cell layer, inner plexiform layer, and inner third of the inner nuclear layer. The other layers are nourished primarily by the choroid.

49. C)   Spherical red blood cells

Ghosts cells represent hemolyzed red blood cells. After a longstanding hyphema or vitreous hemorrhage, the red blood cells lose their normal shape and become more spherical. These cells are more rigid and less able to deform to exit through the trabecular meshwork, resulting in a secondary open angle glaucoma. On slit lamp microscopy, they appear as khaki-colored cells in the anterior chamber.

50. B)   Juvenile xanthogranuloma

Histiocytosis X (Langerhans cell histiocytosis, Langerhans granulomatosis) is characterized by a proliferation of Langerhans cells in an inflammatory background. Immunohistochemically, the cells stain positively for S-100 and vimentin. Ultrastructurally, the cells contain Birbeck granules (containing a central dense core and a thick outer sheath). Three interrelated clinicopathologic entities are known: 1) *eosinophilic granuloma of bone* (benign tumor arising often in the outer part of the upper orbital rim), 2) *Hand-Schüller-Christian disease* (bony lesions in the skull, exophthalmos, and diabetes insipidus), and 3) *Letterer-Siwe disease* (fatal disease with diffuse histiocytosis). Juvenile xanthogranuloma (JXG) does not belong to the histiocytosis X group. JXG is negative for S-100 and contains no Birbeck granules.

Notes

Notes

8

Uveitis

QUESTIONS

1. A 64-year-old white woman presents with complaints of pain, decreased vision, and a red eye for the past 2 days (Fig. 8-1). Her past medical history reveals that she had a trabeculectomy for primary open angle glaucoma in this same eye 6 months before your examination. What would a Gram stain of the vitreous fluid of this patient most likely show?

   A) Gram-negative coccobacilli
   B) Gram-positive rods
   C) Branching pseudohyphal forms
   D) Gram-positive cocci in clusters

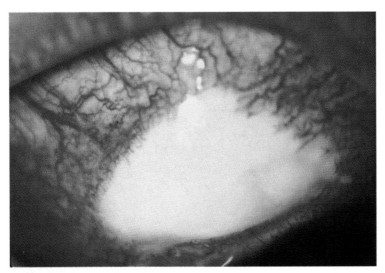

FIGURE 8-1

Questions 2–4

A 69-year-old white man presents with mild discomfort and reports a gradual decrease in the vision of his right eye over the course of 1 week. His past ocular history is remarkable for cataract extraction and posterior chamber intraocular lens (IOL) insertion in this eye 4 months previously. Because of the low grade nature of the inflammation, topical steroids are begun and the inflammation responded favorably. After discontinuing the steroids, the symptoms return and the patient again presents with a granulomatous anterior chamber inflammation, including a small hypopyon and a mild anterior vitritis.

2. What would examination of the white plaque present at the equator of the posterior lens capsule most likely reveal?

   A) *Candida albicans*
   B) *Propionibacterium acnes*
   C) *Staphylococcus epidermidis*
   D) *Mycobacterium tuberculosis*

3. Which one of the following is the most appropriate therapy for this condition?

A) Vitrectomy and intravitreal injection of amphotericin B
B) Observation
C) Vitrectomy, removal of the IOL, and intravitreal injection of gentamicin
D) Vitrectomy, posterior capsulectomy, and intravitreal injection of vancomycin

4. What is the least likely microbial cause for this syndrome?

A) *Propionibacterium granulosum*
B) Achromobacter
C) Klebsiella
D) Corynebacterium

Questions 5–7

A 32-year-old African American woman presents with floaters and blurred vision in her right eye. Slit lamp examination shows nodules on the iris (Fig. 8-2). A recent chest radiograph revealed hilar adenopathy.

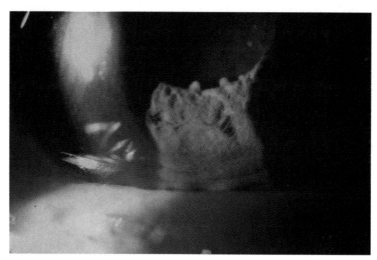

FIGURE 8-2

5. Biopsy of her lacrimal gland would likely reveal:

A) epithelioid cells within necrotic tissue
B) multinucleated giant cells of the Touton type
C) multinucleated giant cells of the Langhans type
D) diffuse lymphocytic infiltration

6. Other ocular manifestations include all of the following EXCEPT:

A) papillitis
B) scleritis
C) follicular conjunctivitis
D) granulomatous keratic precipitates

7. Ocular complications in this condition as a result of steroid treatment include all of the following EXCEPT:

   A) cataract
   B) retinal neovascularization
   C) glaucoma
   D) scleromalacia

Questions 8–9

An 11-year-old white girl presents with reports of floaters in her left eye and a mild decrease in vision. On examination of her anterior chamber, you notice a mild anterior chamber inflammatory reaction and the corneal changes shown in Figure 8-3. Dilated fundus examination reveals whitish fibrous material in the inferior periphery.

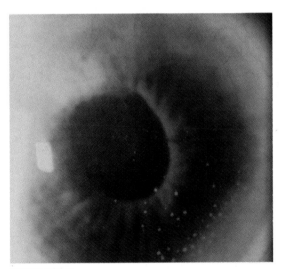

FIGURE 8-3

8. Which one of the following is associated with this condition?

   A) Anterior subcapsular cataracts
   B) HLA-B27
   C) Unilaterality in the majority of cases
   D) Multiple sclerosis

9. Pathologic examination of the "snowbank" would reveal:

   A) lipid exudates
   B) fibroglial and vascular components
   C) an aggregation of epithelioid and multinucleated giant cells
   D) a conglomeration of lipofuscin and chronic inflammatory cells

10. A patient presents with the eye illustrated in Figure 8-4. All of the following conditions can cause this EXCEPT:

    A) Uveitis-glaucoma-hyphema (UGH) syndrome
    B) Herpetic iridocyclitis
    C) HLA-B27 anterior uveitis
    D) traumatic iridocyclitis

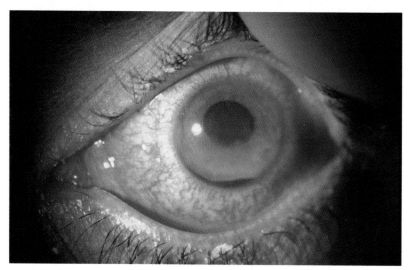

FIGURE 8-4

11. Which one of the following conditions is NOT typically associated with diffusely distributed keratic precipitates?

    A) Fuchs' heterochromic iridocyclitis
    B) Sarcoidosis
    C) Vogt-Koyanagi-Harada
    D) Syphilis

12. Which one of the following conditions is NOT associated with HLA-B27–linked acute iritis?

    A) Behçet's disease
    B) Psoriatic arthritis
    C) Crohn's disease
    D) Reiter's syndrome

Questions 13–15

A 35-year-old man presents with ocular pain, pain in his wrists and feet, pain on urination, and aphthous ulcers. Ocular examination is significant because it reveals a mucoid conjunctival discharge and a mild cellular reaction in the anterior chamber. A peculiar skin lesion is also noted (Fig. 8-5).

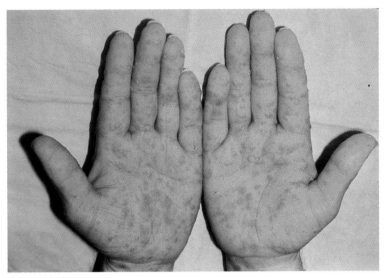

FIGURE 8-5

13. Which one of the following findings would NOT be expected in this patient?

    A) Balanitis
    B) Prostatitis
    C) A recent history of diarrhea
    D) Positive rheumatoid factor

14. Which organism has NOT been implicated in triggering this condition?

    A) Chlamydia
    B) *Ureaplasma urealyticum*
    C) Yersinia
    D) Rochalimaea

15. The classic skin lesion associated with this condition, pictured in Figure 8-5, is:

    A) erythema chronicum migrans
    B) pustular psoriasis
    C) keratoderma blennorrhagicum
    D) eczema

16. A 10-year-old girl with a history of arthralgia and a chronic anterior chamber inflammation of both eyes presents to your office. She has no cells, but mild flare is present in the anterior chamber. Given the natural history of this disease, which one of the following statements is most likely TRUE?

    A) This patient is antinuclear antibody (ANA) negative.
    B) This patient has pauciarticular disease involving the hands and wrists.
    C) This patient has pauciarticular disease involving the lower extremities without involvement of the wrist joints.
    D) This patient is rheumatoid factor positive.

Questions 17–19

A 40-year-old white man is referred for ophthalmologic examination because the vision in one eye could not be refracted better than 20/40. On examination, you note mild unilateral anterior chamber inflammation and stellate keratic precipitates diffusely dispersed over the posterior surface of the cornea. The patient has hazel irides with a mild difference of iris pigmentation between the eyes.

17. Which one of the following statements is most likely TRUE?

    A) The involved eye is darker brown than the uninvolved eye.
    B) Less than 2% of patients with this condition will have bilateral involvement with no obvious heterochromia.
    C) Pathologic specimens of this condition have revealed the presence of plasma cells within the ciliary body.
    D) Posterior synechiae may be prominent.

18. Which one of the following infectious agents has been suggested as having an association with this condition?

    A) Histoplasma
    B) Toxoplasma
    C) Toxocara
    D) Epstein-Barr virus

19. Which of the following topical medications used unilaterally can cause a similar appearance?

    A) dipivefrin
    B) cyclosporine A
    C) latanoprost
    D) brimonidine

20. All of the following major immunoglobulin classes are found in human tears EXCEPT:

    A) IgD
    B) IgE
    C) IgG
    D) IgM

21. Which one of the following statements concerning the classic immune hypersensitivity reactions in diseases that affect the eye is TRUE?

A) The granulomatous response seen in sarcoid uveitis is primarily a Type I hypersensitivity reaction.
B) Phacoanaphylaxis is a Type III hypersensitivity reaction.
C) Hay fever is an example of a Type II hypersensitivity reaction.
D) Type IV hypersensitivity reactions are mediated by cytotoxic antibodies.

Questions 22–23

An elderly African American patient comes with the complaint of a whitish area on her eye for the last several weeks (Fig 8-6). Her eye has been comfortable and no discharge or crusting of her lashes.

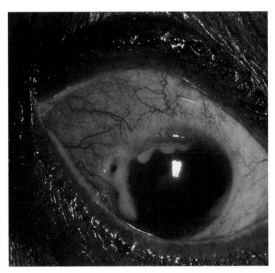

FIGURE 8-6

22. All of the following blood tests would be useful in making the diagnosis EXCEPT:

A) HIV antibodies
B) rheumatoid factor
C) anti-neutrophil cytoplasmic antibody
D) PPD skin test

23. There is a small trickle of fluid from the peripheral corneal defect. What treatment might be most helpful in the acute setting?

A) Aqueous suppressant
B) Application of cyanoacrylate glue
C) Corneal patch graft
D) Topical corticosteroids

24. Which one of the following characteristics regarding serpiginous choroidopathy is TRUE?

    A) Recurrent, indolent course
    B) Primarily affects children
    C) Multifocal lesions
    D) Responds promptly to corticosteroids

25. A 25-year-old man was hammering a nail into a piece of wood in his garage when he noticed a sudden sharp pain in his right eye with only a mild decrease in his vision. He presents to your office 2 days later with reports of gradually increasing pain and a severe loss of vision in that eye. On examination, you notice a small peripheral corneal laceration and a hypopyon. Which one of the following statements concerning endophthalmitis in this setting is TRUE?

    A) The most common infecting organism in these cases is *Staphylococcus aureus*.
    B) A visual acuity of 20/400 or better is likely to be retained in the majority of patients after appropriate treatment and rehabilitation.
    C) Endophthalmitis would be expected to occur in less than 10% of similar trauma cases.
    D) Endophthalmitis with *Bacillus* species has a good visual prognosis.

26. You examine a 78-year-old white man with complaints of decreased vision in his right eye. Three weeks earlier, he had undergone coronary artery bypass surgery with a complicated postoperative course requiring prolonged ventilatory support. He has been receiving hyperalimentation and IV antibiotics since the time of his surgery. On dilated fundus examination of his right eye, you note a fluffy white choroidal lesion under the macula. There is minimal overlying vitritis present. Which one of the following statements concerning the organism most likely responsible for this lesion is TRUE?

    A) The responsible organism grows on blood agar and Sabouraud's glucose within 24 to 48 hours.
    B) This organism exists exclusively as an oval budding cell known as a *blastoconidia*.
    C) Ocular infection caused by this organism is generally accompanied by positive blood cultures.
    D) This organism often colonizes the respiratory tract and is a frequent cause of pneumonia.

27. A 25-year-old homeless man presents to your office with reports of decreased vision and pain in his right eye for the past 2 days. Examination reveals marked conjunctival injection, a 2-mm hypopyon, and dense vitreous opacities on B-scan ultrasound. You suspect endogenous endophthalmitis and, on further questioning, the patient admits to IV drug abuse. Given the patient's history, which one of the following organisms is the LEAST likely to be involved in this patient's endophthalmitis?

    A) *Candida albicans*
    B) *Staphylococcus* species
    C) *Bacillus cereus*
    D) *Haemophilus influenzae*

Questions 28–30

A 27-year-old Japanese exchange student presents to your office with reports of decreased vision in both his eyes. On examination, a small hypopyon OD and a moderate cellular reaction OS is found. Fundus examination of his left eye is shown in Figure 8-7. On further questioning, you elicit a history of arthritis of his knees and wrists, and painful lesions in his mouth and around his genitals. On examination of his lower extremities, you note the lesion seen in Figure 8-8.

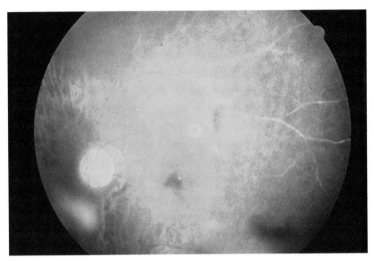

FIGURE 8-7

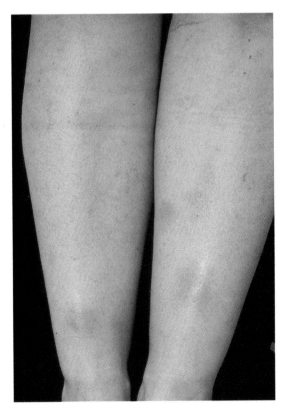

FIGURE 8-8

28. Skin lesions common to this condition include all of the following EXCEPT:

A) acne-like lesions over the back and face
B) erythema nodosum
C) psoriasis
D) thrombophlebitis

29. Which one of the following statements concerning the therapeutic treatment of this condition is TRUE?

A) Oral corticosteroids alone are usually effective in preventing the relapse of ocular inflammation.
B) Periocular steroids alone are usually effective in preventing the relapse of ocular inflammation.
C) Colchicine may be helpful in preventing recurrences.
D) Cyclosporine may be useful in this condition, but the incidence of liver toxicity may limit its use.

30. Which one of the following statements concerning the ocular inflammation associated with this condition is TRUE?

A) Patients generally develop chronic, unremitting ocular inflammation if this condition is not aggressively treated.
B) A granulomatous inflammation is typically present.
C) The retinitis associated with this condition may be confused with a viral retinitis.
D) Inflammation in this condition predominantly affects the choroid.

31. What is the most common cause of acute, non-infectious, hypopyon iritis?

A) Behçet's disease
B) Idiopathic anterior uveitis
C) HLA-B27–associated iritis
D) Sarcoid iridocyclitis

32. In which one of the following is the HLA-B27 antigen LEAST likely to be present?

A) Men with ankylosing spondylitis
B) Young women with pauciarticular juvenile rheumatoid arthritis
C) Men with Reiter's syndrome
D) Men with psoriatic arthritis

33. Which form of uveitis is most common in ocular sarcoidosis?

A) Panuveitis
B) Intermediate uveitis
C) Anterior uveitis
D) Choroiditis

34. Which of the following statements is most accurate regarding the lesions pictured in Figure 8-9?

A) live virus can be recovered from epithelial lesions
B) this disease is usually seen in children or young adults
C) topical corticosteroid drops are effective in eliminating this disease
D) these lesions are frequently bilateral at presentation

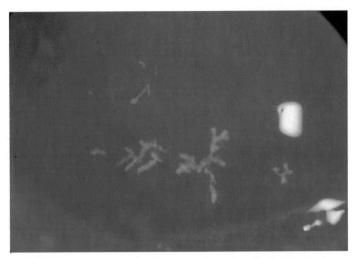

FIGURE 8-9

Questions 35–37 Select the answer that corresponds to the conditions listed.

35. Iris nodules

A) Granulomatous uveitis
B) Nongranulomatous uveitis
C) Both
D) Neither

36. Epithelioid cells

A) Granulomatous uveitis
B) Nongranulomatous uveitis
C) Both
D) Neither

37. Fuchs' heterochromic iridocyclitis

A) Granulomatous uveitis
B) Nongranulomatous uveitis
C) Both
D) Neither

Questions 38-40 (Fig. 8-10 to 8-13)

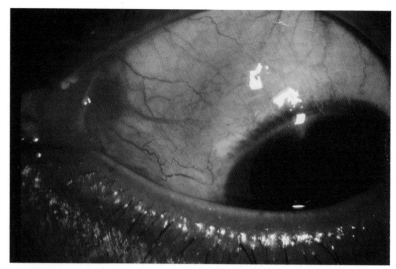

FIGURE 8-10

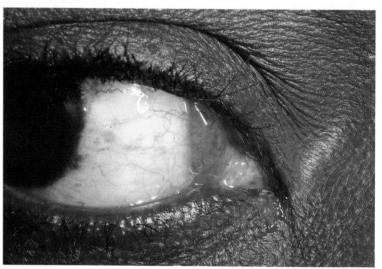

FIGURE 8-11

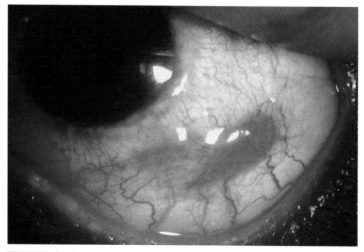

FIGURE 8-12

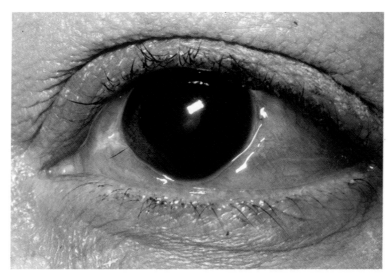

FIGURE 8-13

38. Biopsy of which lesion would show a monotonous proliferation of B cells?

A) Figure 8-10
B) Figure 8-11
C) Figure 8-12
D) Figure 8-13

39. Which would present with pain and localized tenderness?

A) Figure 8-10
B) Figure 8-11
C) Figure 8-12
D) Figure 8-13

40. Human herpesvirus 8 (HHV-8) has been implicated in causing which condition?

A) Figure 8-10
B) Figure 8-11
C) Figure 8-12
D) Figure 8-13

41. What is the most characteristic side effect of oral cyclophosphamide?

A) Secondary infections
B) Secondary malignancies
C) Hemolytic anemia
D) Hemorrhagic cystitis

42. Side effects of systemic corticosteroid therapy include all of the following EXCEPT:

A) Aseptic necrosis of the hip
B) Hypoglycemia
C) Exacerbation of hypertension
D) Gastric ulceration

Questions 43–45 Match the following immunosuppressives to their class.

43. Cyclosporine

 A) Cytotoxic antimetabolite
 B) Cytostatic anti-inflammatory
 C) Immune modulator of interleukin 2
 D) Cytotoxic alkylating agent

44. Prednisone

 A) Cytotoxic antimetabolite
 B) Cytostatic anti-inflammatory
 C) Immune modulator of interleukin 2
 D) Cytotoxic alkylating agent

45. Methotrexate

 A) Cytotoxic antimetabolite
 B) Cytostatic anti-inflammatory
 C) Immune modulator of interleukin 2
 D) Cytotoxic alkylating agent

46. Which one of the following is the most common retinal finding in AIDS?

 A) Cotton wool spots
 B) Cytomegalovirus retinitis
 C) Pneumocystis choroiditis
 D) Acute retinal necrosis

47. The life form of the *Toxoplasma gondii* organism that is responsible for stimulating inflammation is/are:

 A) cyst
 B) bradyzoite
 C) tachyzoite
 D) all of the above

48. Which one of the following statements about the drugs used to treat ocular toxoplasmosis is TRUE?

 A) Pyrimethamine blocks the production of dihydrofolate from para-aminobenzoic acid.
 B) Sulfadiazine inhibits the dihydrofolate reductase enzyme.
 C) Clindamycin can effectively kill Toxoplasma organisms.
 D) Systemic and periocular corticosteroids are contraindicated because they may cause proliferation of Toxoplasma organisms.

49. Juvenile rheumatoid arthritis–associated iridocyclitis is most common in:

    A)   early-onset pauciarticular disease
    B)   late-onset pauciarticular disease
    C)   Still's disease
    D)   late-onset polyarticular disease

50. Schwartz's syndrome is caused by:

    A)   retinal pigment epithelial cells blocking the trabecular meshwork
    B)   forward rotation of the lens–iris diaphragm
    C)   ciliary body and choroidal edema
    D)   photoreceptor outer segments blocking the trabecular meshwork

51. Posner-Schlossman syndrome:

    A)   requires systemic or periocular corticosteroid therapy
    B)   is not associated with late-onset glaucoma
    C)   is painless
    D)   is often self-limited

Questions 52–53 Match the following disease entities with the type of inflammation.

52. Phacoanaphylactic endophthalmitis

    A)   Nongranulomatous inflammation
    B)   Zonal granulomatous inflammation
    C)   Macrophages filled with lens material
    D)   Type I—IgE mediated anaphylaxis

53. Phacolytic glaucoma

    A)   Nongranulomatous inflammation
    B)   Zonal granulomatous inflammation
    C)   Macrophages filled with lens material
    D)   Type I—IgE mediated anaphylaxis

54. Which one of the following regarding acute retinal necrosis is NOT true?

    A)   Severe arteritis is common.
    B)   Herpes zoster virus has been implicated as etiologic agent.
    C)   Posterior pole is involved initially with centrifugal spread.
    D)   Retinal detachments occur frequently.

55. Fuchs' heterochromic iridocyclitis is characterized by:

    A) high rate of posterior capsular rupture during phacoemulsification
    B) filiform hemorrhage with paracentesis
    C) neovascular proliferation in the angle with angle closure
    D) resolution of iridocyclitis with topical corticosteroids

56. Intermediate uveitis is associated with all of the following conditions EXCEPT:

    A) Lyme disease
    B) multiple sclerosis
    C) sarcoidosis
    D) syphilis

57. Complications of pars planitis include all of the following EXCEPT:

    A) calcific band keratopathy
    B) choroidal neovascularization
    C) vitreous hemorrhage
    D) tractional retinal detachment

58. The electroretinogram in the condition pictured in Figure 8-14:

    A) is normal
    B) is flat
    C) reveals diminished scotopic responses
    D) reveals diminished photopic responses

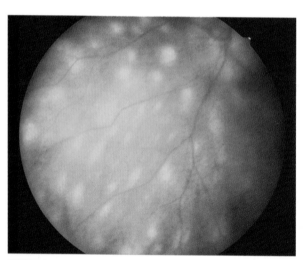

FIGURE 8-14

59. Cystoid macular edema is a common cause of visual loss in all of the following EXCEPT:

    A) Vogt-Koyanagi-Harada syndrome
    B) pars planitis
    C) birdshot retinochoroidopathy
    D) retinal vasculitides

60. The strongest HLA association to ocular disease is between:

    A) HLA-B27 and psoriatic arthritis
    B) HLA-B7 and ocular histoplasmosis syndrome
    C) HLA-B5 and Behçet's disease
    D) HLA-A29 and birdshot retinochoroidopathy

61. Which one of the following regarding diffuse unilateral subacute neuroretinitis is TRUE?

    A) Etiology is unknown.
    B) Treatment is mainly with systemic corticosteroids.
    C) Reduced vision, vitreous cells, and optic disc edema are early findings.
    D) Causative organism is *Ascaris lumbricoides.*

62. Which one of the following statements regarding sarcoidosis is TRUE?

    A) Elevated serum angiotensin converting enzyme level is specific for sarcoidosis.
    B) Blind conjunctival biopsies have a high yield in patients with presumptive diagnosis of sarcoidosis.
    C) Hilar adenopathy is the most common pulmonary finding in sarcoidosis.
    D) Uveitis occurs in 85% of patients with systemic sarcoidosis.

Questions 63–66 A 65-year-old patient presents with a painful, red eye for the past 3 months. The eye is illustrate in Fig. 8–15.

63. Appropriate laboratory evaluation would include:

    A) serum angiotensin converting enzyme
    B) partial sclerectomy for histopathologic evaluation
    C) serum anti-neutrophil cytoplasmic antibody

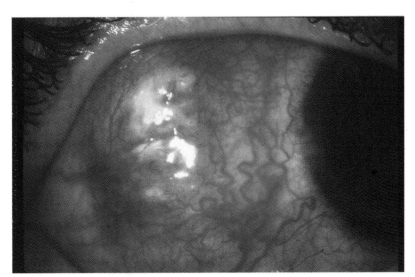

FIGURE 8-15

D)   HLA typing

64.   Appropriate therapy would include all of the following EXCEPT:

A)   colchicine
B)   prednisone
C)   cyclosporine
D)   cyclophosphamide

65.   Which one of the following should never be used to treat this condition?

A)   Topical corticosteroids
B)   Periocular corticosteroids
C)   Both
D)   Neither

66.   All of the following systemic conditions may be associated with Figure 8-15 EXCEPT:

A)   relapsing polychondritis
B)   polyarteritis nodosa
C)   Wegener's granulomatosis
D)   polymyalgia rheumatica

Questions 67–69 A patient with the fundus pictured in Fig. 8-16 is referred for your evaluation.

67.   The work-up of this patient would include:

A)   lumbar puncture
B)   electroretinogram
C)   HIV serology
D)   fluorescein angiogram

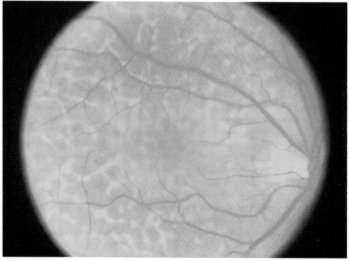

FIGURE 8-16

68. Appropriate treatment would include:

   A) periocular corticosteroids
   B) intrathecal methotrexate, IV cytarabine (Ara-C), and whole brain and eye irradiation
   C) enucleation
   D) no treatment is available for this condition

69. Which one of the following regarding this condition is TRUE?

   A) There is poor prognosis for survival.
   B) Inheritance is autosomal recessive.
   C) Nyctalopia is a common symptom.
   D) Cystoid macular edema is a common complication.

Questions 70–73

This patient has a granulomatous uveitis with multiple serous retinal detachments as shown in Figure 8-17.

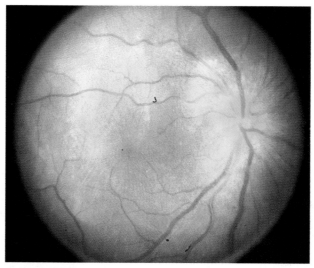

FIGURE 8-17

70. Work-up should include:

   A) VDRL and FTA-Abs
   B) anti-nuclear antibody
   C) B-scan ultrasound
   D) all of the above

71. The most appropriate treatment for this condition would be:

    A) pars plana vitrectomy and internal drainage of subretinal fluid
    B) vortex vein decompression
    C) scleral buckling with external drainage of subretinal fluid
    D) corticosteroids

72. Fluorescein angiography would reveal:

    A) a single "smokestack" of fluorescein leakage into the subretinal space
    B) multiple pinpoint areas of fluorescein leakage into the subretinal space
    C) diffuse retinal venous staining and leakage
    D) well-defined lacy hyperfluorescence with late leakage

73. Differential diagnosis may include all of the following EXCEPT:

    A) posterior scleritis
    B) sympathetic ophthalmia
    C) hypotony
    D) acute neuroretinitis

74. All of the following cutaneous features may be found in Vogt-Koyanagi-Harada syndrome EXCEPT:

    A) vitiligo
    B) poliosis
    C) alopecia
    D) eczema

Questions 75–81 Refer to Fig. 8-18 to 8-23.

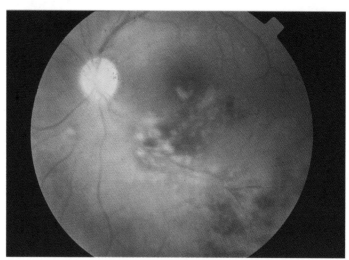

FIGURE 8-18

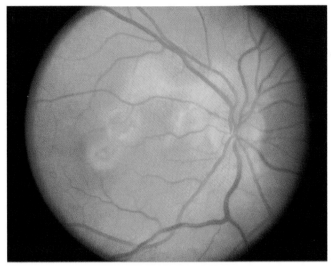

FIGURE 8-19

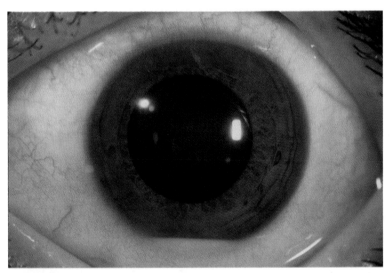

FIGURE 8-20

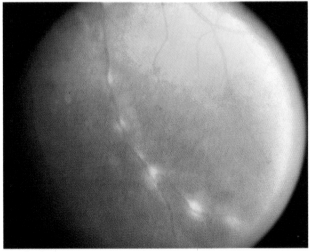

FIGURE 8-21

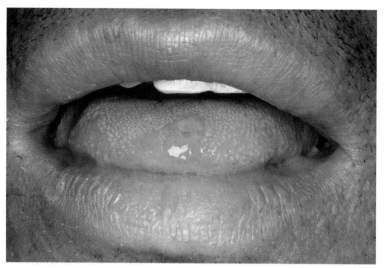

FIGURE 8-22

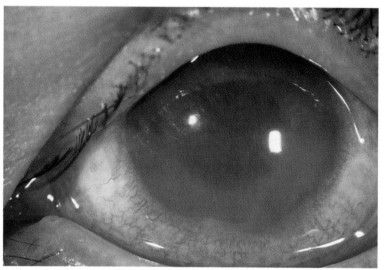

FIGURE 8-23. From Wright K. Textbook of ophthalmology. Baltimore: Williams & Wilkins, 1997.

75. All of the following may be associated with Figure 8-22 EXCEPT:

    A) back pain
    B) diarrhea
    C) cardiac conduction defects
    D) arthritis

76. Painless decrease in vision occurs in the condition shown in which figure?

    A) Figure 8-18
    B) Figure 8-22
    C) Figure 8-19
    D) All of the above

77. Which one of the following serologic tests is correctly matched to the disorder?

   A) Figure 8-19 and FTA-Abs
   B) Figure 8-23 and HLA-B27
   C) Figure 8-21 and angiotensin converting enzyme
   D) Figure 8-22 and HLA-B5

78. Which one of the following therapies is correctly matched to the disorder?

   A) Figure 8-22 and colchicine
   B) Figure 8-19 and laser photocoagulation
   C) Figure 8-21 and triple sulfa and pyrimethamine
   D) Figure 8-22 and amphotericin B

79. The disorder characterized by features in Figures 8-18, 8-20, and 8-23 may also demonstrate which one of the following systemic features?

   A) Hilar adenopathy
   B) Pulmonary artery aneurysm
   C) Kyphoscoliosis
   D) Urethritis

80. Which one of the following are most appropriate in the work-up of the patient in Figure 8-21?

   A) Angiotensin converting enzyme
   B) Dermatologic evaluation
   C) PPD skin test
   D) All of the above

81. Cutaneous abnormalities may occur in all of the following disorders EXCEPT:

   A) Figure 8-18 disorder
   B) Figure 8-19 disorder
   C) Figure 8-21 disorder
   D) Figure 8-22 disorder

82. What is the most common posterior segment opportunistic infection in patients with AIDS?

   A) Pneumocystis choroiditis
   B) Cryptococcal choroiditis
   C) Cytomegalovirus retinitis
   D) Progressive outer retinal necrosis

83. Patients with AIDS and cytomegalovirus retinitis:

   A) have CD4 lymphocyte counts of 100-500 cells/mm^3
   B) have a mean survival of 6 months
   C) have CD4 lymphocyte counts of less than 50 cells/mm^3
   D) have ocular pain and photophobia on presentation

84. Which one of the following is NOT true of ocular toxoplasmosis in patients with AIDS?

    A) Anti-toxoplasma IgM antibodies are elevated more often than in immunocompetent patients.
    B) There are larger areas of retinal necrosis than in immunocompetent patients.
    C) Vitritis is almost always absent because of lymphopenia.
    D) Cerebral toxoplasmosis lesions concurrently present in up to 25% of patients.

85. Which one of the following therapeutic options is appropriate as a first line of therapy for cytomegalovirus retinitis?

    A) Induction with 200 μg intravitreal injections of ganciclovir twice weekly
    B) Induction with 90-120 mg/kg IV foscarnet twice daily
    C) Induction with 5 mg/kg IV ganciclovir twice daily
    D) All of the above

86. IV or intravitreal antiviral induction therapy for cytomegalovirus retinitis is given for:

    A) 2 days
    B) 5 days
    C) 7 days
    D) 14 days

Questions 87–92 Refer to Fig. 8-24 to 8-28. All of these patients have AIDS.

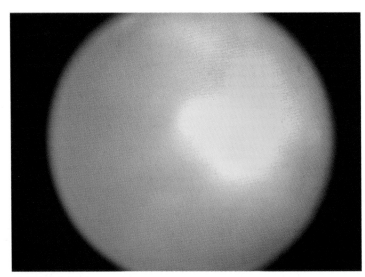

FIGURE 8-24

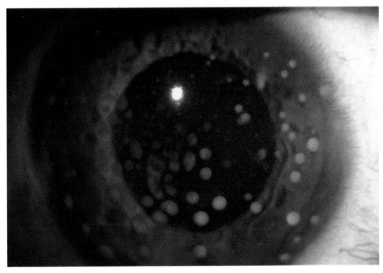

FIGURE 8-25

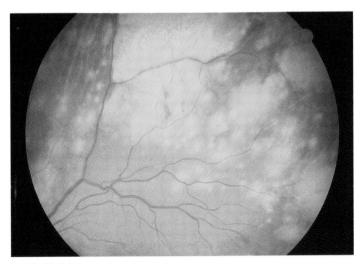

FIGURE 8-26

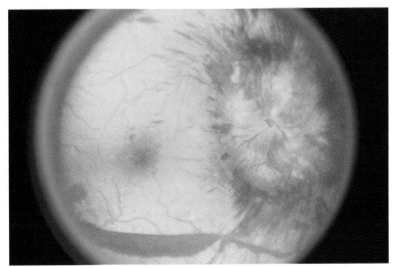

FIGURE 8-27

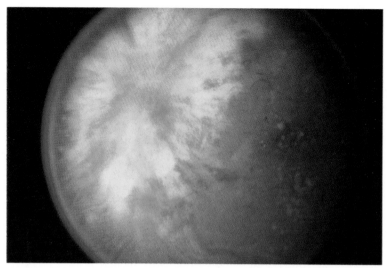

FIGURE 8-28

87. Which disorder(s) can be associated with CD4 counts of less than 50 cells/mm³?

    A) Figure 8-24
    B) Figure 8-26
    C) Figure 8-28
    D) All of the above

88. Elevated intracranial pressure may be found in which one of the following?

    A) Figure 8-24
    B) Figures 8-24 and 8-27
    C) Figure 8-28
    D) Figures 8-27 and 8-28

89. Intravenous ganciclovir is the best therapy for which of the following disorders?

    A) Figure 8-24
    B) Figure 8-26
    C) Figure 8-27
    D) Figure 8-28

90. The anterior segment changes of Figure 8-25 are probably associated with the disorder shown in:

    A) Figure 8-24
    B) Figure 8-26
    C) Figure 8-27
    D) Figure 8-28

91. Cutaneous zoster lesions would most likely be seen in association with the disorder shown in:

    A) Figure 8-24
    B) Figure 8-26
    C) Figure 8-27
    D) Figure 8-28

92.   Retinal detachment may complicate the disorder shown in:

A)   Figure 8-24
B)   Figure 8-26
C)   Figure 8-28
D)   All of the above

Questions 93-94   Figure 8-29 corresponds to a severely immunosuppressed patient with AIDS.

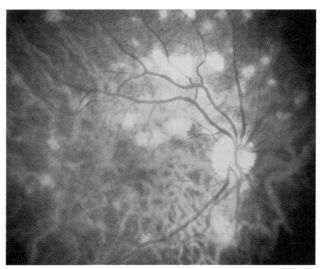

FIGURE 8-29

93.   Which of the following treatments is helpful for this condition?

A)   Pentamidine
B)   Ganciclovir
C)   Albendazole
D)   Amphotericin B

94.   What other organ is commonly involved with this same infection?

A)   nasal mucosa
B)   gastrointestinal tract
C)   lungs
D)   CNS

95.   Choroidal neovascularization occurs in which one of the following disorders?

A)   Sympathetic ophthalmia
B)   Vogt-Koyanagi-Harada syndrome
C)   Serpiginous choroiditis
D)   All of the above

96. The ring-shaped stromal infiltrate seen in herpes simplex keratitis is caused by:

   A)   B cells
   B)   active HSV infection
   C)   antigen–antibody complex precipitation
   D)   giant cell reaction to stromal antigens

97. Which medication has been associated with a sterile hypopyon anterior uveitis in AIDS patients?

   A)   Rifabutin
   B)   Zidovudine (AZT)
   C)   Indinavir (Crixivan)
   D)   Pentamidine

98. What is the predominant cause for damage to ocular structures from infection by *Onchocerca*?

   A)   Infiltration of retinal tissue
   B)   Obstruction of the trabecular meshwork
   C)   Toxins produced by the larvae
   D)   Inflammatory reaction to dead microfilaria

99. Bilateral acute panuveitis with severe visual loss and red, inflamed, painful eyes is best treated with systemic:

   A)   cyclosporine
   B)   corticosteroids
   C)   azathioprine
   D)   chlorambucil

100. What cell type is found in an aqueous specimen in ocular toxocariasis?

   A)   Eosinophils
   B)   T lymphocytes
   C)   Macrophages
   D)   Polymorphonuclear neutrophils

☑ **ANSWERS**

1. A)   Gram-negative coccobacilli

    This patient has filtering bleb–associated endophthalmitis. The most common organisms responsible for this condition include *Streptococcus* species (Gram-positive cocci in pairs or chains) and *Haemophilus influenzae* (Gram-negative coccobacilli). Other organisms, such as *Staphylococcus epidermidis* (Gram-positive cocci in clusters) and Gram-negative species, have been implicated less frequently. Fungal causes are rarely associated with filtering bleb–associated endophthalmitis. The organisms are thought to enter the eye through either intact or leaking conjunctival filtering blebs. Often, Seidel testing is negative. Common presenting symptoms include conjunctival discharge and injection, pain, and decreased vision. The prognosis for eyes with bleb-associated endophthalmitis is generally poor, and the end result is often phthisis.

2. B)   *Propionibacterium acnes*

    This patient's condition is suspicious for chronic postoperative endophthalmitis. Organisms commonly responsible for delayed-onset endophthalmitis after cataract surgery include *Staphylococcus epidermidis*, fungal species such as Candida, and *Propionibacterium acnes*. Endophthalmitis caused by *P. acnes* typically presents from 3 months to 2 years after surgery, whereas *S. epidermidis* generally presents within 6 weeks and Candida within 3 months. The presence of a white plaque within the capsular bag specifically suggests the diagnosis of *P. acnes*. Microscopic examination of plaques removed at the time of vitrectomy has revealed *P. acnes*.

3. D)   Vitrectomy, posterior capsulectomy, and intravitreal injection of vancomycin

    The clinical picture suggests delayed-onset postoperative endophthalmitis caused by *P. acnes*. This condition often responds initially to topical steroids; however, inflammation will recur. Although simple intravitreal injection of vancomycin has resulted in clearing of this infection, recurrences are common. Currently, recommendations for initial therapy include a pars plana vitrectomy with posterior capsulectomy and intravitreal injection of vancomycin. An alternative advocated by some surgeons is a posterior pole vitrectomy, IOL explant, posterior capsulectomy, intravitreal vancomycin, and a sutured IOL.

4. C)   Klebsiella

    In addition to the more common organisms responsible for delayed-onset postoperative endophthalmitis such as *P. acnes, S. epidermidis,* and Candida, other organisms, including *Propionibacterium granulosum,* Achromobacter, and Corynebacterium, have been reported to cause this syndrome. Klebsiella or other Gram-negative bacilli may be seen in endogenous endophthalmitis but would be an unlikely cause of delayed-onset postoperative endophthalmitis.

5. C)   multinucleated giant cells of the Langhans type

The clinical description of a chronic diffuse uveitis with evidence of a choroidal granuloma and hilar adenopathy is highly suggestive of sarcoidosis. A lacrimal gland biopsy is useful in the diagnosis of sarcoidosis, especially if it is enlarged at the time of the biopsy. The gland is involved in approximately 25% of patients. The histologic lesion found in sarcoid biopsies is the noncaseating epithelioid cell tubercle. The tubercle is composed of multinucleated giant cells of the Langhans type surrounded by a rim of lymphocytes. Touton giant cells classically are found in juvenile xanthogranuloma.

6. C)   follicular conjunctivitis

Sarcoid has many protean manifestations affecting almost all of the ocular structures. Inflammation and granulomas may be found as conjunctival nodules, infiltration of the lacrimal gland, anterior uveitis with Koeppe and Busacca nodules, vitreitis, chorioretinal nodules, papillitis, and scleritis. The sequelae of chronic inflammation include keratoconjunctivitis sicca, band keratopathy, synechiae, and glaucoma. Follicular conjunctivitis is commonly found in viral conjunctival infections.

7. B)   retinal neovascularization

Treatment of sarcoid uveitis often requires topical, sub-Tenon's, or systemic corticosteroid therapy. Many ocular and systemic complications may occur as a result of this medication. Ocular complications include cataract formation, steroid-induced glaucoma, scleral thinning, and delayed wound healing. Neovascularization of the retina may occur with sarcoid, but this is a result of inflammation and ischemia, not a consequence of steroid therapy.

8. D)   Multiple sclerosis

This presentation of band keratopathy, a mild anterior chamber reaction, vitreous cells, and a pars plana "snowbank" in a young patient, is highly suggestive of the diagnosis of pars planitis. Multiple sclerosis has been associated with this condition in approximately 5% of cases, and the condition is bilateral approximately 80% of the time. Other associated findings include posterior subcapsular cataracts, anterior chamber synechiae, macular epiretinal membranes, retinal phlebitis, and cystoid macular edema.

9. B)   fibroglial and vascular components

Histologically, the snowbank is composed of fibroglial and vascular elements. It is not an exudate, but a preretinal membrane that forms in response to an inflammatory stimulus. The membrane also contains vascular elements that occasionally bleed and result in a vitreous hemorrhage. The peripheral retinal veins often show a perivascular cuff of lymphocytes, and the vitreous snowballs are composed of epithelioid cells and multinucleated giant cells.

10. A)   Uveitis-glaucoma-hyphema (UGH) syndrome

This patient has a severe anterior uveitis with a hyphema. Any severe uveitis can cause damage to the iris vasculature resulting in anterior chamber bleeding. In particular, VZV iridocyclitis and HLA-B27 (see Fig. 8-4) can result in this picture. A traumatic injury can cause a tear at the iris root in addition to inciting an anterior uveitis. Dispersed blood and fibrin can appear similar to active uveitis. The UGH syndrome is the result of movement of an anterior chamber IOL, which chafes the iris and angle causing inflammation and bleeding. This patient is phakic; therefore, this etiology is not possible.

11. C)   Vogt-Koyanagi-Harada

The following conditions may be associated with diffusely distributed keratic precipitates over the corneal endothelium: Fuchs' heterochromic iridocyclitis, sarcoidosis, syphilis, kerato uveitis, and, rarely, toxoplasmosis. Most inflammatory conditions, including Vogt-Koyanagi-Harada, display keratic precipitates predominantly over the inferior portion of the corneal endothelium. The finding of diffusely distributed keratic precipitates may be a useful diagnostic sign.

12. A)   Behçet's disease

The HLA-B27 genotype is present in approximately 1% to 6% of the general population; however, it may be found in a larger percentage of patients with acute iritis. HLA-B27 is found in almost 90% of patients with ankylosing spondylitis. It also is commonly associated with conditions such as psoriatic arthritis, Crohn's disease, ulcerative colitis, and Reiter's syndrome. Patients with Behçet's disease, however, have an increased incidence of HLA-B5 or subset Bw51.

13. D)   Positive rheumatoid factor

The triad of urethritis, conjunctivitis, and arthritis has described classic Reiter's syndrome. Other associations include keratoderma blennorrhagicum; iritis, keratitis, balanitis, prostatitis, cystitis, spondylitis, fasciitis, tendonitis, oral mucosal lesions, and a recent history of diarrhea. HLA-B27 genotype is present in approximately 75% of cases. Rheumatoid factor is usually not present.

14. D)   Rochalimaea

Reiter's syndrome may occur after dysentery or after nongonococcal urethritis. Ureaplasma urealyticum and *Chlamydia trachomatis* have been associated with the postgenitourinary form. Shigella, Salmonella, and Yersinia have also been shown to be triggers for this condition after episodes of diarrhea or dysentery caused by these agents. Rochalimaea has been implicated as causing cat-scratch fever and neuroretinitis but not this condition.

15. C)   keratoderma blennorrhagicum

Skin involvement may be seen in Reiter's syndrome in approximately 20% of cases. The classic lesion is known as *keratoderma blennorrhagicum* and is pictured in Figure 8-5. When present, this condition is considered a major criterion in making the diagnosis of Reiter's syndrome. The other major criteria include polyarthritis, conjunctivitis, and urethritis. Minor criteria are signs, such as fasciitis, sacroiliitis, spondylitis, keratitis, cystitis, prostatitis, oral mucosal lesions, and diarrhea. Definite diagnosis of Reiter's syndrome is defined by three or more major criteria, or two major criteria and two minor criteria.

16. C)   This patient has pauciarticular disease involving the lower extremities without involvement of the wrist joints.

Juvenile rheumatoid arthritis (JRA) presents in children younger than 16 years of age. Approximately 80% of patients with JRA and iritis are ANA positive and rheumatoid factor negative. The joint involvement in JRA may be polyarticular or pauciarticular (four or fewer joints). When iridocyclitis is present, the joint involvement is most commonly of the pauciarticular type (90% of cases). Systemic JRA with fever and rash is rarely associated with iritis. ANA-positive females with pauciarticular involvement of a lower extremity joint and lack of involvement of the wrists are at highest risk for developing iritis. The anterior chamber inflammation in chronic JRA is characterized by a mild variable degree of anterior chamber cellular reaction with predominance of flare. The conjunctiva is generally quiet.

17. C)   Pathologic specimens of this condition have revealed the presence of plasma cells within the ciliary body.

This patient has Fuchs' heterochromic iridocyclitis. This condition is generally characterized by heterochromia, although up to 15% of cases may have bilateral involvement without obvious heterochromia. Diffuse iris stromal atrophy with variable pigment epithelial layer atrophy accounts for the change in iris color in the involved eye. Because of the pigment loss, brown eyes will appear less brown; blue eyes will appear more blue. This condition is also characterized by small, white, stellate keratic precipitates that are diffusely present over the endothelial surface. Synechiae are almost never present. The inflammatory nature of this disease is supported by the presence of plasma cells and lymphocytes on pathologic examination of ocular tissue.

18. B)   Toxoplasma

This condition is clearly associated with chorioretinal scars consistent with toxoplasmosis; however, whether Toxoplasma is a causative agent is unclear. Not all cases of Fuchs' heterochromic iridocyclitis have chorioretinal scars.

19. C)   latanoprost

The prostaglandin analogues have several proinflammatory side effects, including inciting development of an anterior uveitis and a cystoid macular edema. Unilateral use can also result in changes in iris pigmentation and eyelash growth. The anterior uveitis resolves with topical prednisolone and discontinuation of the causative drug.

20. A)   IgD

IgD has not been detected in any study of human tears. The major immunoglobulin class found in human tears is IgA. IgG and IgM are detectable in only small amounts. IgE is thought to be one of the major mediators of allergic reactions. In contrast, all five immunoglobulins are found routinely in the human conjunctiva within the subepithelial tissue.

21. B)   Phacoanaphylaxis is a Type III hypersensitivity reaction.

There are four general types of hypersensitivity reactions. One of the four types will predominate in any inflammatory response, although several types may be involved at the same time. *Type I* inflammatory responses are antibody mediated. The binding of antibody to mast cells releases histamine, leukotrienes, and other inflammatory mediators. Allergic reactions, such as hay fever, are type I reactions. *Type II* reactions are mediated by cytotoxic antibodies such as those seen with ocular pemphigoid. *Type III* reactions are immune complex mediated. Antibody binds with free floating or fixed antigens and then deposits as a complex, activating the complement cascade. Phacoanaphylaxis fits into this category. Finally, *type IV* reactions are T cell mediated reactions. The granulomatous responses seen in sarcoid or tuberculosis are examples of type IV reactions.

22. A)   HIV antibodies

23. B)   Application of cyanoacrylate glue

This patient has severe rheumatoid arthritis with peripheral ulcerative keratitis. The hands of this patient (Fig. 8-30) show the stereotypic deformities from rheumatoid arthritis. Other conditions to consider include other collagen vascular diseases (Wegener's granulomatosis, polyarteritis nodosa, relapsing polychondritis), Mooren's ulcer, and infections such as tuberculosis and syphilis. Peripheral ulcerative keratitis is not a hallmark of HIV infection or AIDS.

Rheumatoid patients can have spontaneous painless corneal melting. In the acute phase, topical steroids are contraindicated because they can potentiate the corneal collagenases and increase the melting. These patients can be glued temporarily until systemic prednisone and immunosuppressive agents are started. Grafts in an inflamed eye are at high risk for failure or recurrent melting.

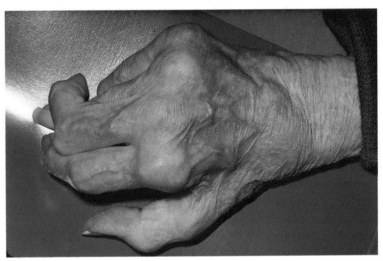

FIGURE 8-30

24. A)   Recurrent, indolent course

Serpiginous choroidopathy (geographic helicoid peripapillary choroidopathy) is a chronic, recurrent, indolent disease of unknown etiology. It usually affects adults with painless loss of vision. Lesions are peripapillary or perimacular and, in the active phase, have inflammation along the edges. Centrifugal spread in a snake-like pattern occurs over months to years. Treatment with steroids or immunosuppressive agents has had variable success.

25. C)   Endophthalmitis would be expected to occur in less than 10% of similar trauma cases.

Posttraumatic endophthalmitis after penetrating trauma typically occurs in fewer than 10% of cases. The most common agents responsible for this infection include *Staphylococcus epidermidis* and *Bacillus* species, although many other organisms have been recovered. The prognosis for visual recovery in this setting is generally poor, especially when *Bacillus cereus* is implicated.

26. A)   The responsible organism grows on blood agar and Sabouraud's glucose within 24 to 48 hours.

This fundus lesion in the setting of a debilitated patient on hyperalimentation and previous antibiotics is highly suggestive of endogenous endophthalmitis often caused by *Candida albicans*. Most cases of Candida endophthalmitis occur without ongoing fungemia or positive blood cultures. All *Candida* species exist in two morphologic forms: a yeastlike form known as *blastoconidia* (pseudohypha) and elongated branching structures (pseudomycelia). *Candida* species typically grow on blood agar and Sabouraud's glucose within 24 to 48 hours. They grow as large creamy-white colonies. A germ tube test from a colony of only 24 hours' duration can result in a presumptive diagnosis of *Candida albicans*. Although this organism is frequently cultured from the respiratory tract, it rarely causes pneumonia.

27. D)   *Haemophilus influenzae*

Endophthalmitis as a complication of IV drug abuse has been widely reported. The most common organisms in these cases are fungal in origin and often occur in the absence of fungemia. Bacterial causes are predominantly a result of *Staphylococcus* species; however, recently *Bacillus cereus* has been reported as an important pathogen. Although *Haemophilus influenzae* can cause infection, it would be unusual in this setting.

28. C)   psoriasis

Patients with Behçet's disease frequently have a variety of associated skin lesions. Lesions resembling erythema nodosum are frequently present over the anterior surface of the lower extremities. These lesions typically resolve over a period of several weeks. Patients may also display typical acne-like lesions, folliculitis, or thrombophlebitis. Cutaneous hypersensitivity is also characteristic of this condition. The behçetine skin test performed by puncturing the skin with an empty hypodermic needle may be useful in making a diagnosis of Behçet's disease. A positive test is indicated by the formation of a pustule at the puncture site within minutes.

29. C)   Colchicine may be helpful in preventing recurrences.

Commonly used agents in the treatment of Behçet's disease include systemic corticosteroids, cytotoxic agents (alkylating agents such as chlorambucil), colchicine, and cyclosporine. Systemic corticosteroids may be initially effective in treating the ocular inflammation in this condition; however, its use has clearly not been found to arrest the long-term progress of this condition. Colchicine is known to inhibit leukocyte migration and has been found to be useful in preventing recurrences. Cyclosporine has also been found to be particularly useful in the treatment of Behçet's disease; however, its use must be carefully monitored because of renal toxicity.

30. C)   The retinitis associated with this condition may be confused with a viral retinitis.

Inflammation in Behçet's disease may affect the anterior and posterior segments and is generally a bilateral process. Recurrent explosive inflammatory episodes are typical with active episodes that range from 2 to 4 weeks. A chronic, lingering inflammatory stage typically does not develop. A nongranulomatous anterior uveitis with formation of a transient hypopyon is common. Posterior inflammation is characterized by recurrent vascular occlusive episodes with retinal hemorrhage and vitreous inflammation. The inflammation is typically confined to the retina and retinal vasculature. Choroidal involvement is rarely seen. The retinitis of Behçet's disease is very suggestive of a viral retinitis and must be considered in the differential.

31. C)   HLA-B27–associated iritis

The most common cause of hypopyon iritis is HLA-B27 associated disease.

32. B)   Young women with pauciarticular juvenile rheumatoid arthritis

Young women with early-onset pauciarticular disease commonly have antinuclear antibodies. The rheumatoid factor is not present in this group. Patients with later-onset pauciarticular disease are predominantly men and have a high incidence of HLA-B27–associated iridocyclitis. The rheumatoid factor–positive polyarticular disease and the rheumatoid factor–negative polyarticular disease are rarely, if ever, associated with uveitis.

33. C)   Anterior uveitis

Two-thirds of patients with sarcoid uveitis have anterior uveitis. Two forms of anterior uveitis exist. One is a chronic, recurrent anterior uveitis that is difficult to treat and control with corticosteroids. The other is an acute granulomatous iridocyclitis that responds well to corticosteroid therapy.

34. A)   live virus can be recovered from epithelial lesions

Varicella zoster epithelial keratitis is depicted. Differences between herpes simplex keratitis are outlined here. An accompanying vesicular eruption is frequently present (Fig. 8-31).

	Acute Varicella Zoster pseudodendrites	**Herpes simplex dendrites**
Active viral replication	Yes	Yes
Appearance	Multiple branching, slightly elevated lesions	Branching, ulcerated lesions with terminal bulbs
Skin rash	Vesicular eruption in V1 dermatome, resolves with scarring	Vesicular eruption affecting lids
Laterality	Unilateral	Usually unilateral, can be bilateral in atopic or immunosuppressed patients

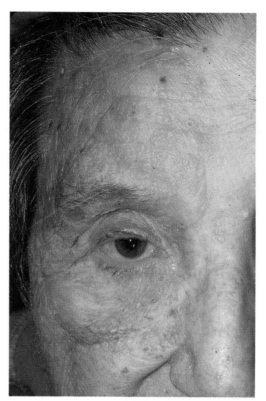

FIGURE 8-31

35. A)   Granulomatous uveitis

36. A)   Granulomatous uveitis

Diffusely distributed keratic precipitates may be seen in herpetic iridocyclitis or in Fuchs' heterochromic iridocyclitis. Herpetic iridocyclitis is typically granulomatous. Fuchs' heterochromic iridocyclitis is chronic and nongranulomatous.

Granulomatous iridocyclitis is often marked by iris nodules and mutton fat keratic precipitates. Histopathologically, the presence of epithelioid cells is pathognomonic for granulomatous inflammation.

38. B)   Figure 8-11

39. A)   Figure 8-10

40. C)   Figure 8-12

Figure 8-10 is a patient with nodular scleritis. Patients present with a deep aching pain. The inflamed vessels are deep in the sclera and do not blanch with topical phenylephrine.

Figure 8-11 shows periocular lymphoma. This pinkish tumor sculpts itself to the scleral surface. These tumors frequently are proliferation of B cells. Excision can be curative. Systemic spread is rare.

Figure 8-12 is conjunctival Kaposi's sarcoma in a patient with AIDS. This tumor has been associated with human herpesvirus 8. No treatment is necessary for ocular lesions unless they are bulky and unsightly. Doxorubicin has been used for systemic treatment. With immune reconstitution, these lesions may regress.

Figure 8-13 is a patient with benign conjunctival chemosis due to sensitivity to airborne allergens.

41.   D)   Hemorrhagic cystitis

Adequate hydration, which may include either oral intake of 2 to 3 liters of fluid or IV intake of 1 to 2 liters of fluid, is important to prevent hemorrhagic cystitis with the use of cyclophosphamide. Oral cyclophosphamide is more likely to produce hemorrhagic cystitis than is IV cyclophosphamide.

42.   B)   Hypoglycemia

Systemic corticosteroid therapy has been associated with numerous complications. Ocular complications include cataracts and glaucoma. Systemic complications include exacerbation of hypertension or diabetes mellitus, osteoporosis, gastric ulceration, hirsutism, weight gain, capillary fragility, and cushingoid appearance.

43.   C)   Immune modulator of interleukin 2

44.   B)   Cytostatic anti-inflammatory

45.   A)   Cytotoxic antimetabolite

Cyclosporine and FK506, a related agent, are potent immune modulators that have very specific activity against the production of interleukin-2 and interleukin-2 receptors and inhibit proliferation of lymphocytes. Prednisone is a cytostatic anti-inflammatory agent that is a nonspecific immunosuppressive.

Cyclophosphamide and chlorambucil are both cytotoxic alkylating agents. They act by creating cross-linkage between DNA strands that result in inhibition of transcription of messenger RNA. Chlorambucil is the slowest acting of all the alkylating agents.

Azathioprine and methotrexate both inhibit purine ring biosynthesis. In addition, methotrexate also inhibits the synthesis of deoxythymidine monophosphate nucleotide.

46.   A)   Cotton wool spots

Cotton wool spots may occur in over 50% of AIDS patients. The cotton wool spots may spontaneously resolve and recur. The most common opportunistic infection of the eye is cytomegalovirus retinitis. Acute retinal necrosis is secondary to herpesvirus retinal infection.

47.   C)   tachyzoite

Toxoplasma organisms tend to be dormant in the cyst form in the intermediate human host. In the encysted form, several dormant organisms may be found. These relatively inactive organisms within the cysts are called *bradyzoites*. Once bradyzoites are released and become free, they are called *tachyzoites*. These metabolically energized protozoans are responsible for stimulation of intraocular inflammation.

48. C)   Clindamycin can effectively kill Toxoplasma organisms.

Pyrimethamine actually inhibits dihydrofolate reductase. Sulfadiazine blocks the production of dihydrofolate from para-aminobenzoic acid. Clindamycin is an antibiotic that can effectively kill Toxoplasma organisms. Systemic and periocular steroids can be used in the treatment of ocular toxoplasmosis in immunocompetent patients.

49. A)   early-onset pauciarticular disease

Pauciarticular early-onset JRA is the entity associated most commonly with chronic, recurrent iridocyclitis. It is seen in young women. The antinuclear antibody is often present in these patients, but rheumatoid factor is uniformly absent. Arthritis of the lower extremities is more common in patients with iridocyclitis.

50. D)   photoreceptor outer segments blocking the trabecular meshwork

Schwartz's syndrome is high IOP associated with a rhegmatogenous retinal detachment. Photoreceptor outer segments migrate transvitreally into the aqueous, block the trabecular outflow pathways, and result in IOP elevation.

51. D)   is often self-limited

Posner-Schlossman syndrome presents with unilateral ocular pain, mild anterior uveitis, and elevated IOP. The episodes that occur are typically self-limited, but they often require the use of topical glaucoma medications to control IOP. Mild topical corticosteroids may be used to control intraocular inflammation. Systemic and periocular corticosteroids are not indicated. Recurrent attacks of this syndrome may lead to eventual optic nerve damage and late-onset glaucoma.

52. B)   Zonal granulomatous inflammation

53. C)   Macrophages filled with lens material

Lens-induced uveitis syndromes may produce granulomatous or nongranulomatous inflammation. Although *phacoanaphylaxis* implies Type I hypersensitivity reactions, the word is a misnomer because it represents a Type III immune hypersensitivity reaction to lens protein that results in a zonal granulomatous inflammation. Macrophages filled with lens materials often clog the trabecular meshwork and result in phacolytic glaucoma. IOLs may produce phacotoxic nongranulomatous inflammation by physically irritating the iris or ciliary body. The UGH syndrome is a type of phacotoxic uveitis.

54. C)   Posterior pole is involved initially with centrifugal spread.

Acute retinal necrosis was first described in healthy, immunocompetent patients. Herpes simplex and zoster viruses have been implicated as causing this condition. Patients present with vitreitis, confluent peripheral necrotizing retinitis, and retinal arteritis with vaso-occlusion. The posterior pole typically is spared until late in the disease. Retinal detachments are common because of the multiple, large areas of retinal necrosis.

55. B) filiform hemorrhage with paracentesis

Fuchs' heterochromic iridocyclitis is typically an insidious, chronic intraocular inflammation that may not respond well to topical corticosteroids. Characteristic findings include diffusely distributed stellate keratitis precipitates and mild anterior segment cell and flare with loss of iris crypts and detail. Blue irides become more blue, and brown irides become less brown in cases of Fuchs' heterochromic iridocyclitis. Gonioscopy will reveal evidence of abnormal bridging vessels in the angle, although neovascular glaucoma with angle closure does not develop. A paracentesis of the anterior chamber may result in a small, splinter-shaped filiform hemorrhage in the angle. Fifty percent of patients with Fuchs' heterochromic iridocyclitis develop cataracts; 60% develop glaucoma. Cataract surgery is not associated with any higher rate of vitreous loss or posterior capsular rupture compared to normal eyes.

56. D) syphilis

Although syphilitic uveitis may mimic any other form of uveitis, intermediate uveitis is a distinctly uncommon presentation. Pars planitis is by far the most common intermediate uveitis entity, a diagnosis of exclusion. Between 5% and 25% of patients with multiple sclerosis may have evidence of periphlebitis and intermediate uveitis.

57. B) choroidal neovascularization

Calcific band keratopathy can develop in young patients with pars planitis. Peripheral retinal neovascularization can result in vitreous hemorrhage and tractional detachments. Progression of tractional detachments can result in rhegmatogenous components, as well. Choroidal neovascularization is not an associated complication of pars planitis. Cystoid macular edema is the most common macular complication of pars planitis and the most common cause of vision loss.

58. C) reveals diminished scotopic responses

Because of the peripheral creamy choroidal infiltrates, retinochoroidopathy, peripheral visual field loss, nyctalopia, and rod dysfunction seen in birdshot retinochoroidopathy, electroretinogram reveals diminished scotopic responses.

59. A) Vogt-Koyanagi-Harada syndrome

Cystoid macular edema is not typically seen in patients with Vogt-Koyanagi-Harada syndrome. Patients with this disorder present with bilateral panuveitis and evidence of disc edema and bilateral multiple serous detachments. In chronic cases, pigmentary changes may be present in the fundus, but cystoid macular edema is not. In addition to the entities listed, any iridocyclitis can cause cystoid macular edema, especially chronic, recurrent cases.

60. D) HLA-A29 and birdshot retinochoroidopathy

The association between HLA-A29 and birdshot retinochoroidopathy is the most consistent of any medical disorder. Approximately 90% of patients with birdshot retinochoroidopathy are HLA-A29–positive (Table 8-1).

TABLE 8-1. Important HLA Associations with Ocular Disease

Disease	Population Studied	HLA Antigen	Percentage of Patients
Birdshot choroidopathy	White	HLA-A29	96%
Ankylosing spondylitis	White	HLA-B27	89%
	Asians	HLA-B27	85%
Behçet's disease	Japanese	HLA-B5	68%
Reiter's syndrome	White	HLA-B27	80%
POHS	White	HLA-B7	77%
	White	HLA-DR2	81%

61. C)   Reduced vision, vitreous cells, and optic disc edema are early findings.

Diffuse unilateral subacute neuroretinitis is thought to be caused by numerous different types of roundworms. *Baylisascaris* species have been implicated most consistently. In early phases of the disorder, reduced vision, vitreous cell, and disc edema are common. As the disorder progresses, eventual optic atrophy, retinal vascular sclerosis, and diffuse pigmentary changes may be seen, resulting in the unilateral wipe-out syndrome. The meticulous evaluation of the fundus for the presence of a small roundworm in the subretinal space, followed by retinal photocoagulation of this worm, can arrest the progression of this disease.

62. C)   Hilar adenopathy is the most common pulmonary finding in sarcoidosis.

Elevated serum angiotensin-converting enzyme levels may be seen in any diffuse granulomatous disease affecting the lung. Blind conjunctival biopsies have a characteristically low yield in patients who have only the presumptive diagnosis of sarcoidosis. If the diagnosis has been made based on elevated angiotensin-converting enzyme levels and a positive chest radiograph, conjunctival biopsies may have yields as high as 60% to 70% for noncaseating granulomas. Pulmonary findings of sarcoid include no changes, hilar adenopathy, and diffuse interstitial lung disease that may progress to severe end-stage pulmonary fibrosis. Ocular involvement occurs in approximately 25% of patients with systemic sarcoidosis. Uveitis may be seen in up to 60% of patients with ocular involvement.

63. C)   serum anti-neutrophil cytoplasmic antibody

64. A)   colchicine

65. B)   Periocular corticosteroids

66. D)   polymyalgia rheumatica

Figure 8-15 shows a patient with severe necrotizing scleritis. Patients will present with severe pain, photophobia, and a red eye. Underlying blue uveal tissue may be seen, giving the redness of the scleritis a violaceous hue. Acute therapy should consist of oral prednisone 1 to 2 mg/kg/day with the eventual addition of cytotoxic immunosuppressives. A thorough investigation for associated systemic vasculitides should be completed. Periocular corticosteroids should be avoided because depo-steroids may enhance collagenase activity in polymorphonuclear leukocytes and result in further scleral melting and necrosis. There is no role for biopsy of the sclera for diagnostic purposes. Although polymyalgia rheumatica is an inflammatory condition, it does not manifest as scleritis.

67. A) lumbar puncture

68. B) intrathecal methotrexate, IV cytarabine (Ara-C), and whole brain and eye irradiation

69. A) There is poor prognosis for survival.

Figure 8-16 shows the characteristic presentation of primary intraocular lymphoma. This leopard skin pattern of yellowish retinal pigment epithelium and subretinal infiltration of lymphomatous cells are typically seen in patients over the age of 70 years. These patients often present initially with vitritis that may be unilateral or bilateral. The initial laboratory evaluation of the vitritis may be noncontributory. However, evaluation of the CNS with MRI, CT scanning with contrast, and lumbar puncture may reveal evidence of CNS lymphoma. Pars plana vitrectomy may be required to establish diagnosis and to stage the neoplasm. Once the diagnosis has been made and staging has been completed, therapy typically consists of combinations of intrathecal methotrexate, IV cytotoxic agents, and whole brain and ocular irradiation. Periocular and systemic steroids may mask the vitritis and reduce the intraocular inflammation, but inflammation would recur on discontinuation of the medications. The prognosis for survival is dismal in patients who have intraocular lymphoma. Primary intraocular lymphoma is a subset of primary CNS lymphoma. Once symptoms of CNS involvement have occurred, median survival drops to approximately 6 months.

70. D) all of the above

71. D) corticosteroids

72. B) multiple pinpoint areas of fluorescein leakage into the subretinal space

73. D) acute neuroretinitis

The patient in Figure 8-17 has Vogt-Koyanagi-Harada syndrome. This diagnosis is one of exclusion, and appropriate laboratory evaluation for this entity should be performed. Vogt-Koyanagi-Harada syndrome is a bilateral granulomatous panuveitis that causes disc edema and bilateral serous retinal detachments with panuveitis in the acute phases of the disease. It is important to rule out infectious entities, including syphilis and possibly tuberculosis. An antinuclear antibody test may also be done to rule out lupus choroidopathy. B-mode echography may be useful in showing the amount of choroidal infiltration, which is quite profound in the posterior pole. This condition is treated with systemic corticosteroids. Fluorescein angiography characteristically reveals multiple pinpoint areas of hyperfluorescence that gradually leak fluorescein into the subretinal space. Retinal vascular staining is uncommon. Differential diagnosis would include posterior scleritis, sympathetic ophthalmia, hypotony, uveal effusion syndrome, and lupus choroidopathy. Acute neuroretinitis would not present with serous retinal detachments.

74.   D)   eczema

Cutaneous manifestations of Vogt-Koyanagi-Harada include alopecia, vitiligo, and *poliosis* (whitening of the lashes). These manifestations confirm the notion that melanin is the immunogenic agent that results in the intraocular inflammation in this condition. Eczema has been associated with atopy.

75.   C)   cardiac conduction defects

76.   C)   Figure 8-19

77.   C)   Figure 8-21 and angiotensin converting enzyme

78.   A)   Figure 8-18 and colchicine

79.   B)   Pulmonary artery aneurysm

80.   D)   All of the above

81.   B)   Figure 8-19 disorder

Figure 8-18 shows branch retinal vein occlusion in a patient with Behçet's disease. Figure 8-20 shows the hypopyon, and Figure 8-2 shows an aphthous ulcer in a patient with Behçet's disease. Figure 8-19 shows a patient with serpiginous retinochoroidopathy. Figure 8-21 shows a patient with retinal periphlebitis, which could be compatible with sarcoidosis, Lyme disease, pars planitis, multiple sclerosis–associated intermediate uveitis, and possibly tuberculosis and Eales' disease. Figure 8-23 shows acute hypopyon/plastic iritis in a patient who is HLA-B27–positive.

Behçet's disease may be associated with painful hypopyon iridocyclitis. However, fibrinous anterior segment inflammation is uncommon. The eye can be remarkably quiet in the presence of a hypopyon in Behçet's disease, unlike in HLA-B27–associated disease, in which pain and photophobia dominate as symptoms. A strong association with HLA-B5 is often present in Behçet's disease. Systemic changes include acne, erythema nodosum, aphthous ulcers, genital ulcers, and interstitial lung changes. A pulmonary artery aneurysm is a pathognomonic chest radiographic finding in a patient with Behçet's disease. Treatment is with systemic and periocular corticosteroids. Colchicine may be useful in reducing recurrences of the disease. Cyclosporine and cytotoxic agents may also be required.

Serpiginous choroidopathy is a condition of unknown etiology with recurrent, progressive episodes of painless visual loss. Inflammation occurs at the edges of previous lesions with centrifugal spread.

Periphlebitis is seen characteristically in sarcoidosis and Eales' disease. Eales' disease is endemic in India and is often associated with pulmonary tuberculosis. The exact etiology of Eales' disease is unknown.

Cutaneous changes are seen in Behçet's disease, sarcoidosis, and Lyme disease. Sarcoid skin changes include erythema nodosum and subcutaneous nodules or granulomata. Lyme disease is associated with erythema chronicum migrans (Fig. 8-32).

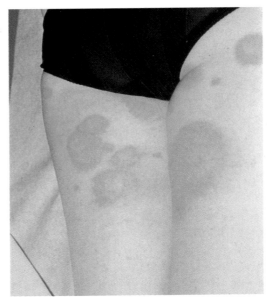

FIGURE 8-32

82. C)   Cytomegalovirus retinitis

83. C)   have CD4 lymphocyte counts of less than 50 cells/mm^3

Patients with cytomegalovirus retinitis and AIDS uniformly have CD4 counts of less than 50. Cytomegalovirus retinitis is by far the most common posterior segment opportunistic infection in patients with AIDS. Toxoplasma retinochoroiditis may be a distant second. Patients with cytomegalovirus retinitis often present with floaters and peripheral visual field loss. Mean survival after the presentation of cytomegalovirus retinitis has improved dramatically with the use of appropriate systemic antiviral therapy and with antiretroviral agents.

84. C)   Vitritis is almost always absent because of lymphopenia.

Ocular toxoplasmosis in AIDS is often associated with significantly more vitreous cells than in cytomegalovirus retinitis. Although some variability exists as to the amount of vitreous inflammation, based on CD4 counts, vitritis is almost always present to some extent.

85. D)   All of the above

86. D)   14 days

Either IV or intravitreal antiviral therapy may be used for the treatment of cytomegalovirus retinitis. Induction is typically carried out for 14 days. Once the retinitis is under control, maintenance therapy is given indefinitely.

87. D)   All of the above

88. B)   Figures 8-24 and 8-27

89. D)   Figure 8-28

90. A)   Figure 8-24

91. B)   Figure 8-26

92. D)   All of the above

Figures 8-24 and 8-25 are from a patient who has AIDS and toxoplasma retinochoroiditis.

Figure 8-26 shows a patient who has progressive outer retinal necrosis and who had cutaneous zoster and AIDS on presentation.

Figure 8-27 shows a patient who has cryptococcal meningitis and bilateral papilledema.

Figure 8-28 shows a patient who has peripapillary cytomegalovirus retinitis.

Toxoplasma retinochoroiditis in patients with AIDS is often marked by intense vitreous inflammation and large areas of retinal necrosis. Treatment consists of triple systemic antitoxoplasma medications. Steroids should be avoided. Up to 25% of patients can have intracranial lesions. Late stages of the disorder may be marked by tractional combined with rhegmatogenous retinal detachments. Mutton fat keratitis precipitates may be dramatic in patients with toxoplasmosis, as is shown in Figure 8-25.

Progressive outer retinal necrosis syndrome is a viral retinitis occurring in patients with AIDS who have a previous history of cutaneous zoster. Herpes zoster virus has been implicated in causing this florid outer retinal necrosis. Treatment consists of IV foscarnet, or foscarnet and ganciclovir. The prognosis is poor. The disease becomes bilateral in nearly all cases. Progression is rapid—within a matter of days. The incidence of retinal detachment is approximately 87%.

Patients with cryptococcal meningitis present with obstructive hydrocephalus, severe headaches, and very high intracranial pressure. This disease may result in florid papilledema as evidenced in Figure 8-27.

93. A)   Pentamidine

94. C)   lungs

Figure 8-29 shows the appearance of *Pneumocystic carinii* infection in an AIDS patient. These patients frequently have CD4 counts of less than 200. Other AIDS-related infections that should be considered include cytomegalovirus, Cryptococcus, fungi, or other protozoa such as Microsporidia.

This protozoan most commonly causes a pneumonitis, but disseminated disease can also result in the yellowish choroidal lesions pictured. Treatment includes trimethoprim/sulfamethoxazole (Bactrim), atovaquone, pentamidine, or dapsone.

95. D)   All of the above

Choroidal neovascularization is common in many posterior uveitides. Choroidal inflammation may enhance production of angiogenic factors, and, when coupled with retinal pigment epithelium–Bruch's membrane disruption, choroidal neovascularization can develop.

96. C)   antigen–antibody complex precipitation

The stromal infiltrate is thought to be similar to the line of precipitation in the Ouchterlony test. Antigens diffuse from one area of the gel and antibodies diffuse from another. The line forms at the meeting point of the diffusing antigen and antibodies.

97. A)   Rifabutin

Recently, rifabutin-associated acute anterior uveitis has been reported in AIDS patients. This can occur weeks to months after starting therapy with rifabutin. Culture of anterior chamber fluid has been negative. Prompt resolution of the uveitis occurs with discontinuation of rifabutin and with topical corticosteroid drops.

98. D)   Inflammatory reaction to dead microfilaria

Onchocerca volvulus infection results in widespread dissemination of the microfilarial larvae. These microfilaria can be seen swimming in the anterior chamber. The live organisms may cause a mild uveitis and obstruct the trabecular meshwork; however, dead organisms incite a vigorous inflammatory reaction, which causes much more ocular damage.

99. B)   corticosteroids

Acute uveitis entities should always be treated with corticosteroids first. Corticosteroids are thus the first line of therapy for all uveitic syndromes. For situations in which topical, periocular, or systemic corticosteroids are ineffective or need to be tapered for steroid-associated side effects, immunosuppressive medications may be useful.

100. A)   Eosinophils

An eosinophilic granuloma occurs with Toxocara intraocular infection. On histopathology, the reaction may be so vigorous that the Toxocara organism may not be visible.

Notes

9

Glaucoma

QUESTIONS

1. Compared with plasma, aqueous humor has an increased concentration of which one of these components?

   A) Protein
   B) Ascorbate
   C) Glucose
   D) Carbon dioxide

2. Which vessel(s) provides the predominant blood supply to the surface nerve fiber layer of the optic nerve head?

   A) Short posterior ciliary artery
   B) Peripapillary choroidal vessels
   C) Pial vessels
   D) Central retinal artery

3. Which one of the following statements is FALSE concerning the condition depicted in Figure 9-1?

   A) It has a worse prognosis than primary open angle glaucoma (POAG).
   B) It may be monocular or binocular.
   C) Lens extraction alleviates the condition.
   D) The IOP is often higher than in POAG.

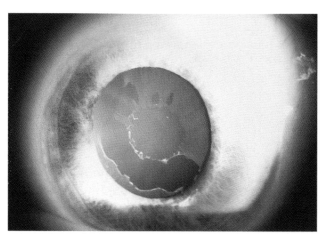

FIGURE 9-1.

4. Which one of the following is NOT a risk factor for POAG?

   A) Topical corticosteroid response
   B) African American heritage
   C) Positive family history
   D) Diabetes mellitus

5. Which drug used during general anesthesia is associated with an increase in intraocular pressure (IOP)?

   A) Halothane
   B) Ketamine
   C) Valium
   D) Phenobarbital

6. Patients with homocystinuria are at increased risk for the following:

   A) lens subluxation
   B) angle closure glaucoma
   C) intravascular thrombosis with general anesthesia
   D) all of the above

7. Indentation tonometry gives falsely low readings under all of the following conditions EXCEPT:

   A) high myopia
   B) decreased central corneal thickness
   C) excessive fluorescein
   D) greater than 3 D of with-the-rule astigmatism

8. The reliability of visual field testing becomes suspect when pupil diameter decreases below:

   A) 4 mm
   B) 3 mm
   C) 2 mm
   D) 1 mm

9. Which test object has four times the area and the same light intensity as the Goldmann II4e target?

   A) III4e
   B) II2e
   C) II4c
   D) V2a

10. A patient is tested on the Humphrey automated perimeter. The machine projects a light at his blind spot and the patient presses the button. What does this patient's response represent?

    A) false-positive response
    B) fixation loss
    C) short-term fluctuation
    D) false-negative response

11. The visual field in Figure 9-2 is caused by a retinal lesion. Which one of the following retinal lesions corresponds to this field? (Note: the fovea is marked by the "X".)

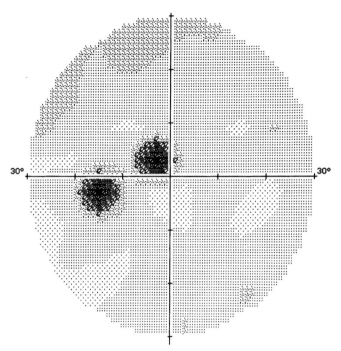

FIGURE 9-2. From Wright K. Textbook of ophthalmology. Baltimore: Williams & Wilkins, 1997.

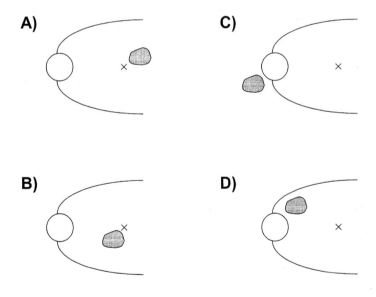

12. Which one of the following signs is most indicative of glaucomatous optic neuropathy?

A)   Figure 9-3A
B)   Figure 9-3B and C
C)   Figure 9-3D
D)   Figure 9-3E

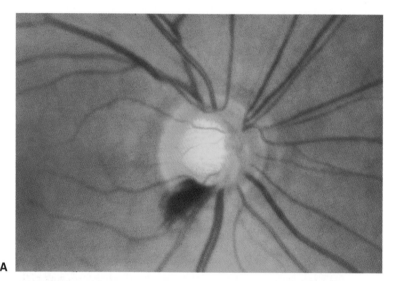

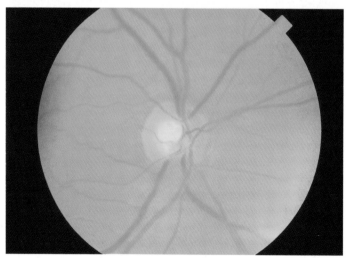

FIGURE 9-3A–B.

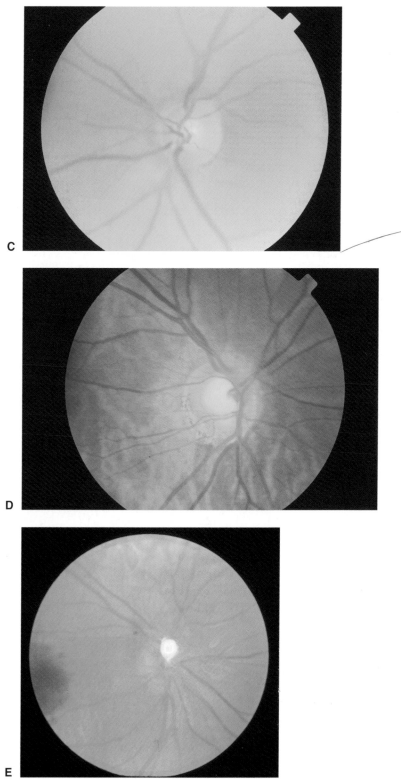

FIGURE 9-3C–E. *(Continued)*

13. Based on histologic studies, what percentage of optic nerve axons may be lost before visual field changes are detected by Goldmann perimetry?

   A) 10%
   B) 15%
   C) 25%
   D) 50%

14. All of the following are well established early signs of glaucomatous damage EXCEPT:

   A) vertical elongation of the cup
   B) peripapillary atrophy
   C) splinter hemorrhage on disc
   D) nerve fiber layer loss

15. All of the following conditions are associated with increased pigmentation of the trabecular meshwork on gonioscopy EXCEPT:

   A) pseudoexfoliation syndrome (PXF)
   B) pigment dispersion syndrome
   C) prior trauma
   D) all of the above

16. Iris transillumination defects are present in all of the following conditions EXCEPT:

   A) oculocutaneous albinism
   B) PXF
   C) plateau iris syndrome
   D) pigment dispersion syndrome

17. All of the following contact lenses for gonioscopy are examples of indirect goniolenses EXCEPT:

   A) Figure 9-4A = Shields, p11b (Koeppe lens)
   B) Figure 9-4B = Shields, p9c (Posner lens)
   C) Figure 9-4C = Shields, p9e (Sussman lens)
   D) Figure 9-4D = Shields, p9b (Goldmann lens)

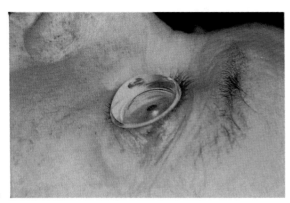

A

FIGURE 9-4A–D. From Shields MB. Color atlas of glaucoma: Williams & Wilkins, 1998.

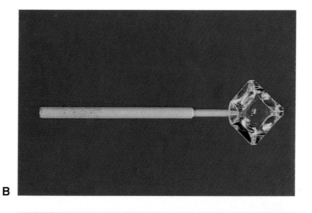

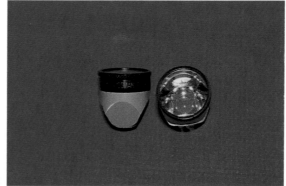

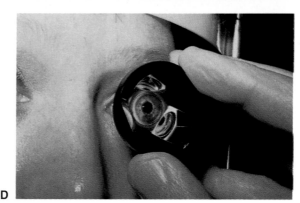

FIGURE 9-4. *(Continued)*

18. The technique LEAST helpful in evaluating the appearance of a glaucomatous optic nerve is:

    A) direct ophthalmoscopy
    B) slit-lamp examination using a contact lens
    C) indirect ophthalmoscopy using a 20-D lens
    D) slit-lamp examination using a 90-D lens

19. Which of the following is LEAST likely to be found in a patient with primary congenital glaucoma?

    A) IOP of 23 mmHg
    B) Cup to disc ratio of 0.4
    C) Corneal diameter of 10.0 mm
    D) Open angle with high iris insertion on gonioscopy

20. With respect to uveitic glaucoma, all of the following are true EXCEPT:

    A) prostaglandins such as latanoprost should be used with caution
    B) argon laser trabeculoplasty (ALT) may be a helpful adjunct if medications are ineffective
    C) miotics are usually avoided
    D) treating the intraocular inflammation is as important as lowering IOP

21. Which one of the following has NOT been suggested to be a possible pathophysiologic mechanism for optic neuropathy in patients suspected of having normal tension glaucoma (low tension glaucoma)?

    A) Nocturnal systemic hypotension
    B) Vasospasm
    C) Shock (hypotensive) optic neuropathy
    D) Systemic hypercholesterolemia

22. Which one of the following conditions does NOT have the same pathogenesis of glaucoma as the others?

    A) Sturge-Weber syndrome
    B) Thyroid eye disease
    C) Aniridia
    D) Carotid-cavernous sinus fistula

23. Which surgical procedure would be initially used to manage primary congenital glaucoma with a markedly cloudy cornea?

    A) Trabeculectomy with mitomycin C
    B) Cyclophotocoagulation
    C) Goniotomy
    D) Trabeculotomy

24. Which one of the following is the MOST common cause of glaucoma in eyes being treated for the condition depicted in Figure 9-5?

    A) Tumor cells invading the angle
    B) Neovascularization
    C) Acute angle closure
    D) Uveitis

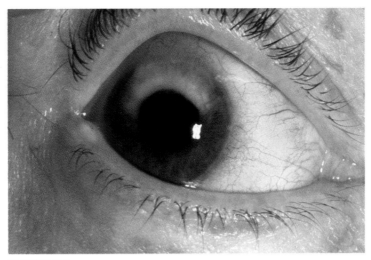

FIGURE 9-5.

25. Which one of the following chemical burns is MOST likely to be associated with an acute elevation of IOP?

    A) Chlorine bleach
    B) Sulfuric acid
    C) Hydrogen peroxide
    D) Sodium hydroxide

26. With respect to corticosteroid glaucoma, all of the following are true EXCEPT:

    A) in most cases, after discontinuing the steroid, the IOP returns to normal over a few days to several weeks
    B) the rise in IOP may be delayed for years after starting the steroid
    C) most cases are caused by long-term oral administration of steroids
    D) patients with POAG are more susceptible to steroid-induced IOP elevations

27. Glaucomatous optic neuropathy is associated with damage to which types of retinal cells?

    A) Amacrine cells
    B) Ganglion cells
    C) Bipolar cells
    D) Photoreceptors

28. What is the best initial therapy for malignant glaucoma?

    A) Pilocarpine 2%
    B) Laser iridotomy
    C) Mydriatic-cycloplegic therapy
    D) Lens removal

29. The condition shown in Figure 9-6 may be associated with which one of the following choices?

  A)   Visual loss
  B)   Papilledema
  C)   Autosomal recessive inheritance
  D)   Bilaterality in 25%

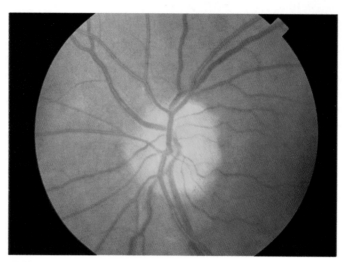

FIGURE 9-6.

30. The MOST important treatment for a patient with diabetic neovascular glaucoma and good vision is:

  A)   atropine and topical steroids
  B)   aqueous suppressants
  C)   adequate blood sugar and blood pressure control
  D)   panretinal photocoagulation

31. Which one of the following types of glaucoma is LEAST likely to respond to medical therapy alone?

  A)   Phacolytic glaucoma
  B)   Pigmentary glaucoma
  C)   Lens particle glaucoma
  D)   Pseudoexfoliation

32. The eye condition LEAST likely to be associated with aqueous misdirection syndrome is:

  A)   angle closure glaucoma
  B)   uveitis
  C)   myopia
  D)   nanophthalmos

33. Topical beta-adrenergic antagonists are known to be associated with all of the following side effects EXCEPT:

    A) increased plasma high-density lipoprotein cholesterol levels
    B) bronchospasm and airway obstruction
    C) weakened myocardial contractility
    D) exercise intolerance

34. A patient who has recently undergone panretinal photocoagulation after a central retinal vein occlusion presents with corneal edema, neovascularization of the iris, and an IOP of 58 mmHg. All of the following medications are appropriate to use EXCEPT:

    A) atropine
    B) dorzolamide
    C) apraclonidine
    D) pilocarpine

35. Ocular side effects of pilocarpine include all of the following EXCEPT:

    A) hyperopia
    B) retinal detachment
    C) exacerbation of pupillary block
    D) lacrimation

36. Which one of the following is NOT considered a possible side effect of the hyperosmotic agents?

    A) Congestive heart failure
    B) Subdural hemorrhage
    C) Worsening of obstructive pulmonary disease
    D) Mental confusion

37. What is the most likely cause of allergic conjunctivitis in a glaucoma patient? List in order of probability.

    1. Latanoprost
    2. Dorzolamide
    3. Brimonidine
    A) $1 > 2 > 3$
    B) $3 > 2 > 1$
    C) $3 > 1 > 2$
    D) $2 > 3 > 1$

38. Which statement about carbonic anhydrase inhibitors is FALSE?

    A) Aqueous production in the eye is not significantly reduced until more than 90% of the carbonic anhydrase activity is inhibited.
    B) Carbonic anhydrase inhibitors cause reduced excretion of urinary citrate or magnesium, therefore predisposing to formation of kidney stones.
    C) Carbonic anhydrase inhibitors may cause idiosyncratic and transient acute myopia.
    D) Metabolic acidosis is greater with oral acetazolamide than with IV injection of acetazolamide.

39. What is the most common cause of bleb failure?

    A) Bleb encapsulation (Tenon's cyst formation)
    B) Episcleral fibrosis
    C) Late bleb leak
    D) Closure of the internal sclerostomy

40. Which one of the following is the MOST important medication to discontinue as far before glaucoma surgery as possible?

    A) Pilocarpine
    B) Echothiophate
    C) Dipivefrin
    D) Timolol

41. Medical management of bleb leaks involves all of the following EXCEPT:

    A) bandage soft contact lens
    B) autologous blood injection
    C) aqueous suppressants
    D) 5-fluorouracil (5-FU)

42. Use of 5-FU following filtration surgery has been associated with all of the following EXCEPT:

    A) conjunctival wound leaks
    B) suprachoroidal hemorrhage
    C) hypotony maculopathy
    D) retinal detachment

43. Apraclonidine (Iopidine), an alpha$_2$-adrenergic agonist, has all of the following side effects EXCEPT:

    A) systemic hypotension
    B) superior lid retraction
    C) dry mouth
    D) blanching of conjunctival vessels

44. Dorzolamide (Trusopt) lowers IOP by:

    A) increasing uveoscleral outflow
    B) decreasing aqueous production
    C) increasing conventional (trabecular meshwork) outflow
    D) decreasing episcleral venous pressure

45. What combination of medications is MOST effective in lowering IOP?

    A) Timolol and a carbonic anhydrase inhibitor
    B) Echothiophate and pilocarpine
    C) Pilocarpine and dipivefrin
    D) Timolol and dipivefrin

46. Prostaglandin analogs lower IOP predominantly by which one of the following mechanisms?

A) Increased uveoscleral outflow
B) Enhanced aqueous outflow by stimulation of ciliary muscle contraction
C) Reduced vitreous volume
D) Reduced aqueous production

47. Which one of the following statements about ALT is TRUE?

A) ALT achieves its effect by creating physical openings in the trabecular meshwork through which aqueous humor can pass from the anterior chamber into Schlemm's canal.
B) The chance of post-treatment IOP rise is not influenced by the number of laser burns applied in each treatment session.
C) The best location for laser burns with respect to minimizing complications of post-treatment IOP rise and peripheral anterior synechiae formation is the posterior trabecular meshwork.
D) Repeating ALT in eyes in which ALT was initially effective and in which IOP control was eventually lost may provide pressure control in one-third to one-half of cases, although 10% to 15% may have a sustained elevation of IOP.

48. Laser trabeculoplasty is most likely to be helpful in an eye with which one of the following types of uncontrolled glaucoma?

A) Pigmentary glaucoma
B) Angle recession glaucoma
C) Iridocorneal endothelial syndrome
D) Inflammatory glaucoma

49. Complications of ALT include all of the following EXCEPT:

A) iritis with posterior synechiae
B) postoperative IOP spike
C) synechial angle closure
D) cataract formation

50. Which are the most appropriate laser settings for ALT?

A) Spot size: 50 μ, duration: 0.1 seconds, energy: 700mW
B) Spot size: 50 μ, duration: 0.5 seconds, energy: 500mW
C) Spot size: 500 μ, duration: 0.1 seconds energy: 200mW
D) Spot size: 500 μ, duration: 0.5 seconds energy: 800mW

51. The advantages of selective laser trabeculoplasty (SLT) over ALT include all of the following EXCEPT:

A) SLT is more effective at lowering IOP
B) SLT uses a potentially repeatable laser
C) SLT selectively targets pigmented TM cells
D) General structure of TM intact post-SLT.

52. In which condition would a laser peripheral iridectomy NOT be indicated?

    A) Iris bombé
    B) Neovascular glaucoma
    C) Acute angle closure glaucoma
    D) Prophylaxis in an eye with narrow angles

53. Compared with the argon laser, the Nd:YAG laser is associated with which one of the following with respect to iridotomies?

    A) Late closure of the iridotomy
    B) Fewer total applications
    C) Less frequent bleeding with application
    D) More extensive histologic damage to the treatment site

54. In contrast to trabeculectomy without mitomycin, the use of mitomycin intraoperatively during trabeculectomy may be associated with:

    A) lower surgical success rate
    B) higher long-term risk of endophthalmitis
    C) higher risk of retinal detachment
    D) more inflammation and a more vascular-appearing bleb

55. Which one of the following procedures has the highest incidence of hypotony?

    A) Full-thickness sclerectomy
    B) Trabeculectomy with mitomycin C
    C) Seton
    D) Trabeculectomy with 5-FU

56. The adjunctive use of antifibrotic agents in trabeculectomy is indicated in all of the following situations EXCEPT:

    A) previously failed filtering surgery
    B) young myopic patients
    C) aphakic/pseudophakic patients
    D) neovascular glaucoma

57. The following are true about the drugs used to modulate wound healing post glaucoma surgery, EXCEPT:

    A) BAPN (beta-aminoproprionitrile), an inhibitor of lysyl oxidase, blocks collagen cross-linking
    B) 5-FU inhibits fibroblast proliferation by acting selectively on the S phase of the cell cycle
    C) mitomycin-C is an alkylating agent that decreases DNA synthesis by causing DNA cross-linking
    D) colchicine acts by inhibiting fibroblast migration and proliferation

58. Which of the following is a theoretical advantage of nonpenetrating glaucoma surgery (nonpenetrating deep sclerectomy/viscocanalostomy)?

    A) Lower incidence of postoperative complications
    B) Technically easier
    C) Better IOP reduction when compared to standard trabeculectomy
    D) None of the above

Questions 59–61

A 34-year-old lawyer is struck in the eye by a golf ball launched by an ophthalmologist. The ophthalmologist rushes the lawyer to his office and examines his eye. A 20% hyphema is present in the anterior chamber. No rupture of the globe is present.

59. The traumatized eye is at risk for developing all of the following types of glaucoma EXCEPT:

A) angle closure glaucoma
B) open angle glaucoma
C) angle recession glaucoma
D) phacolytic glaucoma

60. Because the IOP is elevated in the traumatized eye, proper management of the hyphema could include all of the following EXCEPT:

A) corticosteroids
B) beta blockers
C) aminocaproic acid
D) miotic agents

61. The hyphema clears within a week; however, the eye remains hypotonus for several months while retaining good vision. Suddenly, while on vacation in a remote region of the country, the lawyer experiences extreme pain and blurred vision in the previously traumatized eye. Hours later, he is examined in an emergency room of a local rural hospital; his eye has an IOP of 62 mmHg by Schiotz tonometry. Treatment with timolol drops and acetazolamide tablets is instituted, and the lawyer rushes home to the care of his ophthalmologist. What is the most likely cause for this sudden elevation in IOP?

A) Angle recession glaucoma
B) Ghost cell glaucoma
C) Recurrent hyphema
D) Spontaneous closure of a cyclodialysis cleft

Questions 62–64

A mother brings in her 7-month-old son for evaluation of excessive tearing from both of his eyes. On examination, the patient is noted to be photophobic, have bilateral corneal enlargement, and have corneal clouding.

62. What is the best course of action to take?

A) Send the patient home and instruct the mother on how to perform nasolacrimal sac massage.
B) Perform corneal scrapings and treat as a corneal ulcer.
C) Examine the patient under general anesthesia.
D) Perform B-scan ultrasonography.

63. This patient may experience visual loss for all of the following reasons EXCEPT:

    A)   anisometropic amblyopia
    B)   hyperopic astigmatism
    C)   corneal scarring
    D)   optic nerve damage

64. Initial treatment options for this patient include all of the following EXCEPT:

    A)   goniotomy
    B)   trabeculotomy
    C)   medical therapy
    D)   trabeculectomy

65. Indications for surgical intervention after traumatic hyphema include all of the following EXCEPT:

    A)   corneal blood staining
    B)   prolonged presence of a large clot after 15 days
    C)   rebleeding
    D)   IOP greater than 45 mmHg despite maximum tolerated topical and systemic medications

Questions 66–67

A 65-year-old phakic hyperopic woman undergoes trabeculectomy for uncontrolled POAG. On the first postoperative day, her IOP is 10 mmHg, a diffuse bleb is present, and the anterior chamber is deep. However, on the second postoperative day, the chamber is shallow with peripheral iridocorneal apposition and an IOP of 22 mmHg.

66. Appropriate management includes all of the following EXCEPT:

    A)   Topical cycloplegic medications
    B)   Peripheral laser iridotomy
    C)   Pars plana vitrectomy
    D)   Topical corticosteroids

67. The patient is seen on postoperative day 3 and is noted to have a completely flat anterior chamber, no bleb, and an IOP of 45 mmHg. At this point, appropriate medical management includes each of the following EXCEPT:

    A)   topical cycloplegic medications
    B)   systemic and topical aqueous suppressants
    C)   miotic medications
    D)   topical corticosteroids

68. A 72-year-old phakic African American man undergoes glaucoma filtration surgery for POAG. Adjunctive mitomycin C is used intraoperatively. Postoperatively, the IOP remains at 2 to 3 mmHg, and he develops choroidal effusions. Surgical intervention should be considered for all of the following EXCEPT:

A) impending failure of the bleb
B) continued hypotony beyond 4 weeks
C) kissing choroidals
D) flat anterior chamber with corneal decompensation

69. All of the following may be associated with the abnormality depicted in Figure 9-7 EXCEPT:

A) inflammation
B) pseudoexfoliation
C) neoplasm
D) Fuchs' heterochromic iridocyclitis

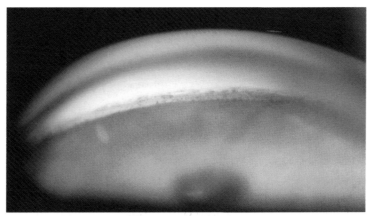

FIGURE 9-7.

Questions 70–71

A 60-year-old man from India presents with a painful red eye. He has had poor vision in this eye for years, but he feels it has worsened over the past 2 weeks. He denies any ocular trauma. On examination, he is noted to have epithelial edema, heavy flare and cell (large cells), and a dense, brunescent cataract. The IOP is 56 mmHg.

70. What is the most likely diagnosis?

A) Phacomorphic glaucoma
B) Phacolytic glaucoma
C) Phacoanaphylactic glaucoma
D) Uveitic glaucoma

71. What is the definitive management of this condition?

    A) Trabeculectomy
    B) Anterior chamber washout
    C) Extracapsular cataract extraction
    D) Posterior pole vitrectomy

72. According to the Laser Glaucoma Trial, all of the following are true EXCEPT:

    A) ALT is at least as effective at reducing IOP as one glaucoma medical agent, timolol.
    B) the majority of patients treated with laser first did not require any additional medical therapy to maintain IOP control
    C) Laser-treated eyes had a slightly lower IOP than medication-treated eyes
    D) ALT is a safe alternate and may be offered as initial therapy to POAG patients

Questions 73–74

A 67-year-old Asian woman calls complaining of 3 hours of acute right eye pain, blurred vision, and redness of her eye. She has a cloudy cornea with epithelial edema, shallow anterior chamber, 4-mm nonreactive pupil, and IOPs of 62 mmHg OD and 17 mmHg OS. Gonioscopy of the left eye reveals a narrow potentially occludable angle with virtually no angle structures visible. She has never had any previous similar episodes.

73. Other findings expected on examination include:

    A) keratic precipitates
    B) glaukomflecken
    C) optic nerve pallor and cupping
    D) optic nerve hyperemia and swelling

74. Which one of the following treatments should be attempted first?

    A) Peripheral iridectomy
    B) Laser trabeculoplasty
    C) Trabeculectomy
    D) Seton implant

75. Primary angle closure glaucoma occurs most commonly in patients with shallow anterior chambers. Among the following, which does NOT contribute to a shallow anterior chamber?

    A) Mature lens
    B) Hyperopia
    C) Ocular hypertension
    D) Iris bombé

76. Secondary angle closure glaucoma may be associated with each of the following conditions EXCEPT:

A) intraocular tumor
B) scleral buckle for retinal detachment
C) nanophthalmos
D) Schwartz's syndrome

Questions 77–78

A 72-year-old African American man had a cataract extraction with posterior chamber IOL in the right eye 7 years ago, and 5 years ago he developed a retinal detachment, which was repaired with a scleral buckle. He developed intractable glaucoma in that eye with an open angle on gonioscopy. Despite having undergone two sessions of laser trabeculoplasty and now being on maximum-tolerated medical therapy with a visual acuity of 20/200, the IOP remains at 28 mmHg. Slit-lamp examination reveals 360° of scarred and non-mobile conjunctiva, and there is almost total cupping of the nerve.

77. Which one of the following procedures would be MOST indicated at this point in this patient's management?

A) Transscleral cyclophotocoagulation
B) Trabeculectomy with antimetabolite
C) Laser trabeculoplasty
D) Laser iridotomy

78. If a drainage implant were placed in this patient's eye, which type of implant would be indicated?

A) Double-plate Molteno implant
B) Krupin implant
C) Anterior chamber tube shunt
D) Ahmed implant

79. A 65-year-old man undergoes extracapsular cataract surgery. Postoperatively, he has a peaked pupil, hypotony, and incarceration of iris into the wound with leakage. Two weeks later, a grayish white membrane with a scalloped, thickened leading edge was noted on the posterior corneal surface. Treatment of involved iris tissue with argon laser turns this membrane white. Appropriate treatment for this condition includes which one of the following?

A) X-irradiation to involved tissues
B) Beta-irradiation to involved tissues
C) Photocoagulation of involved iris tissues with cryotherapy to remaining membranes on corneal tissues
D) Excision of involved iris tissues with cryotherapy to remaining membranes on corneal tissues

80. A diabetic patient has had a complicated retinal detachment repaired with silicone oil instillation. Which one of the following is true concerning the peripheral iridectomy?

    A) It prevents pupillary block that can occur from neovascularization of the iris.
    B) It allows for a much-needed alternate pathway for light entry into the eye.
    C) It prevents pupillary block glaucoma that can occur with silicone oil.
    D) The iridectomy should have been performed superiorly.

81. Which of the following statements is/are true with respect to the Collaborative Initial Glaucoma Treatment Study (CIGTS)?

    A) The study was designed to address the question of medical therapy versus early filtration surgery on the long-term progression of glaucoma.
    B) Patients in the early surgery group were more likely to lose visual acuity and visual field during the first few years of follow-up study.
    C) After 4 years of follow-up, both groups (medical versus early surgery group) were similar in visual acuity and visual field.
    D) All of the above are true.

82. A 75-year-old white man underwent intracapsular cataract extraction 25 years ago. Approximately 15 years ago, he underwent secondary anterior chamber lens placement. Two years ago, this eye underwent penetrating keratoplasty. Over the past year, he has had recurrent uveitis in this eye, and on referral evaluation in your office, his IOP is 25 mmHg. Gonioscopy reveals an open angle and a small hyphema. The MOST appropriate management of his eye would be:

    A) aminocaproic acid
    B) topical corticosteroids
    C) panretinal photocoagulation
    D) surgical removal of his anterior chamber lens

83. A young man is seen in your office over a 5-year period with several episodes of unilateral elevation of IOP to the 40 to 50 mmHg range. During these episodes, fine keratic precipitates and faint flare are noted. A mild ciliary flush is noted. No iris changes are noted. Each episode seems to respond well to topical corticosteroids and topical and systemic aqueous suppression. What is the most likely cause of his episodic glaucoma?

    A) Fuchs' heterochromic iridocyclitis
    B) Juvenile rheumatoid arthritis
    C) Posner-Schlossman syndrome
    D) Sarcoidosis

84. Features associated with the disease shown in Figure 9-8 include all of the following EXCEPT:

    A) 20% to 60% incidence of glaucoma
    B) poor pupillary dilation
    C) weak zonules
    D) peripheral iris transillumination defects

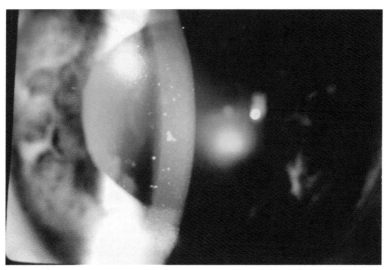

FIGURE 9-8.

85. All of the following are true with respect to prostaglandin analogs EXCEPT:

    A) unoprostone isopropyl (Rescula) reduces IOP by increasing uveoscleral outflow
    B) latanoprost (Xalatan) is a prodrug that becomes biologically active after being hydrolyzed by corneal esterase
    C) bimatoprost (Lumigan) is a prostamide analog
    D) conjunctival hyperemia is a reported side effect of the prostaglandin analogs

86. A 46-year-old woman with a long history of insulin-dependent diabetes mellitus presented with a nonclearing vitreous hemorrhage in her left eye. She underwent a vitrectomy to clear the hemorrhage. One week after surgery, she presented with left eye pain, an IOP of 58 mmHg, and the slit-lamp appearance shown in Figure 9-9. The most likely diagnosis is:

    A) hemolytic glaucoma
    B) phacolytic glaucoma
    C) ghost cell glaucoma
    D) hyphema

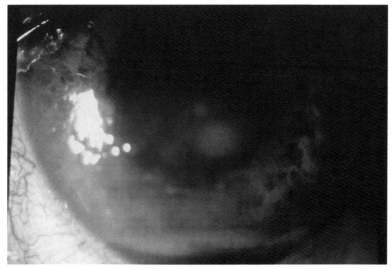

FIGURE 9-9.

Questions 87–88

A 64-year-old pseudophakic woman presented with severe pain in her left eye 6 days after a standard trabeculectomy. Her visual acuity was hand motions, and IOP was 33 mmHg. The anterior chamber of the left eye was shallow.

87. The diagnosis of this patient's condition could include each of the following EXCEPT:

   A) malignant glaucoma
   B) excessive filtration
   C) delayed suprachoroidal hemorrhage
   D) incomplete iridectomy with obstruction of sclerostomy

88. This patient is later found to have large choroidal detachments (Fig. 9-10) with central touch. Which one of the following risk factors has NOT been shown to be associated with this condition?

   A) Preoperative elevated IOP
   B) Aphakia
   C) Hyperopia
   D) Previous vitrectomy

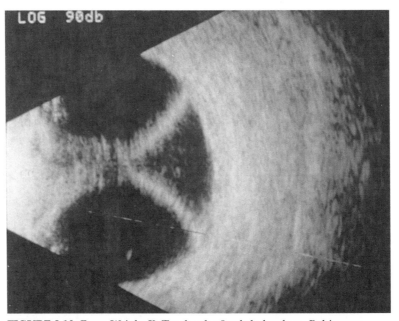

FIGURE 9-10. From Wright K. Textbook of ophthalmology. Baltimore: Williams & Wilkins, 1997.

89. An elderly patient underwent an uncomplicated trabeculectomy of the right eye. The next day, the IOP was 1 mmHg and the patient had the slit-lamp appearance shown in Figure 9-11. The bleb is flat. The retina and choroid appear normal. What is the MOST likely cause of these findings?

A) Malignant glaucoma
B) Choroidal detachments
C) Bleb leak
D) Excessive filtration

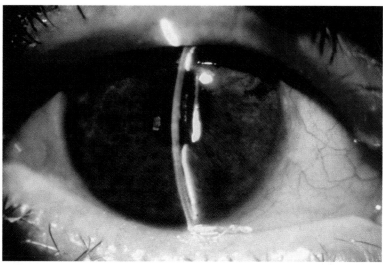

FIGURE 9-11.

90. Ocular tumors can cause glaucoma through a variety of mechanisms. Malignant melanomas of the anterior uveal tract might cause glaucoma through each of the following mechanisms EXCEPT:

A) direct extension of the tumor in the trabecular meshwork
B) obstruction of the trabecular meshwork by macrophages laden with melanin
C) seeding of tumor cells into the outflow channels
D) increase in episcleral venous pressure

91. Reported side effects of the prostaglandin (PG) analog drops include all of the following EXCEPT:

A) Conjunctival hyperemia
B) Cystoid macular edema (CME)
C) Conjunctival melanosis
D) Increased iris pigmentation

92. Two months ago, a 68-year-old man suffered a central retinal vein occlusion in his left eye. He comes in with a red, painful eye and florid rubeosis (Fig. 9-12). What is the most appropriate treatment for this patient?

    A) Panretinal photocoagulation
    B) Seton implantation
    C) Diode cyclophotocoagulation
    D) Laser iridotomy

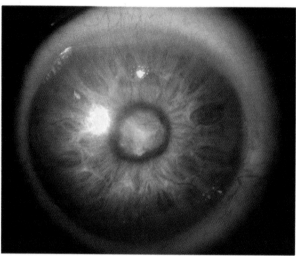

FIGURE 9-12.

93. According to the Ocular Hypertension Treatment Study (OHTS) all of the following are risk factors for glaucoma EXCEPT:

    A) African American race
    B) thick corneas
    C) increasing age
    D) optic nerve anatomy

Questions 94-97 Visual field defects (Figs. 9-13 to 9-19)

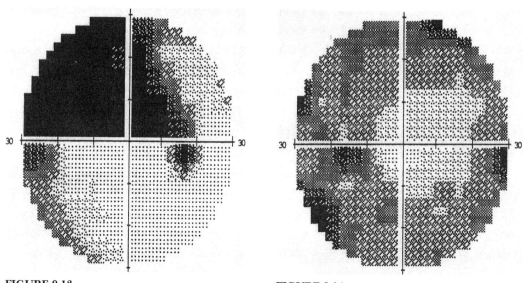

FIGURE 9-13.   FIGURE 9-14.

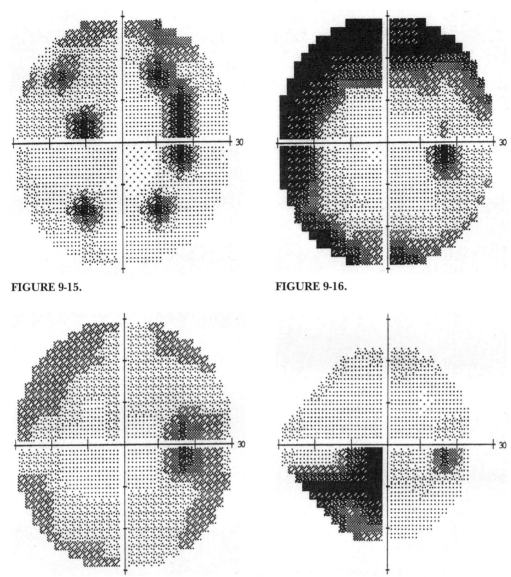

FIGURE 9-15.

FIGURE 9-16.

FIGURE 9-17.

FIGURE 9-18.

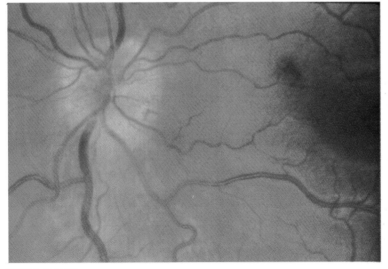

FIGURE 9-19.

94. A patient with which field corresponds to the greatest optic nerve damage?

A) Figure 9-13
B) Figure 9-14
C) Figure 9-16
D) Figure 9-18

95. The visual field in Figure 9-15 was seen in a patient with a healthy-appearing optic nerve and retina. What might account for the findings?

A) A patient pushing the button too frequently
B) Poor head positioning
C) Field test with both eyes open
D) Failure to press the button at the beginning of the test

96. Which field best corresponds to the optic nerve appearance in Figure 9-20?

A) Figure 9-17
B) Figure 9-13
C) Figure 9-14
D) Figure 9-18

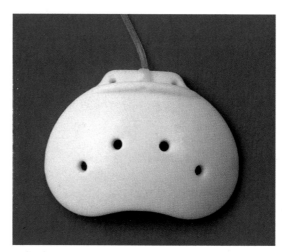

FIGURE 9-20.

97. Figure 9-18 was found upon visual field testing in a 72-year-old man with intact neuroretinal rims on optic nerve evaluation. Which etiology is most likely?

A) POAG
B) Myopia with peripapillary atrophy
C) CNS vascular event
D) Low tension glaucoma

98. Glaucoma implant surgery (aqueous shunt devices) would be indicated in the following circumstances EXCEPT:

A) previously failed filtration surgery with anti-metabolites
B) uveitic glaucoma
C) congenital glaucoma patient with poor visual potential
D) glaucoma patient with previous vitrectomy with scleral buckle

99. All of the following are potential complications of tube shunt procedures EXCEPT:

A) corneal neovascularization
B) conjunctival melt
C) hypotony
D) diplopia

100. The following measures can be taken to limit postoperative hypotony with the device in Figure 9-20 EXCEPT:

A) two-stage procedure
B) collagen plugs
C) pressure-sensitive valve
D) ligature occlusion of tube

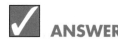 **ANSWERS**

1. B)   Ascorbate

    Compared with plasma, aqueous is slightly hypertonic and acidic. Aqueous has a marked excess of ascorbate (15 times greater than that of arterial plasma) and a marked deficit of protein (0.2% in aqueous as compared to 7% in plasma).

2. D)   Central retinal artery

    The four divisions of the optic nerve head correlate roughly with a four-part blood supply (Fig. 9-21). The surface fiber layer is supplied mainly by branches of the central retinal artery. The prelaminar region is supplied by capillaries of the short posterior ciliary arteries. The lamina cribrosa region is also supplied by vessels that come directly from the short posterior ciliary arteries to form a dense plexus in the lamina. The retrolaminar region is supplied by both the ciliary and retinal circulations, with the former coming from recurrent pial vessels. The central retinal artery provides centripetal branches from the pial region.

    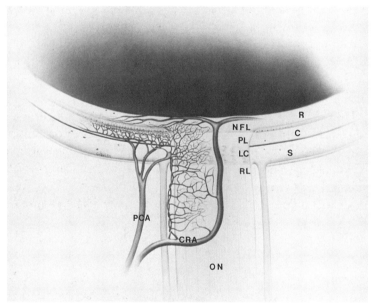

    FIGURE 9-21. LC = lamina cribrosa, S = sclera, C = choroid, R = retina, PCA = posterior ciliary artery, NFL = nerve fiber layer, PL = prelamina, RL = retrolamina, CRA = central retinal artery, ON = optic nerve. From Wright K. Textbook of ophthalmology. Baltimore: Williams & Wilkins, 1997.

3. C)   Lens extraction alleviates the condition.

    PXF is an age-related disease involving an accumulation of abnormal fibrillar extracellular material within ocular and systemic tissues. Glaucoma occurs more commonly in eyes with PXF than in those without it. In fact PXF has been recognized as the most common identifiable cause of glaucoma. The glaucoma is a secondary open angle glaucoma and can be unilateral or bilateral. IOPs can be quite elevated and are often higher than in POAG. Glaucoma associated with PXF tends to respond less well to medical therapy than does POAG, to be more difficult to treat, to require surgical intervention more often, and to have a worse overall prognosis. Unfortunately, lens extraction is not curative, although the pressure may be lowered by a few mm of Hg following simple cataract extraction.

4. A)   Topical corticosteroid response

POAG is a multifactorial disease that may occur on the basis of inherited risk factors. Risk factors for POAG include family history of glaucoma (five to six times greater risk), African American heritage (five to eight times higher incidence than in whites), and age over 50 (the risk of glaucoma increases with each decade of life to nearly a 15% incidence in the population over 80 years of age). It is seen with greater frequency in patients with diabetes mellitus, high myopia, retinal detachment, and central retinal vein occlusion. Patients with POAG and relatives of POAG patients have a higher incidence of elevated IOP in response to topical or systemic corticosteroids, but this is not a risk factor for POAG; rather, it is a risk factor for steroid-induced secondary open angle glaucoma.

5. B)   Ketamine

In most cases, patients have a decrease in IOP with general anesthesia. In particular, halothane and the inhalational anesthetics can decrease IOP. Ketamine and trichloroethylene, however, can cause IOP to increase. Tranquilizers and barbiturates may cause a slight decrease in IOP.

6. D)   all of the above

Homocystinuria is a rare autosomal recessive condition. Affected patients are generally tall with osteoporosis, scoliosis, and chest deformities. About 50% of the time there is associated mental retardation. These patients are at increased risk of thrombotic vascular occlusions, and this should be taken into consideration if general anesthesia is planned. Lens dislocation occurs in 90% of patients and is generally inferior and bilateral. Homocystinuria may lead to angle closure glaucoma if the lens dislocates into the anterior chamber.

7. C)   excessive fluorescein

If the fluorescein rings are too narrow, the IOP is underestimated. If they are too thick, the IOP is overestimated. Use of excessive fluorescein causes thick mires and an overestimation of IOP. The thickness of the cornea affects IOP readings. If the cornea is thin, the IOP is underestimated. In high myopia, there is decreased scleral rigidity, which may lead to an underestimation of IOP. If corneal astigmatism is greater than 3 D, IOP is underestimated for with-the-rule astigmatism and overestimated for against-the-rule astigmatism.

8. B)   3 mm

A pupillary diameter of less than 3 mm can cause general depression of the field. It is best to test the field with a pupil larger than 3 mm. Patients taking pilocarpine may need to refrain from taking the medication for 24 hours before the test or be dilated at the time of their examination.

9. A)   III4e

    On the Goldmann perimeter, the test objects can be varied in both size and intensity by using different filters. The size of the test object is represented by the Roman numeral (I–V). Each increment of the Roman numeral doubles the diameter (and quadruples the area) of the test object. Light intensity can be altered using different neutral density filters. Filters 1–4 are in increments of 5 dB each. Filters a–e are in increments of 1 dB each. The III4e test object will have twice the diameter and four times the area of the II4e test object.

10. B)   fixation loss

    The Humphrey automated perimeter has a number of ways to test the reliability of the test taker. A fixation loss occurs when the patient responds as if seeing a light when a target is displayed in his blind spot. A false-negative response occurs when the patient fails to respond to a suprathreshold stimulus at a location that would be expected to be seen. This response may indicate a patient who is falling asleep or losing interest. Intermittently, the perimeter will pause and the motorized light will change position, but no stimulus will be presented. If the patient presses the button, a false-positive response is recorded. A nervous or trigger-happy patient may have a high false-positive rate. Short-term fluctuation describes the change in sensitivity when the same point is retested.

11. B)

    The center of the visual field corresponds to the fovea. The visual field shows a lesion located superior to the fovea of the left eye between the fovea and the blind spot. Superior defects correspond to lesions inferior to the fovea in the retina.

12. C)   Figure 9-3D

    Figure 9-3D shows narrowing (notching) of the rim. For the early detection of glaucomatous optic nerve damage, the most important variable appears to be focal narrowing or notching of the neuro-retinal rim. Other important variables are optic cup size in relation to optic disc size, disc asymmetry, and presence of disc hemorrhages. However, disc hemorrhages can occur in other conditions (e.g., anterior ischemic optic neuropathy [AION]) and disc asymmetry may be a normal finding if the difference is slight (<0.2 difference).

13. D)   50%

    It is known that pathologic changes of the optic nerve precede visual field changes. In fact, up to 50% of optic nerve axons can be lost before any change is detected on the Goldmann visual field. This observation has stimulated interest in measuring the retinal nerve fiber layer thickness via computer. Different technologies have been developed and are being refined, most notably scanning laser polarimetry (GDx) and optical coherence tomography (OCT). These technologies will likely be useful but will never replace the need for a careful ophthalmoscopic exam and clinical assessment.

14. B)   peripapillary atrophy

    Focal enlargement of the cup appears as localized notching of the rim. The cup can become vertically oval if narrowing of the rim occurs at either the superior or inferior pole of the disc. Splinter hemorrhages usually clear over several weeks but are often followed by localized notching of the rim. Glaucomatous optic atrophy is associated with loss of axons in the nerve fiber layer, which can be best evaluated with red-free illumination. Peripapillary atrophy is not considered to be a sign of early glaucomatous damage. Other conditions such as ocular histoplasmosis or myopia can result in peripapillary atrophy.

15. D) all of the above

In a young normal eye, it is unusual to see any trabecular pigment band. This is because insufficient pigment has filtered through the trabecular meshwork to form a visible pigmented line. If pigmentation is apparent, it is usually most prominent in the inferior angle. The two most common conditions in which the pigment band is very prominent are pigment dispersion syndrome/pigmentary glaucoma and PXF/pseudoexfoliation glaucoma. Lesser amounts of trabecular pigmentation can be seen in iritis, diabetes, or following intraocular surgery, trauma, or laser.

16. C) plateau iris syndrome

In oculocutaneous albinism there is diffuse transillumination of the iris. Patients with exfoliation syndrome have peripupillary transillumination defects. Peripheral discrete or confluent iris transillumination defects may be seen in pigment dispersion syndrome. Plateau iris syndrome does not customarily produce transillumination defects.

17. A) Figure 9-4A = Shields, p11b (Koeppe lens)

In direct gonioscopy, the angle is visualized directly through the contact lens. In indirect gonioscopy, the light rays are reflected by a mirror in the contact lens. The Zeiss four-mirror lens is an example of an indirect gonioprism, where all four mirrors are inclined at 64°. The Sussman lens is a hand-held Zeiss-type gonioprism. The Goldmann mirror is inclined at 62° for gonioscopy. The Koeppe lens is the prototype diagnostic direct goniolens.

18. C) indirect ophthalmoscopy using a 20-D lens

The small image obtained using indirect ophthalmoscopy does not allow for adequate evaluation of the optic nerve details. Careful examination with the direct ophthalmoscope can provide important information about the pallor of the optic cup; however, the most effective methods include stereoscopic examination using the slit lamp in combination with a posterior-pole contact lens, a 90-D lens, or a Hruby lens.

19. C) Corneal diameter of 10.0 mm

Although congenital glaucoma has an incidence of 1 in 12,500 births, it accounts for about 5% of students in schools for the visually handicapped. It is bilateral in two-thirds of patients; two-thirds of these patients are male; and about 10% of congenital glaucoma is familial (autosomal recessive). Symptoms include tearing, photophobia, and blepharospasm. Signs include:

1. IOP over 21 mmHg
2. optic nerve cup:disk ratio greater than 0:3 (present in only 2.6% of normal newborns)

3. horizontal corneal diameter greater than 12.5 mm with or without corneal edema or breaks in Descemet's membrane (Fig. 9-22)
4. open angle with anterior iris insertion (either flat insertion into the trabecular meshwork or, less commonly, concave insertion with the plane of the iris posterior to scleral spur and anterior iris stroma sweeping upward and inserting into the meshwork)
5. no iris abnormality other than that previously described (i.e., no hypoplasia or corectopia)

Important diagnoses to exclude include neural crest dysgenesis (aniridia, Peter's anomaly, Axenfeld-Rieger), phakomatoses, metabolic abnormalities (Lowe's, homocystinuria, mucopolysaccharidoses), inflammatory conditions (congenital rubella, herpes simplex iridocyclitis), neoplasms (retinoblastoma, juvenile xanthogranuloma), congenital diseases (X-linked megalocornea, Down syndrome, Patau's syndrome, Zellweger syndrome, Rubinstein-Taybi syndrome, persistent hyperplastic primary vitreous [PHPV], retinopathy of prematurity), trauma, and steroid use.

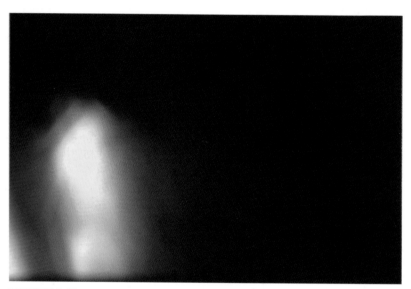

FIGURE 9-22

20. B) argon laser trabeculoplasty (ALT) may be a helpful adjunct if medications are ineffective

Ocular inflammation can lead to glaucoma via a variety of mechanisms including 1) obstruction of the trabecular meshwork by inflammatory debris, 2) increased viscosity of aqueous humor, 3) neovascularization, 4) uveal effusion, 5) pupillary block, and 6) formation of peripheral anterior synechiae. Treatment depends on the underlying condition, but in most cases, inflammation is suppressed by some combination of topical, periocular, or oral corticosteroids. Occasionally, other immunosuppressive agents are needed. Elevated IOP is managed by topical and oral glaucoma medications as needed. Miotics are generally avoided because they lead to increased pain and congestion and promote the formation of posterior synechiae. Prostaglandin agents are used with caution because they may exacerbate uveitis. ALT is not very helpful in eyes with active inflammation.

21. **D)** Systemic hypercholesterolemia

Normal tension glaucoma is not one disease but rather a collection of disease processes characterized by characteristic glaucomatous visual field loss without elevated IOPs. Nocturnal systemic hypotension caused by excessively large late evening or bedtime doses of antihypertensive agents has recently been suggested to cause low tension glaucoma on the basis of compromised optic nerve blood supply. Vasospasm and shock may also compromise optic nerve blood supply. Systemic hypercholesterolemia has not been implicated in the pathophysiology of low tension glaucoma.

22. **C)** Aniridia

The common pathogenesis of glaucoma in the Sturge-Weber syndrome, thyroid eye disease, and carotid-cavernous sinus fistula is an increase in episcleral venous pressure through elevated venous outflow pressure or orbital congestion. The glaucoma associated with aniridia is caused by congenital agenesis of the angle structures.

23. **D)** Trabeculotomy

Management of congenital glaucoma involves surgery, either goniotomy (70% success) or trabeculotomy (70% to 80% success). A goniotomy requires that the cornea be clear enough to view the meshwork. In the scenario presented, a trabeculotomy ab externo is the procedure of choice because of the cloudy cornea. In general, for primary congenital glaucoma, if repeated attempts at goniotomy and/ or trabeculotomy fail, filtering surgery with mitomycin C or seton placement is considered. Topical medication, such as beta-blockers, miotics, or carbonic anhydrase inhibitors can temporize and potentially clear the cornea enough to allow goniotomy to be performed. Cyclophotocoagulation and other cyclodestructive procedures usually are reserved for eyes that have undergone other unsuccessful surgeries.

24. **B)** Neovascularization

Malignant melanomas can be associated with normal, elevated, or depressed IOP. Elevated IOP occurs more frequently with melanomas of the iris/ciliary body than with choroidal melanomas. Glaucoma may occur by a variety of mechanisms, including 1) obstruction of the trabecular meshwork by melanin-containing macrophages (melanomalytic glaucoma), 2) direct extension of tumor into the trabecular meshwork, 3) angle closure from anterior displacement of the lens-iris diaphragm or peripheral anterior synechiae, 4) inflammation, and 5) neovascularization of the angle. Neovascularization of the angle appears to be the most common cause of elevated IOP, especially among eyes treated with radiation.

25. **D)** Sodium hydroxide

Glaucoma is most often associated with alkali burns but can also be seen after severe alkali burns. IOP rises initially because of scleral shrinkage and release of prostaglandins. Later, IOP rises because of inflammation, posterior synechiae causing pupillary block, or acute lens swelling. Finally, IOP may continue to be high due to direct injury to the trabecular meshwork. Filtering surgery may be needed but can be difficult due to conjunctival scarring. A cyclodestructive procedure or seton valve may be required.

26. C)   most cases are caused by long-term oral administration of steroids

Most cases of corticosteroid glaucoma are caused by drops or ointments instilled in the eye. Steroid creams, lotions, and ointments applied to the face or eyelids may reach the eye in sufficient quantity to raise IOP, as may systemically administered corticosteroids. There have been case reports of increased IOP following the use of steroid inhalers for asthma or steroid nasal spray for allergic rhinitis. The IOP elevation may occur within a week of initiating treatment or may be delayed for years. The first step in managing steroid glaucoma is to discontinue the drug. In most cases, the IOP will return to normal within a few days to several weeks. The residual glaucoma can be treated with glaucoma medicines, laser, or surgery. Corticosteroids are thought to raise IOP by lowering outflow facility perhaps due to an accumulation of glycosaminoglycans in the trabecular meshwork.

27. B)   Ganglion cells

The optic nerve carries axons from ganglion cells into the inner retina. The nerve fiber layer is comprised of these ganglion cell axons.

28. C)   Mydriatic-cycloplegic therapy

Malignant glaucoma, or aqueous misdirection, occurs when aqueous is secreted into and sequestered in the vitreous cavity, pushing the lens, hyaloid face, and iris forward, thus collapsing the anterior chamber and blocking the trabecular meshwork. The IOP often rises to 20 to 60 mm Hg, and the anterior chamber is shallow both centrally and peripherally. The common clinical features include 1) shallow or flat anterior chamber, 2) increased or normal IOP, 3) poor response to miotics, 4) favorable response to cycloplegics-mydriatics. Mydriatic-cycloplegics help by pulling the lens-iris diaphragm posteriorly.

29. A)   Visual loss

Optic nerve drusen occurs in 2% of optic nerve specimens on histopathology and is bilateral in 50%. Pathologic studies have revealed intra-axonal calcification of mitochondria. The nerve head may be elevated, but no axonal swelling or edema exists. Optic nerve drusen may be inherited in an autosomal dominant fashion and occur more frequently in whites. Visual loss can occur and is thought to result from axonal compression, subretinal hemorrhage, or choroidal neovascular membrane formation. Systemic conditions associated with optic nerve drusen include Paget's disease, Ehlers-Danlos, sickle cell, and pseudoxanthoma elasticum.

30. D)   panretinal photocoagulation

Initial treatment of a patient with an acute episode of neovascular glaucoma includes a topical beta-blocker, an alpha agonist, and/or carbonic anhydrase inhibitor as well as atropine and topical steroids. Carbonic anhydrase inhibitors may be less effective in the presence of marked corneal edema. Miotics, prostaglandins, and epinephrine should be avoided. In most cases, it is important to proceed rapidly with panretinal photocoagulation to prevent total angle closure. Following panretinal photocoagulation, new vessels may regress within a few days to a few weeks. If IOP remains elevated despite panretinal photocoagulation and medicines, filtering surgery, seton valve placement, or cyclodestruction may be needed.

31. A) Phacolytic glaucoma

Phacolytic glaucoma results when mature or hypermature cataracts leak soluble lens protein through microscopic defects in the lens capsule. This heavy-molecular weight protein directly obstructs the outflow of aqueous. Macrophages engorged with this material may also obstruct the outflow channels. Although it is desirable to first bring the IOP under medical control with hyperosmotics, carbonic anhydrase inhibitors, and topical beta-blockers, definitive therapy requires removal of the lens. Lens particle glaucoma may occur after trauma to the lens capsule or after cataract surgery with retained cortical material. The lens material may resorb spontaneously. Medical management is used to control IOP; however, surgical removal of the lens material may be necessary if medical management fails.

32. C) myopia

Patients at particular risk for aqueous misdirection are those with crowded anterior segments (i.e., angle closure, nanophthalmos). Postoperative inflammation may cause swelling of the ciliary body and ciliary processes leading to aqueous misdirection. Myopia is not associated with an increased risk of aqueous misdirection.

33. A) increased plasma high-density lipoprotein cholesterol levels

Blockade of beta$_1$-adrenergic receptors slows the pulse rate and weakens myocardial contractility, which can affect the time of exhaustion with heavy exercise. Blockade of beta$_2$-adrenergic receptors produces contraction of bronchial smooth muscle. Topical timolol has been shown to decrease plasma high-density lipoprotein cholesterol levels. Carteolol is a topical nonselective beta-adrenergic antagonist that has intrinsic sympathomimetic activity and has been shown to have less adverse effect on plasma lipids. Betaxolol is relatively beta$_1$-selective and may have less of an effect on the respiratory muscles.

34. D) pilocarpine

Aqueous suppressants have the best chance of controlling the IOP. Because the trabecular outflow has been occluded by neovascularization, miotic medications will be ineffective and may, in fact, reduce the uveoscleral outflow, further elevating the IOP. Miotics are also less effective in eyes with severely increased IOP.

35. A) hyperopia

Ocular side effects of pilocarpine include conjunctival vascular congestion, miosis, induced myopia, cataract formation, and temporal or periorbital headaches. Rarely, pilocarpine can be associated with retinal detachment. Pilocarpine does not cause hyperopia.

36. C) Worsening of obstructive pulmonary disease

Hyperosmotic agents may aggravate congestive heart failure by an increase in extracellular volume. Backache; headache; mental confusion; and subdural, even subarachnoid, hemorrhages have also been reported.

37. B) $3 > 2 > 1$

Prostaglandin analogs such as latanoprost (Xalatan) more commonly produce conjunctival hyperemia than true allergic conjunctivitis. From 1% to 5% of patients taking dorzolamide (Trusopt) may have allergic symptoms. Up to 20% of patients taking brimonidine (Alphagan) may show such symptoms.

38. D) Metabolic acidosis is greater with oral acetazolamide than with IV injection of acetazolamide.

Metabolic acidosis is greater with IV injection of acetazolamide. Acute myopia is the only ocular reaction commonly associated with carbonic anhydrase inhibitors.

39. B) Episcleral fibrosis

The most frequent cause of failure after filtration surgery is bleb scarring due to episcleral fibrosis. This excessive healing response is largely due to the proliferation of fibroblasts and the production of collagen and glycosaminoglycans. The antimetabolite 5-FU has been used to modulate wound healing after filtration surgery. 5-FU inhibits fibroblast proliferation to prevent episcleral fibrosis. Mitomycin C, an antitumor antibiotic isolated from *Streptomyces caespitosus,* also suppresses cellular proliferation. Both antimetabolites have been used to modify wound healing in glaucoma surgery.

40. B) Echothiophate

Echothiophate is a strong, relatively irreversible cholinesterase inhibitor. This drug causes a disruption of the blood–aqueous barrier, which may cause increased inflammation after intraocular surgery in eyes pretreated with echothiophate. Indirect agents also block other cholinesterases, including plasma pseudocholinesterase, which deactivates succinylcholine. Patients may be paralyzed for extended periods of time after anesthesia with succinylcholine and need to be warned about this. For these reasons, it is usually advisable to discontinue the drug several weeks before surgery. Many surgeons also like to discontinue dipivefrin several days before surgery to lessen conjunctival and episcleral injection.

41. D) 5-fluorouracil (5-FU)

Bandage soft contact lenses, autologous blood injections, and aqueous suppressants have all been used in the management of bleb leaks. Bleb leaks are more common in eyes with thin cystic blebs and after treatment with antimetabolites.

42. D) retinal detachment

In addition to inhibiting fibroblast proliferation, 5-FU also inhibits the growth of epithelial cells of the conjunctiva and cornea. It is associated with several undesirable complications including conjunctival wound leaks, corneal epithelial defects, thin-walled ischemic blebs, hypotony, and suprachoroidal hemorrhage. It has not been associated with increased risk of retinal detachment.

43. A) systemic hypotension

Apraclonidine hydrochloride is a para-amino derivative of clonidine hydrochloride, an alpha$_2$-adrenergic agonist that is used clinically as a potent systemic antihypertensive agent. Several studies have shown the lack of effect of apraclonidine on blood pressure and pulse. However, a transient dry mouth or dry nose is commonly reported. Ocular side effects include eyelid retraction, mydriasis, and conjunctival blanching.

44. B) decreasing aqueous production

Dorzolamide is a topical carbonic anhydrase inhibitor that works in an analogous fashion to systemic carbonic anhydrase inhibitors (acetazolamide, methazolamide) by inhibiting carbonic anhydrase on the ciliary epithelium and decreasing aqueous production. Dorzolamide's main side effects are burning or blurring on instillation and a bitter or metallic taste in the mouth. It appears to produce far fewer systemic side effects than do the oral agents.

45. A) Timolol and a carbonic anhydrase inhibitor

The combined effect of timolol and a miotic or timolol and a carbonic anhydrase inhibitor is significantly greater than the effect of any of the medications alone. The combination of timolol and an epinephrine compound, however, has less additional IOP-lowering effect. Because epinephrine stimulates and beta-blockers inhibit beta-adrenergic receptors, one drug may interfere with the action of the other. When an epinephrine compound and a miotic are given in combination therapy, the reduction in IOP is usually not to the same degree as timolol and a carbonic anhydrase inhibitor in combination. When other miotics are administered in combination with pilocarpine, they not only fail to increase the IOP-lowering effect but also may interfere with the action of pilocarpine.

46. A) Increased uveoscleral outflow

The prostaglandin analogs, of which latanoprost is a member, appear to lower IOP by increasing uveoscleral outflow. Aqueous outflow follows both conventional and nonconventional pathways. The conventional pathway, which accounts for 85% to 90% of aqueous outflow, consists of the trabecular meshwork, Schlemm's canal, and episcleral/conjunctival veins. The nonconventional pathway's principal route is via the uveal tract and sclera. This accounts for about 10% to 15% of total outflow. Whereas conventional outflow is dependent on the baseline level of IOP, the nonconventional pathway is not.

47. D) Repeating ALT in eyes in which ALT was initially effective and in which IOP control was eventually lost may provide pressure control in one-third to one-half of cases, although 10% to 15% may have a sustained elevation of IOP.

The technique of creating laser holes through the trabecular meshwork is known *as laser trabeculopuncture* (trabeculotomy). This technique is the earliest attempt to treat glaucoma using laser technology, but it has not been successful in people or in animal models. The risk of posttreatment IOP rise increases with increasing numbers of laser burns. For this reason, some clinicians treat 180° of the angle with 50 laser burns in each session. Laser burns should be placed in the anterior trabecular meshwork.

48. A) Pigmentary glaucoma

Laser trabeculoplasty effectively lowers IOP in patients with POAG, pigmentary glaucoma, or pseudoexfoliation. It is ineffective and may actually worsen the IOP in eyes with inflammatory glaucoma, recessed angles, or membranes in the angle, and in young patients with developmental defects.

49. D) cataract formation

ALT has been associated with the complications of iritis, postoperative IOP spike, and anterior synechiae formation but not with cataract formation.

50. A) Spot size: 50 μm, duration: 0.1 seconds, energy: 700mW

A large spot size and long duration provide more of a coagulative effect than might be employed for shrinking iris tissue for an iridoplasty. The smaller spot size and shorter duration provide greater energy for a given area of tissue treated. This is more appropriate for the ALTP applied to a very small, thin structure with disruptive rather coagulative effect.

51. A) SLT is more effective at lowering IOP

SLT works by irradiating and targeting only the melanin-containing cells in the trabecular meshwork, without causing thermal damage to adjacent nonpigmented trabecular meshwork cells and underlying trabecular beams. When treated with SLT, a primarily biologic response is induced in the trabecular meshwork. This response involves the release of cytokines, which trigger macrophage recruitment and other changes leading to IOP reduction. The laser beam bypasses surrounding tissue, leaving it undamaged by light. This is why, unlike ALT, SLT is repeatable several times. ALT patients can receive two treatments in a lifetime, whereas SLT patients can receive two treatments a year. Even though SLT is a promising new technology, further studies need to be done to prove that SLT is in fact better than ALT at decreasing IOP pressure; at best, SLT is currently equivalent to ALT at reducing IOP.

52. B) Neovascular glaucoma

In acute angle closure, the iris occludes the trabecular meshwork. This may be relieved, in some cases, by a peripheral iridectomy. Prophylactic iridectomies in eyes with narrow angles may prevent a subsequent attack of angle closure. In iris bombé, synechiae between the iris and the lens block the normal flow of aqueous through the pupil into the anterior chamber. Because of this obstruction, fluid accumulates in the posterior chamber, causing the iris to bow forward and obstruct the angle. A laser peripheral iridectomy creates an alternate pathway for aqueous humor to flow from the posterior to the anterior chamber. Neovascular glaucoma is caused by the growth of new vessels into the angle. This growth requires panretinal photocoagulation to cause regression of the vessels, not a peripheral iridectomy.

53. B) Fewer total applications

The continuous-wave argon laser was the unit most commonly used for creating iridotomies in the early days of laser surgery; however, the pulsed Nd:YAG laser is probably the more commonly used today. Iridotomies created with an argon laser have more extensive early edema and tissue destruction at the margins of treatment histologically as compared with those created with the Nd:YAG laser. Argon laser has the disadvantage of more iritis, pupillary distortion, and late closure of the iridotomy. Clinically, the Nd:YAG laser has the disadvantage of frequent bleeding.

In general, Nd:YAG laser iridotomies require fewer total applications with a marked reduction in total energy as compared with argon laser iridotomies. In some cases, it may be advantageous to use both lasers: the argon for its coagulative effects and the Nd:YAG for its disruptive properties.

54.   B)   higher long-term risk of endophthalmitis

Mitomycin C is a potent antineoplastic agent that intercalates with DNA and prevents its replication. It is toxic to fibroblasts and vascular endothelial cells and hence gives rise to diffuse, thin, avascular blebs. Recent reports suggest that these thin blebs may carry a higher risk of endophthalmitis than is associated with filtering surgery without the use of mitomycin C. Studies comparing mitomycin with intraoperative or postoperative 5-FU suggest roughly equal outcomes with regard to successful filtration surgery; however, well-controlled, long-term trials still need to be done.

55.   A)   Full-thickness sclerectomy

The incidence of hypotony is highest with full-thickness procedures such as a posterior lip sclerectomy. Because of this, these procedures are performed less commonly today. Partial thickness procedures, including trabeculectomies with antimetabolites, have lower rates of hypotony. Setons are intermediate in incidence depending on the type of implant and whether a ligature or other device is used to occlude the drainage tube.

56.   B)   young myopic patients

Although originally advocated for use in high risk eyes such as those with aphakia/pseudophakia, neovascular glaucoma, or a history of previously failed surgeries, antifibrotic agents are now routinely used by many surgeons. Antifibrotic agents should be used with caution in young myopic patients due to the risk of hypotony.

57.   D)   colchicine acts by inhibiting fibroblast proliferation and migration

Colchicine affects collagen cross-linking and thereby decreases scar formation.

58.   A)   Lower incidence of postoperative complications

Nonpenetrating glaucoma surgery includes deep sclerectomy with collagen implant and deep sclerectomy with injection of viscoelastic into Schlemm's canal (viscocanalostomy). The surgery involves creating a superficial scleral flap and a deeper scleral dissection underneath to leave behind a thin layer of sclera and Descemet's membrane. Preliminary data comparing nonpenetrating procedures to standard trabeculectomy shows better IOP reduction after standard trabeculectomy but a lower incidence of postoperative complications such as hypotony after nonpenetrating procedures. However, the nonpenetrating surgeries are technically more difficult.

59.   D)   phacolytic glaucoma

Blunt trauma may produce angle recession glaucoma, a form of secondary open-angle glaucoma. The contusion and hyphema can eventually cause the formation of peripheral anterior synechiae, with the development of a chronic angle-closure glaucoma. Phacolytic glaucoma develops from the obstruction of the trabecular meshwork by macrophages laden with lens material leaking from a mature lens.

60. D)   miotic agents

Miotic agents should be avoided in the treatment of hyphema because they can cause breakdown of the blood–aqueous barrier, increase inflammation, and worsen the discomfort of ciliary spasm associated with the traumatic injury.

61. D)   Spontaneous closure of a cyclodialysis cleft

Cyclodialysis clefts occur after traumatic injuries. Chronic hypotony usually results. These clefts close spontaneously weeks to months later, usually resulting in a sudden increase in the IOP. Usually, the trabecular outflow system will begin functioning more normally a short period of time after the pressure spike has occurred.

62. C)   Examine the patient under general anesthesia.

This is classic for bilateral infantile glaucoma. If possible, the diagnosis may be made in the office through IOP measurement, cycloplegic refraction (induced myopia), and optic nerve examination. In most cases, however, the patient needs to be taken to the operating room to confirm the diagnosis and to initiate surgical correction while under the same anesthesia.

63. A)   anisometropic amblyopia

Most cases of primary congenital glaucoma are bilateral. The signs include:

an enlarged eye (buphthalmos)
megalocornea
corneal edema
Haab's striae
corneal scarring and decompensation
immature angle and TM
elevated IOP
cupped optic nerve
myopia and astigmatism (secondary to enlargement of the globe and K
   irregularity)

64. D)   trabeculectomy

Congenital glaucoma is a surgical disease. The basic abnormality is a localized dysgenesis of the superficial angle structures, and both trabeculotomy and goniotomy may alleviate this problem. IOP-lowering medications are useful in the management of pediatric glaucoma: they may clear corneal edema, which in turn facilitates surgery; the lower IOP may lessen optic nerve damage until surgery can be performed; and the IOP-lowering medications may be used in the postoperative course if additional lowering of IOP is required. Trabeculectomy may be an option, but given that these young patients tend to heal exuberantly, its success may be limited. Judicious use of antimetabolites, however, may improve the success of trabeculectomy in the pediatric population.

65. C) rebleeding

Rebleeding is not an indication to operate unless elevated pressure and corneal blood staining are threatened.

66. C) Pars plana vitrectomy

There are multiple causes for shallowing of the anterior chamber after glaucoma filtration surgery. In this case, the IOP is not grossly elevated and the anterior chamber is not completely flat. Therefore, aqueous misdirection syndrome is unlikely. Pars plana vitrectomy has a role in the management of aqueous misdirection syndrome, but it is not the initial choice of therapy. Pupillary block is a likely cause and may respond to cycloplegia or to laser iridotomy.

67. C) miotic medications

The most likely diagnosis in this clinical setting is aqueous misdirection (ciliary block glaucoma, malignant glaucoma). Patients at greatest risk include those with shallow anterior chambers: older patients, women, and hyperopes. Maximum cycloplegia and aqueous suppression may help to break the cycle of aqueous being misdirected into the vitreous cavity. Reformation of the anterior chamber with viscoelastic material may also help rotate the ciliary body posteriorly to break the misdirection. Half of eyes with aqueous misdirection may be successfully managed medically. Pseudophakic eyes can, on occasion, be treated successfully with Nd:YAG laser to disrupt the posterior capsule and/or anterior hyaloid face. The rest will require surgical intervention (pars plana vitrectomy with or without lensectomy). A wound leak would present with a shallow chamber and flat bleb; however, the IOP would be low.

68. B) continued hypotony beyond 4 weeks

Hypotony and choroidal effusions can occur after glaucoma filtration surgery, especially if antimetabolites are used. The therapeutic window of mitomycin C is especially small, meaning that the optimal therapeutic dose is not far from the toxic dose. Overfiltration can occur if excessive doses of mitomycin C are used intraoperatively. Drainage of choroidal effusions should be considered with apparent failure of the bleb. Drainage of choroidal effusions should also be considered with worsening cataract or corneal decompensation.

69. D) Fuchs' heterochromic iridocyclitis

An intensely pigmented meshwork may be caused by pseudoexfoliation, pigment dispersion syndrome, inflammation (uveitis), malignant melanoma, trauma, surgery, and hyphema. The meshwork may also be more pigmented in individuals with darkly pigmented irides and may become more pigmented with age. Patients with Fuchs' heterochromic iridocyclitis typically have abnormal vessels present in the angle without peripheral anterior syndrome (PAS), but they do not have a hyperpigmented meshwork.

70. B) Phacolytic glaucoma

71. C)   Extracapsular cataract extraction

Phacolytic glaucoma occurs when lens proteins leak through an intact lens capsule, inducing a heavy macrophage response. The trabecular meshwork is obstructed with high molecular weight lens proteins and bloated macrophages. It usually occurs in older patients with a mature, hypermature, or even Morgagnian cataract. The lens needs to be removed to cure this problem. Phacomorphic glaucoma occurs in patients with large crystalline lenses, causing pupillary block and secondary angle closure. Phacoanaphylactic glaucoma occurs after a traumatic injury ruptures the lens capsule, allowing a granulomatous inflammation and secondary glaucoma.

72. B)   the majority of patients treated with laser first did not require any additional medical therapy to maintain IOP control

The Glaucoma Laser Trial study has demonstrated that ALT is a reasonable alternative to medication (timolol) in the initial treatment of POAG. However, 2 years into the study, 56% of laser-treated eyes needed supplemental medical therapy to control IOP. Laser-treated eyes had a lower mean IOP.

73. D)   optic nerve hyperemia and swelling

In acute angle closure glaucoma, hydropic degeneration and impaired axoplasmic flow cause swelling and hyperemia of the optic nerve. Glaukomflecken and optic nerve pallor and cupping would indicate previous episodes of angle closure glaucoma, which the patient denies. Cell and flare may be seen with prolonged attacks, but keratic precipitates are rarely seen.

74. A)   Peripheral iridectomy

Large lenses in hyperopic eyes can cause pupillary block and subsequent angle closure glaucoma. In these situations, a peripheral iridectomy may relieve the pupillary block and relieve the angle closure attack. If the cornea does not clear sufficiently for a laser peripheral iridectomy, a surgical iridectomy may be necessary. Trabeculoplasty has no role in angle closure episodes. Trabeculectomy and seton implants may be needed in the future, but they are not the initial therapy of an angle closure attack.

75. C)   Ocular hypertension

Elevated IOP does not necessarily result in shallowing of the anterior chamber. The other conditions may result in shallowing of the anterior chamber or narrowing of the angle.

76. D)   Schwartz's syndrome

Schwartz's syndrome is the name given to open angle glaucoma after rhegmatogenous retinal detachment. The elevated IOP results from obstruction of outflow by inflammation, pigment released from the retinal pigment epithelium (RPE), glycosaminoglycans released by the photoreceptors, or photoreceptor outer segments. It usually resolves after repair of the retinal detachment (RD). Scleral buckles may interfere with venous drainage of the uveal tract, leading to swelling and anterior rotation of the ciliary body with resultant angle closure. In nanophthalmos, uveal effusions resulting from obstruction of venous blood flow through abnormally thick sclera cause rotation of the ciliary body anteriorly with resultant angle closure. Intraocular tumors may push the angle closed from posteriorly with the development of chronic angle closure.

77. A) Transscleral cyclophotocoagulation

Transscleral cyclophotocoagulation is useful in many types of refractory glaucoma, such as glaucoma in aphakia or pseudophakia, neovascular glaucoma, glaucoma associated with inflammation, and glaucoma in eyes with multiple failed filtering procedures. Observations in animal and human eyes suggest that the most likely mechanism of IOP-lowering is reduced aqueous production through destruction of ciliary epithelium. Performing a trabeculectomy in an eye with 360° of scarred or nonmobile conjunctiva would be very difficult and is likely to fail. Although repeating trabeculoplasty is helpful in some eyes that have had a good response to initial treatment, most studies have shown a much lower success rate with repeat trabeculoplasty, and it is unlikely that the pressure-lowering response would be adequate for this patient. This patient has an open angle configuration, so an iridotomy would have no further IOP-lowering effect.

78. C) Anterior chamber tube shunt

In eyes with coexistent vitreoretinal disease and glaucoma that have previously undergone scleral buckling surgery, placement of an implant device is difficult because of the lack of adequate scleral surface area for securing the seton. In those cases, a silicone tube may be used to shunt fluid from the anterior or posterior chamber to the fibrous capsule surrounding the episcleral encircling element. This procedure allows for drainage of aqueous to a preformed reservoir of large surface area.

79. D) Excision of involved iris tissues with cryotherapy to remaining membranes on corneal tissues

Epithelial downgrowth has been reported most commonly as a complication of cataract surgery, but it can occur after penetrating keratoplasty, glaucoma surgery, penetrating trauma, and partial removal of epithelial cysts of the anterior segment. It is more likely when surgery is associated with hemorrhage, inflammation, vitreous loss, or incarcerated tissue. It usually results in intractable secondary angle closure glaucoma unless successfully treated. The treatment is difficult and usually unrewarding. All the techniques attempt to close the fistula and destroy the epithelium inside the eye. The extent of iris involvement can be outlined using the argon laser. Irradiation and photocoagulation have been abandoned as ineffective. Excision of involved iris tissue with cryotherapy to remaining corneal membranes is currently the best technique, although good vision is maintained in only a few cases. Prevention is much more effective than the treatment of established disease.

80. C) It prevents pupillary block glaucoma that can occur with silicone oil.

A large inferior peripheral iridectomy (Fig. 9-23) is mandatory when silicone oil is placed into an eye. The oil is lighter than water, and to prevent pupillary block glaucoma, an inferior peripheral iridectomy is performed.

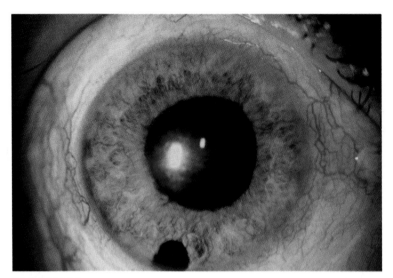

FIGURE 9-23.

81. D) All of the above are true.

A standard medical treatment for newly diagnosed glaucoma is to use drops and/or laser treatment to lower the pressure inside the eye. Recent studies have questioned this approach, suggesting that the risk of vision loss from glaucoma could be reduced by instead having immediate filtration surgery. The CIGTS was designed to address this question by comparing the effects of medical treatment to early filtration surgery in newly diagnosed open angle glaucoma.

The CIGTS found that increased IOP was significantly decreased in both the medically and surgically treated groups, with the surgery group having a larger decrease. However, in the surgery group, the need for subsequent cataract surgery was significantly higher, and patients were more likely to lose visual acuity and visual field during the first few years of follow-up study. After 4 years, patients in both groups were similar in visual acuity and visual field. Few patients developed serious vision loss from glaucoma after either treatment.

The CIGTS investigators concluded that the study results provided no reason to change current treatment approaches to glaucoma. The CIGTS researchers also compared the impact of these two treatments on the patients' health-related quality of life. Their findings provided no reason to change current treatment approaches to glaucoma.

82. D) surgical removal of his anterior chamber lens

Uveitis-glaucoma-hyphema syndrome is rarely seen today, but it was a common complication of older, rigid, haptic anterior chamber lenses that suffered from poor design, poor finishing characteristics, or excessive mobility, allowing them to chafe the iris surface. Pseudophakic bullous keratopathy was also more common with these types of lenses. Modern flexible haptic anterior lenses are better tolerated and less apt to cause these complications. Therefore, because this patient's anterior chamber lens is causing problems, it should be replaced or, at least, removed. If it were well-tolerated, surgical replacement would not be necessary.

83.   C)   Posner-Schlossman syndrome

The clinical picture described resembles Posner-Schlossman syndrome. Fuchs' heterochromic iridocyclitis can present with a similar picture but with iris hypochromia and gray-white nodules on the anterior iris.

84.   D)   peripheral iris transillumination defects

PXF syndrome is bilateral in 50% of patients and manifests itself in older-age patients. It is recognized by the presence of dandruff-like particles on the pupillary border, anterior lens capsule, zonules, and other areas in the anterior segment. (Figure 9-8 shows PXF particles on the posterior corneal surface as well as PXF on the anterior lens capsule). The material is distributed widely, including the conjunctiva, orbital tissues, skin, and viscera, supporting the concept that PXF is a systemic disease. Associated eye findings include a Krukenberg spindle, decreased corneal endothelial cell density, a heavily pigmented trabecular meshwork, narrow angle, poor pupillary dilation (iris muscle degeneration and/ or lack of iris stroma elasticity due to accumulation of PXF), nuclear sclerotic cataract, zonular weakness leading to forward subluxation or dislocation of the lens, and peripupillary (not peripheral) transillumination defects. An accumulation of pigment may also be seen along Schwalbe's line (Sampaolesi's line). From 20% to 60% of patients can have an associated open angle glaucoma.

85.   A)   unoprostone isopropyl (Rescula) reduces IOP by increasing uveoscleral outflow

The prostaglandin analogs are a relatively new class of anti-glaucoma agents. Unlike latanoprost and travoprost, which lower IOP by increasing uveoscleral outflow, bimatoprost decreases IOP by increasing uveoscleral and trabecular outflow. Unoprostone appears to lower IOP by increasing trabecular outflow only. Latanoprost and travoprost are pro-drugs that penetrate the K and become biologically active after being hydrolyzed by corneal esterase. Neither bimatoprost nor unoprostone appears to be a pro-drug. An ocular side effect unique to this class of drugs is the darkening of the iris and periocular skin. Other side effects include hypertrichosis of the eyelashes, conjunctival hyperemia, exacerbation of herpes keratitis, CME, and uveitis.

86.   C)   ghost cell glaucoma

The candy stripe is a tip-off to ghost cell glaucoma. Two conditions are necessary for the development of this unique form of glaucoma: vitreous hemorrhage (red blood cells degenerate and become rigid in the vitreous) and a break in the anterior hyaloid face (to allow the cells to enter the anterior chamber). The crenated khaki-colored ghost cells layer out in the anterior chamber and can be distinguished from fresher red cells, creating the effect of a candy stripe. Ghost cells cannot escape easily from the meshwork and hence produce intertrabecular obstruction and raise the IOP.

In hemolytic glaucoma, hemoglobin-laden macrophages block the meshwork, whereas in phacolytic glaucoma, macrophages are engorged with lens protein. Hyphema can also produce elevated IOP, especially in the setting of sickle cell hemoglobinopathies, which include sickle cell trait.

87.   B)   excessive filtration

A pressure rise during the early postoperative period associated with a flat or shallow anterior chamber can be seen with malignant (ciliary block) glaucoma, an incomplete iridectomy with obstruction of the sclerostomy, or a delayed suprachoroidal hemorrhage. Excessive filtration is usually manifested by hypotony and a flat anterior chamber. Other causes of postoperative hypotony with a flat anterior chamber include choroidal detachments and a conjunctival defect.

88.   C)   Hyperopia

Delayed suprachoroidal hemorrhages after filtering surgery typically present during the first few postoperative days with severe pain, occasional nausea, and a marked reduction in vision. The IOP is usually elevated, the anterior chamber is shallow or flat, and large choroidal detachments are present. Risk factors associated with this condition include aphakia, pseudophakia, myopia, previous vitrectomy, and preoperative IOP greater than 30 mmHg.

89.   C)   Bleb leak

A low, often unrecordable IOP is common during the early postoperative period and is typically associated with a shallow anterior chamber. If there is an obvious hole in the conjunctiva, one would see brisk Seidel positivity and a flat bleb. Spontaneous closure of the defect often is possible with a pressure patch; however, if this technique is not effective, a Simmons' scleral compression shell may help close the leak. Other treatment options for bleb leak include defect suturing, trichloroacetic acid, soft contact lens, and autologous blood injection.

Fluid commonly collects in the suprachoroidal space in hypotonous eyes, leading to serous choroidal detachments. The fluid in the detachments is high in protein (67% of plasma concentration). Most serous choroidal detachments resolve spontaneously along with the normal rise in IOP during the first few postoperative days or weeks. In other cases, there may be no apparent conjunctival defect, but filtration may simply be excessive as a result of a large fistula or filtering bleb. Malignant glaucoma is associated with an elevated IOP and a flat anterior chamber.

90.   D)   increase in episcleral venous pressure

Episcleral venous pressure may be elevated by conditions that obstruct the superior vena cava, thyroid eye disease, or arteriovenous fistulas. It is not caused by intraocular tumors. In addition to direct extension or seeding of outflow pathways, melanomas may elevate IOP by pigment dispersion, inflammation, hemorrhage, angle closure, or neovascularization of the angle. Melanomalytic glaucoma results from blockage of the trabecular meshwork by macrophages that have engulfed material released from the tumor.

91.   C)   Conjunctival melanosis

The PG analogs represent a new class of glaucoma drugs aimed at decreasing IOP by increasing uveoscleral outflow of aqueous humour. The most frequent side effects include increased iris hyperpigmentation, iris cyst formation, eyelash hypertrichosis, conjunctival hyperemia, and CME. Systemic side effects are rare.

92. A)   Panretinal photocoagulation

The patient pictured has developed neovascular glaucoma after a central retinal vein occlusion. The definitive treatment is to destroy areas of ischemic retina in the eye by panretinal photocoagulation or cryotherapy. Seton implantation would be fraught with complications in this hot, inflamed eye. Diode cyclophotocoagulation is not the first line of therapy for this condition.

93. B)   thick corneas

The primary goal of the Ocular Hypertension Treatment study was to determine whether reducing elevated IOP delayed or prevented the onset of glaucoma and subsequent vision loss in people at risk of developing the disease. The study showed that reducing IOP with eye drops was effective at delaying (and possibly preventing) the onset of POAG. The investigators also reported several factors predictive of those who would develop POAG, mainly age, race, IOP, optic nerve anatomy, and central corneal thickness. By considering these factors, the clinician may identify those at risk for developing glaucoma and who are more likely to benefit from early medical treatment. Thin corneas are a risk factor for the development of glaucoma. IOP obtained by applanation tonometry is underestimated in patients with thin corneas, that is, the true IOP is actually greater than that measured.

Figure 9-13 demonstrates a superior arcuate/altitudinal defect. Figure 9-14 shows generalized depression as might be seen with the development of a cataract. Figure 9-15 is a field with scattered, isolated defects, which may be due to retinal lesions or patient artifact. Figure 9-16 shows peripheral construction. The patient in Figure 9-17 has an enlarged blind spot. Figure 9-18 has a inferior quadrantanopia respecting the horizontal and vertical midlines.

94. A)   Figure 9-13

This patient has almost complete loss of his superior visual field. Loss of central fixation is also indicative of more advanced glaucomatous damage. These patients would benefit from reducing their IOP as low as possible.

95. D)   Failure to press the button at the beginning of the test

A number of artifacts can result depending on patient understanding of and compliance with the testing procedure. Isolated depressed quadrantic defects result if the patient misses the early portion of the test in which the machine attempts to determine the threshold for each quadrant. A trigger-happy patient would have a field with high false-positive errors and a high mean deviation. If both eyes are open for a field, no blind spot will be plotted.

96. A)   Figure 9-17

In acute papilledema, visual acuity is usually normal unless macular edema is present. Color vision and pupillary responses are also normal. The visual field generally shows only an enlargement of the blind spot. The earliest loss of visual field in chronic papilledema is typically in the inferior nasal quadrant.

97. C)   CNS vascular event

Retinal and optic nerve lesions produce field defects that do not generally respect the vertical midline. In most patients, the presence or absence of glaucomatous field defects can usually be predicted from the appearance of the optic nerve head. The presence of a field defect that respects the vertical midline should always arouse suspicion of a neurologic lesion (e.g., cerebrovascular accident, tumor), especially when the disc and field changes do not correspond. Some studies have shown that patients with low tension glaucoma have scotomas with steeper slopes, greater depth, and closer proximity to fixation than POAG patients with higher IOP.

98. C)   congenital glaucoma patient with poor visual potential

Aqueous shunt devices are reserved for those glaucoma cases in which standard filtration surgery would fail or has already failed. Therefore, glaucoma implant surgery is indicated in the following situations:

> failed trabeculectomy
> active uveitis
> neovascular glaucoma
> inadequate conjunctiva
> impending need for PK

A tube shunt can be placed in the presence of a scleral buckle. In post vitrectomy cases, the tube can be placed through the pars plana. It may not be wise to perform incisional surgery in an eye with poor visual potential given the risks and, at times, complicated postoperative course of tube shunt surgery.

99. A)   corneal neovascularization

The following are complications of glaucoma implant procedure: hypotony, shallow chamber, migration/expulsion of tube, conjunctival melts, corneal edema, diplopia, and elevated IOP.

100. C)   pressure-sensitive valve

The Baerveldt implant, as shown in Figure 9-20, does not have a pressure-sensitive valve, so hypotony in the early postoperative period has to be managed by other means. Hypotony is common when drainage implants are installed in a one-stage procedure without complete tube occlusion. The absence of any resistance to aqueous outflow invariably results in reduction of IOP to below physiologic levels. A two-stage procedure has been recommended to limit early hypotony. During the first operation, the scleral plate is sutured to the globe without connecting the tube into the anterior chamber. This procedure is followed by a second operation 2 to 8 weeks later, during which the tube is inserted into the anterior chamber. An alternative to limit overfiltration after one-stage installation involves the temporary occlusion of the tube lumen with a ligature, or with semipermeable, biodegradable collagen lacrimal plugs.

Notes

Notes

10

Cornea

QUESTIONS

1. All of the following are included in the differential diagnosis of this condition shown in Figure 10-1 EXCEPT:

   A) herpes simplex virus (HSV)
   B) molluscum contagiosum
   C) allergic drug reactions
   D) Stevens-Johnson syndrome

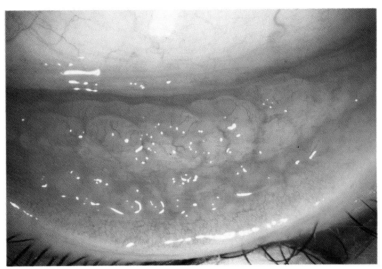

FIGURE 10-1

2. Which disease is NOT caused by *Chlamydia trachomatis*?

   A) Ligneous conjunctivitis
   B) Adult inclusion conjunctivitis
   C) Lymphogranuloma venereum
   D) Trachoma

3. All of the following may cause a false-positive Venereal Disease Research Laboratories (VDRL) and rapid plasma reagin (RPR) test for syphilis EXCEPT:

   A) rheumatoid arthritis
   B) anticardiolipin antibody
   C) systemic lupus erythematosus
   D) Wegener's granulomatosis

4. Based on the appearance of the corneal infiltrate in Figure 10-2, which laboratory test would be LEAST helpful in aiding in the diagnosis?

   A) Culture on Sabouraud agar
   B) Calcofluor white stain
   C) Lowenstein-Jensen agar
   D) Giemsa stain

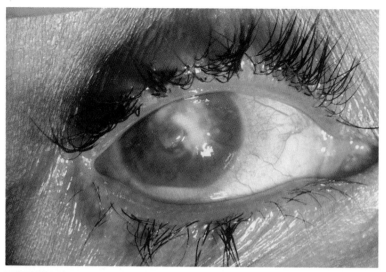

FIGURE 10-2

5. Which one of the following associations between a microorganism and a useful medium for growth is CORRECT?

    A) Moraxella—blood agar in 5% to 10% carbon dioxide
    B) Fungi—Sabouraud's dextrose agar with cycloheximide
    C) *Mycobacterium tuberculosis*—Loeffler's medium
    D) Haemophilus—blood agar

6. Which one of the following medications is most commonly used to treat cases of filamentous fungal keratitis caused by *Fusarium* spp?

    A) Flucytosine
    B) Natamycin
    C) Amphotericin B
    D) Miconazole

7. All of the following are appropriate therapy for primary HSV epithelial keratitis EXCEPT:

    A) trifluridine 1% ophthalmic solution every 2 hours while awake
    B) acyclovir 800 mg five times daily
    C) débridement of corneal lesions
    D) valacyclovir 500 mg twice a day

8. Which one of the following regarding megalocornea is TRUE?

    A) Most common inheritance is autosomal dominant
    B) Associated with progressive corneal enlargement
    C) Corneal diameter greater than 10 mm
    D) Associated with Down syndrome

Questions 9–11 Select the condition(s) associated with the given finding.

9. Associated with congenital cardiac defects:

   A) Peters' anomaly
   B) Axenfeld syndrome
   C) both
   D) neither

10. Can result from mutation at the PAX6 gene:

    A) Peters' anomaly
    B) Rieger syndrome
    C) both
    D) neither

11. Associated with glaucoma:

    A) Axenfeld syndrome
    B) Peters' anomaly
    C) both
    D) neither

12. Which one of the following is NOT included in the differential diagnosis of blue sclera?

    A) Hurler's syndrome
    B) Osteogenesis imperfecta
    C) Turner's syndrome
    D) Marfan's syndrome

13. All of the following are associated with conjunctival cicatrization EXCEPT:

    A) atopic keratoconjunctivitis
    B) ocular cicatricial pemphigoid
    C) Stevens-Johnson syndrome
    D) superior limbic keratoconjunctivitis

14. Which one of the following is a characteristic of sclerocornea?

    A) This disease is secondary to an inflammatory process.
    B) Most cases are unilateral.
    C) Most affected patients are women.
    D) This process is nonprogressive.

15. All of the following may be considered part of the iridocorneal endothelial (ICE) syndrome EXCEPT:

    A) Chandler's syndrome
    B) essential iris atrophy
    C) Cogan-Reese syndrome
    D) posterior embryotoxon

16. A 2-year-old boy presents with poor vision in both eyes, mental retardation, a thin upper lip, and low-set ears. The patient's mother is currently being treated with disulfiram for her substance abuse problem. Findings of your examination might include all of the following EXCEPT:

    A) Peters' anomaly
    B) tortuous retinal vessels
    C) optic nerve hypoplasia
    D) sclerocornea

17. Which one of the following is found with Rieger's anomaly?

    A) Autosomal dominant inheritance
    B) Maxillary hypoplasia
    C) Hypospadias
    D) Peg-shaped teeth

18. Which one of the following is NOT in the differential of a baby whose cornea is shown in Figure 10-3?

    A) Congenital hereditary stromal dystrophy
    B) Peter's anomaly
    C) Congenital glaucoma
    D) Iridocorneal endothelial syndrome

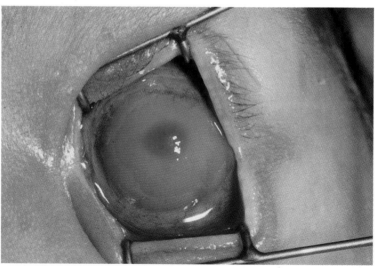

FIGURE 10-3

19. Which one of the following represents a choristoma?

    A) Dermolipoma
    B) Keratoacanthoma
    C) Hemangioma
    D) Lymphangioma

20. Which of the following OCCURS with the condition pictured in Figure 10-4?

    A) The steepest meridian of the cornea is adjacent to this lesion.
    B) These are benign with no malignant potential.
    C) They can grow rapidly.
    D) Patients may also have congenital cardiac defects.

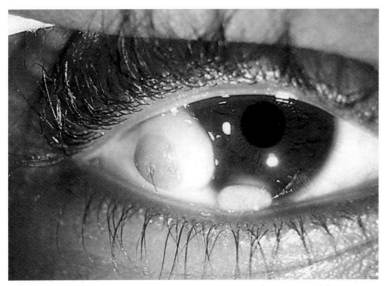

FIGURE 10-4. Courtesy of Helen K. Wu, MD.

21. Which structure is not found in the lesion in Figure 10-4?

    A) Skin
    B) Muscle
    C) Sebaceous glands
    D) Hair

22. All are true of Goldenhar's syndrome EXCEPT:

    A) iris colobomas may be present
    B) upper eyelid colobomas may be present
    C) preauricular skin tags may be present
    D) it can have an autosomal dominant inheritance

23. Erythema multiforme major (Stevens-Johnson syndrome) is associated with which of the following etiologic factors?

    A) Mycoplasma pneumonia
    B) Sulfonamides
    C) Coxsackievirus
    D) All of the above

24. Which one of the following is NOT associated with enlarged corneal nerves?

    A) Refsum's disease
    B) Congenital glaucoma
    C) Ichthyosis
    D) Multiple endocrine neoplasia (MEN), type I

Questions 25–27 (Fig. 10-5A-D)

25. Which condition is caused by a virus?

    A) Figure 10-5A
    B) Figure 10-5B
    C) Figure 10-5C
    D) None of the above

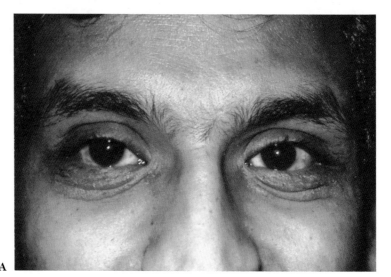

A

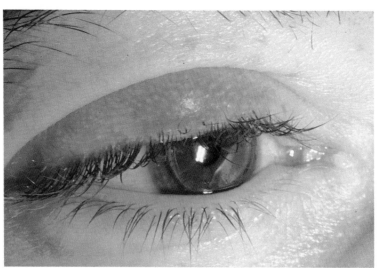

B

FIGURE 10-5

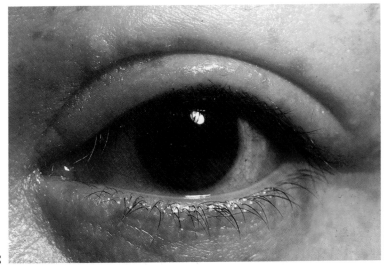

C

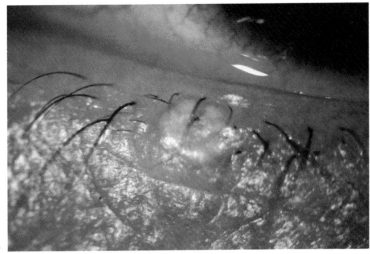

D

FIGURE 10-5 *(Continued)*

26. Which treatment can be successful for the patient in Figure 10-5D?

    A) Acyclovir
    B) Steroid ointment
    C) Excision
    D) Doxycycline

27. All of the conditions are associated with the condition pictured in Figure 10-5A EXCEPT:

    A) rheumatoid arthritis
    B) asthma
    C) hay fever or seasonal allergies
    D) eczema

28.   Which organism is NOT a usual commensal found on the lids and lashes?

A)   *Moraxella catarrhalis*
B)   *Haemophilus influenzae*
C)   *Propionibacterium acnes*
D)   *Staphylococcus epidermidis*

29.   Which one of the following statements is CORRECT for the condition in Figure 10-6?

A)   Phthirus pubis is a normal commensal of adult meibomian glands.
B)   *Demodex folliculorum* is transmitted by sexual contact.
C)   Physostigmine acts as a respiratory poison to Phthirus pubis.
D)   *Demodex folliculorum* is responsible for collarettes along the base of eyelashes.

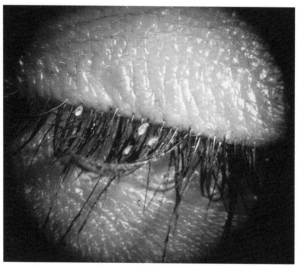

FIGURE 10-6

30.   All of the following medications commonly cause the condition pictured in Figure 10-7 EXCEPT:

A)   atropine
B)   neomycin
C)   ketorolac
D)   apraclonidine

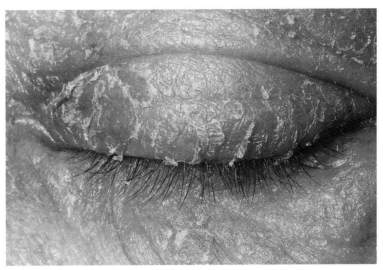

FIGURE 10-7

31. All of the following bacteria are commonly known to cause the clinical condition shown in Figure 10-8 EXCEPT:

    A) Streptococcus
    B) Staphylococcus
    C) Nocardia
    D) Haemophilus

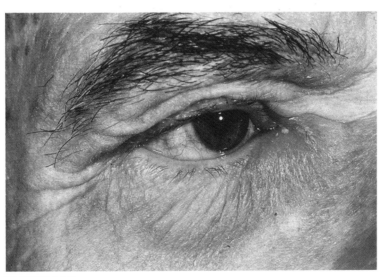

FIGURE 10-8

Questions 32–33

A 60 year-old man presents to your office complaining of a "spot" in his right eye, as shown in Figure 10-9.

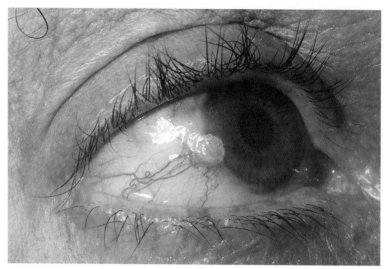

FIGURE 10-9

32.   Which of the following is not appropriate treatment for this lesion?

A)   Local excision with wide margins followed by cryotherapy
B)   Topical prednisolone drops
C)   Local radiotherapy with a ruthenium 106 plaque sutured to the scleral bed following excision
D)   Mitomycin C

33.   The lesion pictured in Figure 10-9:

A)   is always benign
B)   is contagious and easily spread to others
C)   affects only the superficial epithelium
D)   can produce keratin

34.   Which one of the following statements regarding conjunctival lymphoma is TRUE?

A)   Microscopic examination without cellular atypia would confirm the benign nature of the lesion.
B)   It always arises from systemic metastasis.
C)   The initial presentation is frequently painful loss of vision.
D)   A salmon-colored lesion on the bulbar conjunctiva is characteristic.

35.   All of the following statements about mucoepidermoid carcinoma of the conjunctiva are true EXCEPT:

A)   it usually occurs in elderly patients
B)   it represents a more aggressive variant of basal cell carcinoma
C)   it should be suspected in a recurrent squamous cell carcinoma of the conjunctiva
D)   it has a tendency to invade the globe

36. Patients with ocular cicatricial pemphigoid:

    A)   have immunoglobulins bound to the conjunctival basement membrane
    B)   may have increased numbers of goblet cells
    C)   benefit from limbal stem cell transplants
    D)   frequently present with scleritis

Questions 37–39

A 24-year-old student presents after noticing a localized area of redness in his right eye near his caruncle as shown in Figure 10-10. He has had similar previous episodes that have resolved spontaneously.

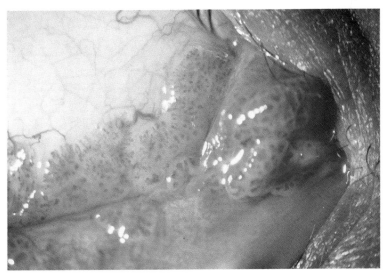

FIGURE 10-10

37. What would the lesion likely show histopathologically?

    A)   Spindle-shaped atypical cells with dark nuclei
    B)   Acanthotic epithelium over fibrovascular cores
    C)   Small caliber vascular channels in collagenase stroma
    D)   Lined nonkeratinizing stratified squamous epithelium

38. Which therapy might be most appropriate at this time?

    A)   Observation
    B)   Simple excision
    C)   Photocoagulation
    D)   Excision with frozen section controls

39. Which virus has been implicated in causing this lesion?

    A)   Epstein-Barr virus
    B)   Human papilloma virus
    C)   HSV
    D)   Molluscum contagiosum virus

40. What is the most common malignant epithelial tumor of the conjunctiva?

   A) Basal cell carcinoma
   B) Squamous cell carcinoma
   C) Malignant melanoma
   D) Squamous papilloma

41. Regarding conjunctival intraepithelial neoplasia, which one of the following is TRUE?

   A) It rarely occurs in the interpalpebral zone.
   B) Treatment is by enucleation.
   C) Abnormal vascularization is rare.
   D) The entire thickness of the epithelium may be involved.

42. Which one of the following is NOT a cause of secondary acquired conjunctival melanosis?

   A) Pregnancy
   B) Topical epinephrine drops
   C) Addison's disease
   D) Scleritis

Questions 43–46 (Fig. 10-11 to 10-14)

   A) Figure 10-11
   B) Figure 10-12
   C) Figure 10-13
   D) Figure 10-14

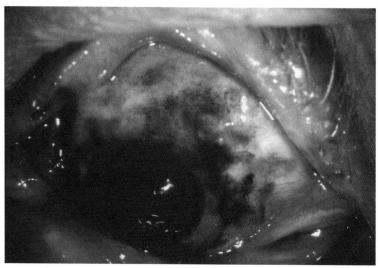

FIGURE 10-11

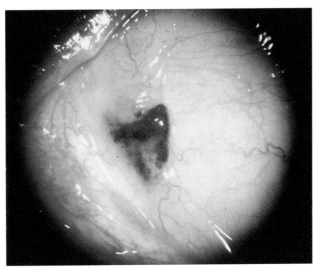

FIGURE 10-12

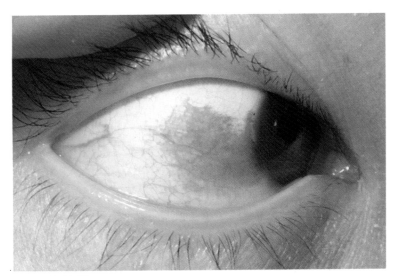

FIGURE 10-13

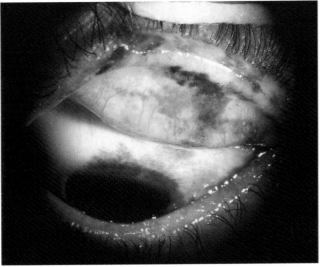

FIGURE 10-14

43. Which has the lowest neoplastic potential?

44. Which often occurs bilaterally?

45. Which may enlarge during adolescence or with pregnancy?

46. Which requires a systemic disease work-up?

Questions 47–49

A 47-year-old farmer presents with the lesion pictured in Figure 10-15. He states it has been present for at least 2 years, and it has been gradually increasing in size.

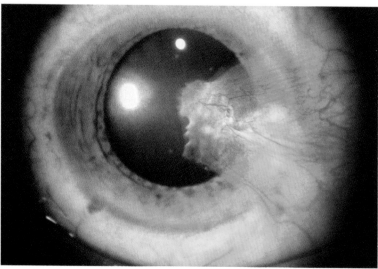

FIGURE 10-15

47. This lesion may lead to all of the following EXCEPT:

A) an adjacent dellen
B) flattening in the involved meridian with change in central astigmatism
C) destruction of Bowman's layer
D) distant metastasis

48. Possible treatment options, if this was a recurrent lesion, would likely include all of the following EXCEPT:

A) simple excision, leaving bare sclera
B) excision with amniotic membrane graft
C) excision with mitomycin C application and conjunctival autograft
D) excision with conjunctival autograft

49. Which is correct regarding the lesion pictured in Figure 10-15?

    A)   Histopathology shows fibrovascular ingrowth just beneath Bowman's layer.

    B)   A pigmented iron line (Ferry's line) is found at the corneal edge of the lesion.

    C)   Prolonged actinic exposure is a risk factor.

    D)   Recurrence after treatment is rare.

Questions 50–51

50. Which one of the following regarding the condition shown in Figure 10-16 is TRUE?

    A)   Corneal sensation is reduced.

    B)   Resection of the adjacent conjunctiva may be indicated.

    C)   Treatment with a silver nitrate stick is beneficial.

    D)   A Fox shield at bedtime is helpful.

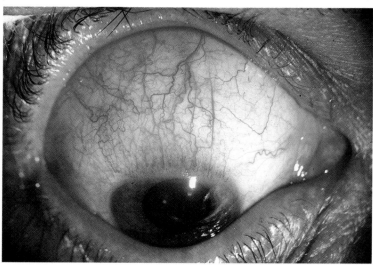

FIGURE 10-16

51. Which systemic finding might be found in association with this condition?

    A)   Increased urine catecholamine

    B)   Macular skin rash

    C)   Hyperextensible joints

    D)   Decreased thyroid stimulating hormone

52. Which of the following is appropriate treatment of the condition shown in Figure 10-17?

    A)   Topical moxifloxacin

    B)   Skin testing for allergens

    C)   Change from hard contact lenses to soft contact lenses

    D)   Topical mast cell stabilizers or corticosteroid drops

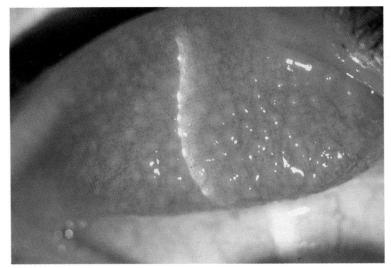

FIGURE 10-17

Questions 53–55 Corneal staining patterns in Figure 10-18.

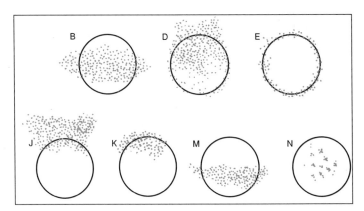

FIGURE 10-18

53. Which pattern can be found in a patient with thyroid eye disease and proptosis?

    A)   Figure 10-18M
    B)   Figure 10-18D
    C)   Figure 10-18N
    D)   Figure 10-18E

54. Which pattern is most typical of Thygeson's keratopathy?

    A)   Figure 10-18K
    B)   Figure 10-18E
    C)   Figure 10-18N
    D)   Figure 10-18B

55. Figure 10-18J corresponds to which condition below?

A) Superior limbic keratitis
B) Epidemic keratoconjunctivitis (EKC)
C) Rosacea keratoconjunctivitis
D) Exposure keratopathy

Questions 56–57 (Fig. 10-19)

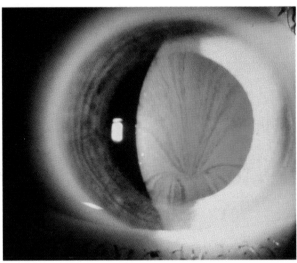

FIGURE 10-19

56. All of the following drugs can cause a corneal appearance as in Figure 10-19 EXCEPT:

A) amiodarone
B) lithium
C) chloroquine
D) indomethacin

57. Which metabolic disease can manifest as shown in Figure 10-19?

A) Fabry's disease
B) Tay-Sachs disease
C) Alport's syndrome
D) Refsum's disease

58. Which one of the following is MOST accurate regarding a 54-year-old man with cystinosis?

A) All other siblings would have similar findings.
B) He is likely of short stature and has renal dysfunction.
C) He is unlikely to develop epithelial erosions.
D) The cystine deposits begin centrally within the anterior stroma and progress to involve the entire cornea.

Questions 59–60

A 15-year-old girl presents with muscle tremors and a brownish ring near the limbus shown in Figure 10-20.

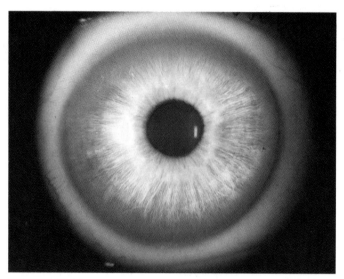

FIGURE 10-20

59. The deposits shown in the photograph are localized to which layer of the cornea?

    A)   Epithelium
    B)   Bowman's layer
    C)   Posterior stroma
    D)   Descemet's membrane

60. Which one of the following statements regarding this disease is TRUE?

    A)   It is an isolated, nonhereditary disease.
    B)   The corneal findings can be used to monitor therapy.
    C)   It is caused by a defect in the kidneys.
    D)   The corneal findings are pathognomonic for this patient's disease.

Questions 61–62

61. The findings in Figure 10-21 can be found in which condition?

    A)   Adult inclusion conjunctivitis
    B)   Vernal keratoconjunctivitis
    C)   Trachoma
    D)   Staphylococcal marginal keratitis

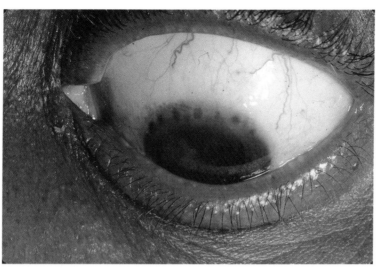

FIGURE 10-21

62. All of the following ocular findings may accompany this condition EXCEPT:

    A)   superior corneal pannus
    B)   conjunctival scarring
    C)   superior conjunctival follicles
    D)   leukoplakia

Questions 63–64

63. Which one of the following statements regarding the disease process shown in Figure 10-22 is FALSE?

    A)   The deposits consist of calcium hydroxyapatite and are found mainly in Bowman's layer.
    B)   This patient may have deposition of copper in the liver, kidneys, and brain.
    C)   Patients with this disease may be on long-term topical steroids.
    D)   This disease may be associated with chronic mercurial exposure.

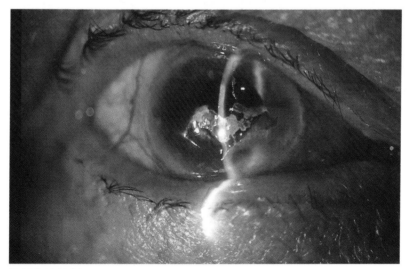

FIGURE 10-22

64. Which topical agent might be used to treat this condition?

    A) Ethylenediaminetetraacetic acid (EDTA)
    B) Penicillamine
    C) Corticosteroids
    D) Acetylcysteine

65. Which one of the following statements regarding spheroidal degeneration of the cornea is FALSE?

    A) It is usually bilateral.
    B) Pathologically, it appears as lipid deposition in the cornea.
    C) Patients usually remain asymptomatic.
    D) Actinic exposure is implicated in the pathogenesis of spheroidal degeneration.

66. Which one of the following is the MOST ACCURATE statement regarding the condition shown in the Figure 10-23?

    A) It is often associated with a systemic autoimmune disease.
    B) With-the-rule astigmatism may be induced.
    C) Thinning is more apparent than real.
    D) Epithelium remains intact.

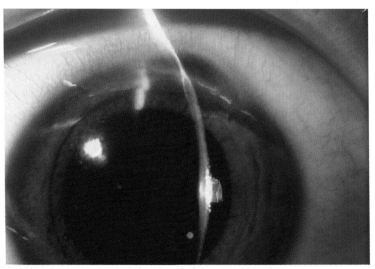

FIGURE 10-23

67. Which one of the following statements regarding the clinical condition found in this 73-year-old woman (Fig. 10-24) is TRUE?

    A) Biopsy of the adjacent conjunctiva may show increased plasma cells.
    B) Corneal perforation will occur rapidly.
    C) Systemic immunosuppressives will be necessary.
    D) It is a painless, slowly progressive process.

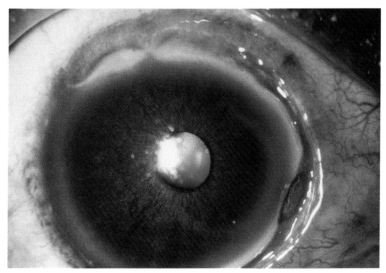

FIGURE 10-24

68. Which is TRUE of pellucid marginal degeneration?

    A) Decreased vision results from lipid deposition.
    B) Protrusion of the cornea is at the point of maximal thinning.
    C) This is a bilateral condition.
    D) Women are affected more than men.

Questions 69–71

69. Which one of the following is NOT characteristic of the condition shown on corneal topography (Fig. 10-25)?

    A) Apical scarring
    B) Scissoring of the red reflex on retinoscopy
    C) Spontaneous perforation
    D) Fleischer ring

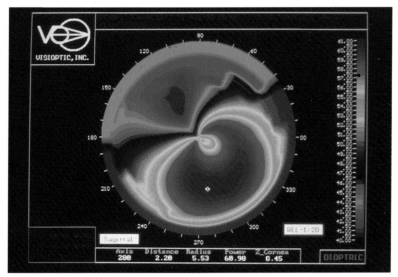

FIGURE 10-25

70. All of the following are accepted treatment measures for visual rehabilitation in this condition EXCEPT:

    A) spectacle correction
    B) hard contact lens fitting
    C) penetrating keratoplasty
    D) photorefractive keratectomy

71. This same patient comes back with a dramatic decrease in vision and this corneal appearance (Fig 10-26). What is the initial treatment?

    A) Hypertonic saline
    B) Antibiotic drops
    C) Corneal transplantation
    D) Excimer phototherapeutic keratectomy

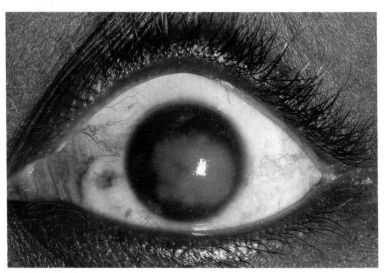

FIGURE 10-26

72. Which of the following is TRUE concerning circumscribed posterior keratoconus?

    A) Men are more commonly affected than women.
    B) Descemet's membrane and endothelium are absent in the area of the defect.
    C) It is unilateral with sporadic occurrence.
    D) It is a progressive disease process.

73. The following statements about pellucid marginal degeneration are true EXCEPT:

    A) it typically occurs in patients over age 60 years
    B) it typically causes irregular astigmatism
    C) it more commonly affects the inferior cornea
    D) it is frequently bilateral

74. Which one of the following is TRUE regarding congenital hereditary endothelial dystrophy?

    A)   Nystagmus is absent in the recessive form of the disease.

    B)   There are usually associated systemic abnormalities.

    C)   The recessive form is nonprogressive, whereas the dominantly inherited form is slowly progressive.

    D)   Corneal clouding is present at birth in both forms of the disease.

75. Which one of the following concerning congenital hereditary stromal dystrophy is FALSE?

    A)   Autosomal dominant inheritance

    B)   Pain, tearing, photophobia

    C)   Central anterior stromal flaky, feathery opacity

    D)   Cornea of normal thickness

76. Which one of the following is the most common corneal dystrophy?

    A)   Lattice stromal dystrophy

    B)   Macular stromal dystrophy

    C)   Granular stromal dystrophy

    D)   Meesmann's dystrophy

Questions 77–78

A 24-year-old woman presents with ocular irritation, foreign body sensation, decreased vision in the right eye, and the findings shown in Figure 10-27.

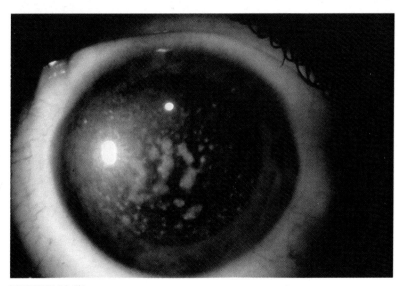

FIGURE 10-27

77. What would histopathologic examination of the corneal specimen show?

    A) Amyloid deposits
    B) Cholesterol and neutral fats
    C) Acid mucopolysaccharides
    D) Hyaline

78. Which one of the following statements regarding the disease shown in Figure 10-27 is TRUE?

    A) Both of the patient's siblings are likely affected.
    B) The disease is caused by a defect in the synthesis of keratan sulfate.
    C) Epithelial erosions are a frequent, recurring problem.
    D) In the majority of cases, only the central cornea is affected.

Questions 79–80

A 27-year-old woman presents with foreign body sensation in her eye and has the findings shown in Figure 10-28.

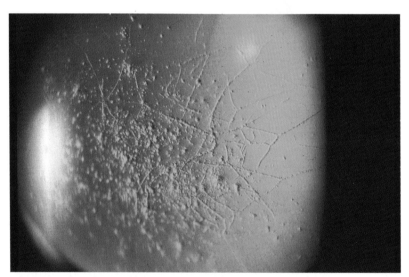

FIGURE 10-28

79. Which of the following is true?

    A) Initially, deposits are concentrated in the periphery.
    B) The corneal findings are best shown by specular reflection.
    C) The deposits are found in the posterior stroma.
    D) Skin findings and nerve palsies are manifestations of systemic involvement.

80. All of the following stains will highlight the deposits seen in this disease EXCEPT:

    A) thioflavin T
    B) Congo red
    C) alcian blue
    D) crystal violet

81. Each of the following statements regarding granular corneal dystrophy is true EXCEPT:

A) the corneal findings precede symptoms by several years
B) the intervening cornea is characteristically clear between lesions
C) recurrent erosions are common
D) the deposits consist of hyaline which stain with Masson trichrome

Questions 82–86 Match the condition(s) with the associated finding.

A) Figure 10-29
B) Figure 10-30
C) Both
D) Neither

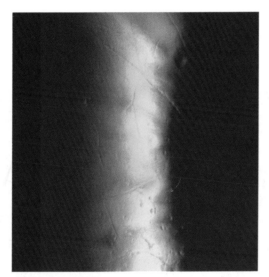

FIGURE 10-29

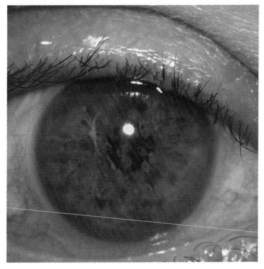

FIGURE 10-30

82. Progressive disorder?

83. Recurrence of disease in grafts?

84. Autosomal recessive inheritance?

85. Epithelial erosions occur frequently?

86. Vision severely affected in most cases?

Questions 87–88

A 34-year-old man presents with a report of decreased visual acuity in both eyes. He has had many episodes of pain and redness that last several days. His father has the same condition. His right eye is shown in Figure 10-31.

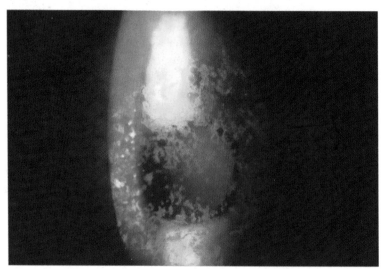

FIGURE 10-31

87. Which one of the following statements regarding these findings is TRUE?

   A) The opacities are at the level of the stroma.
   B) The lesions are among the most common to recur after penetrating keratoplasty.
   C) This condition is not progressive.
   D) Recurrent erosions are rare.

88. Histopathology would show:

   A) disruption and absence of Bowman's layer
   B) "peculiar substance" replacing Bowman's layer
   C) birefringence and dichroism
   D) staining of these lesions with oil red O

89. All of the following statements regarding the condition pictured in Figure 10-32 are true EXCEPT:

    A) it is the most common anterior corneal dystrophy
    B) it is the most common dystrophic cause of recurrent corneal erosions
    C) it occurs as a unilateral disease
    D) symptoms are more common after age 30

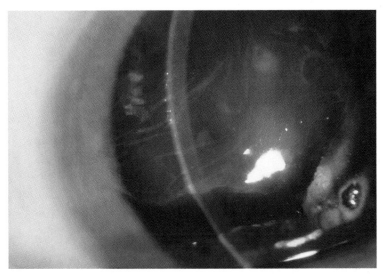

FIGURE 10-32

Questions 90–92

A 72-year-old woman presents with blurred vision in both eyes that is worse upon awakening and clears somewhat throughout the day. She denies eye pain. Both eyes have a similar clinical appearance, which is shown in Figure 10-33.

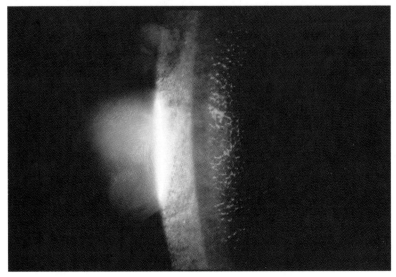

FIGURE 10-33

90. Which of the following might be found in this disease?

   A) Multilaminar Descemet's membrane studded with excrescences
   B) Heavy pigment deposition in the trabecular meshwork
   C) Breaks in Descemet's membrane
   D) Deposition of proteoglycans in the corneal stroma

91. Which diagnostic modality provides the most definitive diagnosis?

   A) Pachymetry
   B) Corneal topography
   C) Specular microscopy
   D) Corneal biopsy

92. The statement MOST correct about treatment and prognosis is:

   A) Bandage contact lens may be used to treat ruptured bullae.
   B) Hypertonic drops and lowering of IOP are long-term solutions for corneal edema.
   C) Penetrating keratoplasty carries a poor prognosis.
   D) Anterior stromal puncture may be used to treat ruptured bullae outside the visual axis.

93. A patient undergoes cataract surgery and has the appearance shown in Figure 10-34 the day after surgery. All of the following are possible causes for this EXCEPT:

   A) retained viscoelastic material within the anterior chamber
   B) endothelial toxicity from intracameral antibiotics
   C) anterior chamber phacoemulsification of a dense nucleus
   D) Descemet's detachment

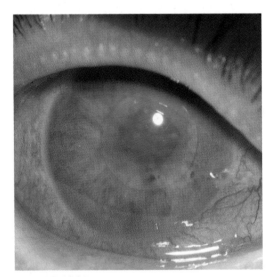

FIGURE 10-34

94. All of the following corneal dystrophies are linked to chromosome 5q31 EXCEPT:

A) Meesmann dystrophy
B) lattice dystrophy
C) Reis-Buckler's dystrophy
D) Avellino dystrophy

95. Which is NOT true regarding the condition shown in Figure 10-35:

A) it is associated with trachoma, anterior basement membrane dystrophy, and severe rosacea
B) the lesions are most frequently located in the midperipheral cornea
C) nodular collagenous material is present between the epithelium and Bowman's layer
D) best treated by excimer laser phototherapeutic keratectomy

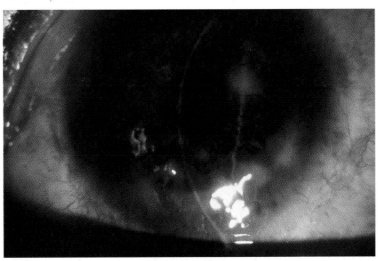

FIGURE 10-35

96. A 65-year-old woman had cataract surgery. She comes back for her 1-week visit; her eye is shown in Figure 10-36. What should be done to help this resolve?

A) Start her on fortified antibiotic drops.
B) Increase the frequency of her topical steroid drop.
C) Discontinue her fluoroquinolone drop.
D) Scrape lesion and look for hyphae on microscopy.

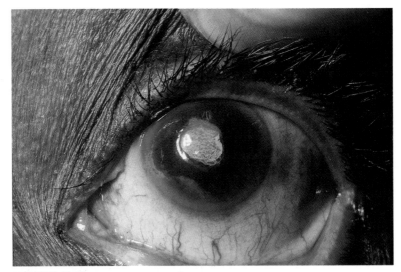

FIGURE 10-36

A 42-year-old man presents with photophobia and tearing. Both eyes have a similar appearance. His right eye is shown in Figure 10-37.

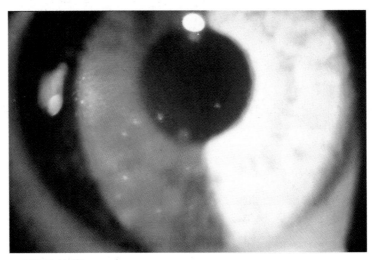

FIGURE 10-37

97. All the following are true EXCEPT:

    A)   corneal sensation is reduced
    B)   it may be treated with topical cyclosporine
    C)   there is typically a chronic recurrent course
    D)   it is associated with histocompatibility antigen HLA-DR3

98. A 32-year-old woman presents 1 week after experiencing redness, discharge, and itching in both her eyes with a concurrent upper respiratory infection with decreased vision. Her right eye is shown in Figure 10-38. All are possible treatments EXCEPT:

A) cool compresses
B) topical steroid therapy
C) débridement
D) lubrication

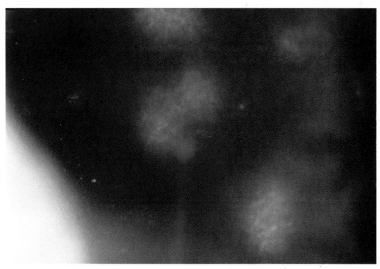

FIGURE 10-38

Questions 99–101

A 37-year-old woman presents with 2 days of redness, tearing, and the sensation of grittiness in her eye. Her cornea is pictured in Figure 10-39.

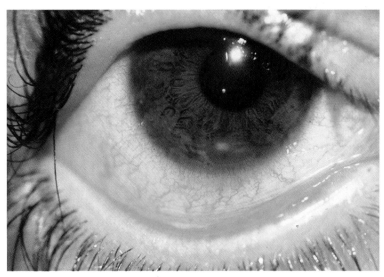

FIGURE 10-39

99. What organism is associated with this condition?

   A)   Herpes simplex
   B)   *Propionibacterium acnes*
   C)   *Staphylococcus aureus*
   D)   Hepatitis C

100. What accompanying condition might this patient have?

   A)   Blepharitis
   B)   Lagophthalmos
   C)   Skin rash
   D)   Arthritis

101. Which treatment would rapid resolve this condition?

   A)   Prednisolone acetate
   B)   Hypertonic sodium chloride
   C)   Trifluridine
   D)   Gatifloxacin

102. Which one of the following organisms is capable of traversing intact corneal epithelium and establishing bacterial keratitis as shown in Figure 10-40?

   A)   *Staphylococcus aureus*
   B)   *Staphylococcus epidermidis*
   C)   *Pseudomonas aeruginosa*
   D)   *Haemophilus influenzae*

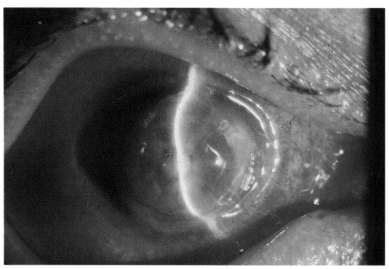

FIGURE 10-40

Questions 103–104

A 23-year-old medical student underwent photorefractive keratectomy for mild myopia. He did well during the procedure but postoperatively complained of severe pain. At 3 days postoperatively, the epithelial defect had not healed and appeared unchanged in size with ragged borders. One week postoperatively, he presented as shown in Figure10-41.

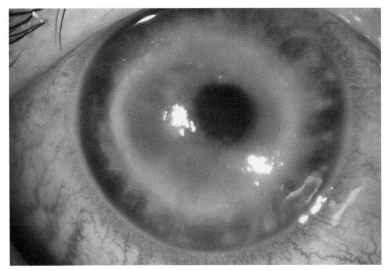

FIGURE 10-41

103. Which one of the following is LEAST likely in the differential diagnosis?

A) Bacterial keratitis
B) Fungal keratitis
C) Toxic medicamentosa
D) Disciform keratitis

104. All of the following are important initial diagnostic steps to perform EXCEPT:

A) corneal scraping for smear and culture
B) questioning about use of topical medications
C) corneal biopsy
D) testing corneal sensation

Questions 105–109

A) Herpes simplex keratitis
B) Herpes zoster keratitis
C) Both
D) Neither

105. Corneal anesthesia?

106. Active viral replication in epithelial lesions?

107. Sectoral iris atrophy?

108. Ulcerated epithelial lesion?

109. Vesicular skin rash?

110. Which one of the following regarding Schnyder's crystalline corneal dystrophy is INCORRECT?

    A) Opacities recur in corneal transplants.
    B) It is composed of cholesterol crystals.
    C) There are associated lipid arcus.
    D) It is an indicator of elevation of systemic lipid levels.

Questions 111–112

A 32-year-old man presents with a 3-day history of redness and photophobia of his right eye. He vaguely remembers having redness of this same eye 6 months ago that resolved spontaneously. He denies trauma. His appearance at the slit lamp is shown in Figure 10-42.

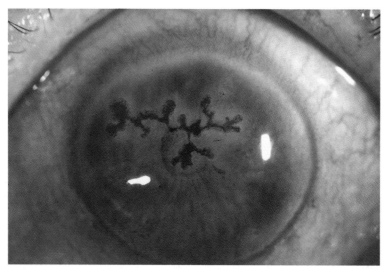

FIGURE 10-42

111. Which one of the following is MOST accurate about this condition?

    A) His previous episode of ocular redness is irrelevant.
    B) Edges of these lesions stain with rose bengal.
    C) Histopathology would show intracytoplasmic inclusions.
    D) Treatment is necessary for resolution.

112. This same patient presents 2 years later as shown (Fig 10-43). All of the following statements regarding treatment are true EXCEPT:

A) oral acyclovir will expedite recovery

B) the lowest effective dose of a topical anti-inflammatory (steroid) should be used

C) topical antivirals should be used concomitantly with topical steroids

D) patients with peripheral lesions and mild inflammation who maintain good visual acuity may be observed

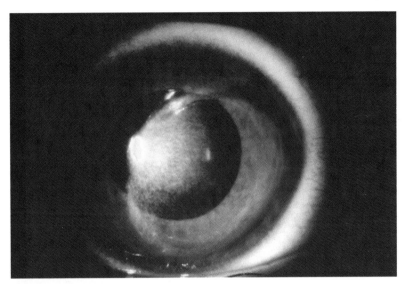

FIGURE 10-43

Questions 113–114

A 17-year-old contact lens wearer developed pain, redness, photophobia, and decreased visual acuity in her right eye 2 days ago. She states that she cares for and cleans her lenses meticulously and wears them no more than 8 hours a day. She does admit to being on a camping trip for 3 days about 2 weeks ago. Her left eye is pictured in Figure 10-44.

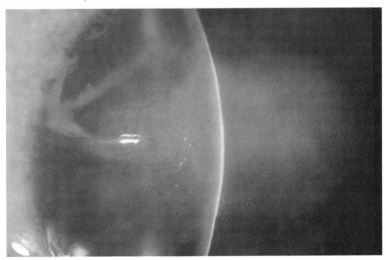

FIGURE 10-44

113. Which one of the following regarding this condition is TRUE?

    A)   Patients complain of a dull, aching pain.
    B)   Enlarged corneal nerves are pathognomonic.
    C)   These organisms grow best in thioglycolate broth.
    D)   Simple mechanical débridement may be curative when confined to the corneal epithelium.

114. Corneal biopsy may be expected to show:

    A)   Gram-negative rods
    B)   double-walled cysts
    C)   acid-fast pleomorphic rods
    D)   branching hyphae

115. A 25-year-old soft contact lens wearer presents with severe pain in her right eye after wearing her daily disposable contact lens overnight for 1 week. Pictured is her right eye. (Fig. 10-45). The least appropriate therapy is:

    A)   topical moxifloxacin
    B)   topical cefazolin
    C)   topical gatifloxacin
    D)   topical vancomycin and tobramycin

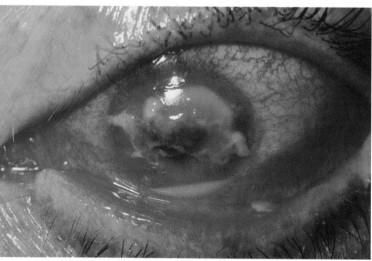

FIGURE 10-45

116. Which is the MOST common cause of bilateral interstitial keratitis?

    A)   Congenital syphilis
    B)   Tuberculosis
    C)   Cogan's syndrome
    D)   Acquired syphilis

Questions 117–118

117. Which one of the following is a cause for the condition pictured in Figure 10-46?

A) Sjögren's syndrome
B) Cranial nerve V paralysis
C) Chemical splash
D) Bell's palsy

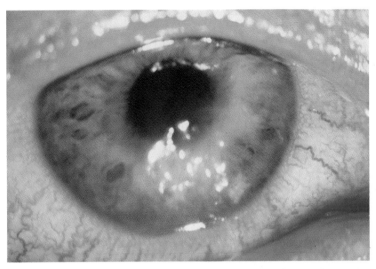

FIGURE 10-46

118. Which one of the following treatments would be most effective for this condition?

A) Tarsorrhaphy
B) Bandage contact lens
C) Penetrating keratoplasty
D) Anterior stromal micropuncture

Questions 119–120

A 72-year-old woman presents to your office with a report of red eyes and foreign body sensation for several months. She also recently notes the onset of dysphagia. Her slit lamp appearance is shown (Fig. 10-47).

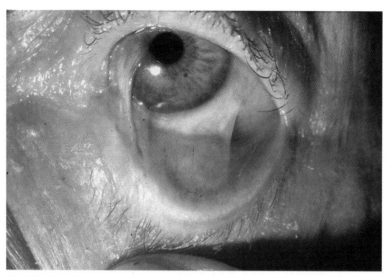

FIGURE 10-47

119. All of the following statements are true EXCEPT:

    A)   she should be asked about use of topical medications
    B)   conjunctival scrapings may reveal eosinophils
    C)   corneal scarring and vascularization are successfully treated with penetrating keratoplasty
    D)   immunoglobulins are deposited along the conjunctival basement membrane

120. Which treatment would be MOST effective for this condition?

    A)   Dapsone
    B)   Topical steroid drops
    C)   Lysis of membranes
    D)   Topical cyclosporine

121. Which one of the following is NOT a cause of cicatrizing conjunctivitis?

    A)   Trachoma
    B)   Chemical burns
    C)   Stevens-Johnson syndrome
    D)   Staphylococcal hypersensitivity

122. All of these conditions may cause the corneal picture in Figure 10-48 EXCEPT:

    A)   prolonged patching
    B)   dry eyes
    C)   superior limbic keratoconjunctivitis
    D)   floppy eyelid syndrome

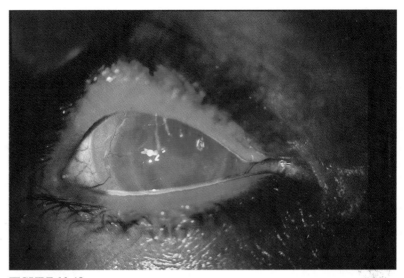

FIGURE 10-48

123. This cornea has markedly decreased sensation (Fig. 10-49). The patient denies a history of trauma. Which one of the following statements is LEAST correct?

A)   This condition may be surgically induced.
B)   Long-term steroids are helpful.
C)   Patching may be beneficial.
D)   Tarsorrhaphy is often helpful in refractory cases.

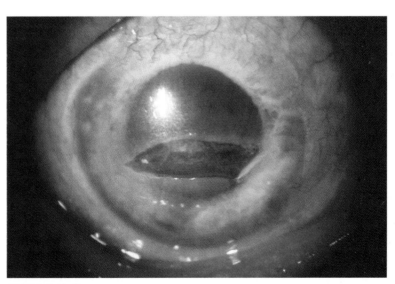

FIGURE 10-49

Questions 124–125

A healthy 18-year-old black man presents with a total hyphema after being struck in the right eye with a tennis ball. Visual acuity is hand motions, and the IOP is normal (Fig. 10-50).

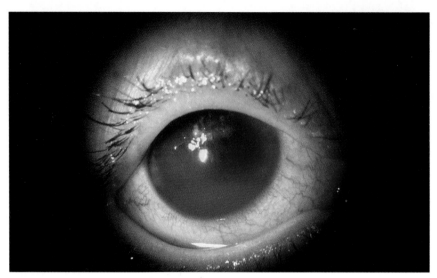

FIGURE 10-50

124. Which one of the following would be appropriate in the management of this patient?

   A)   Topical steroids and a cycloplegic
   B)   Bed rest, elevation of the head of the bed, bilateral patches
   C)   Oral aminocaproic acid
   D)   All of the above

125. If this patient's intraocular pressure (IOP) had been elevated and a small amount of corneal blood staining resulted, what would be the MOST appropriate next step?

   A)   Anterior chamber washout
   B)   Topical carbonic anhydrase inhibitor
   C)   Continued observation
   D)   Injection of tissue plasminogen activator into the anterior chamber

126. Superficial phototherapeutic keratectomy is indicated in treating symptoms in the following conditions EXCEPT:

   A)   Reis-Buckler's dystrophy
   B)   granular dystrophy
   C)   epithelial basement membrane dystrophy
   D)   Fleck dystrophy

Questions 127–128

A 28-year-old man was splashed in the eyes with a chemical solvent while at work. He noted immediate pain and decreased vision despite aggressive irrigation. His right eye is pictured in Figure 10-51.

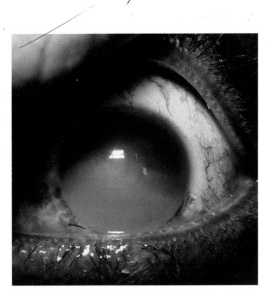

FIGURE 10-51

127. Which one of the following statements concerning this injury is TRUE?

A) Acid burns cause loss of ground substance and collagen swelling.
B) The worst damage from alkali burns occurs immediately.
C) Burns at the limbus and burns at the palpebral conjunctiva have a similar prognosis.
D) Severe uveitis and glaucoma may occur.

128. All of the following statements concerning treatment are true EXCEPT:

A) irrigation should be started immediately and continued in the emergency room
B) débridement of necrotic conjunctiva should be performed
C) topical steroids are used long-term to decrease the inflammatory response
D) prognosis for penetrating keratoplasty is best after the inflammatory process has quieted

Questions 129–130

A healthy 20-year-old white man presents with sudden onset of tearing, redness, and irritation of his right eye (Fig. 10-52). He does not complain of floaters, blurred vision, or pain with eye movement. Visual acuity is 20/20 in both eyes.

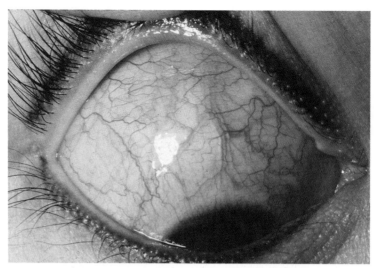

FIGURE 10-52

129. Which one of the following would be LEAST helpful in your diagnosis?

    A)   Recent history of upper respiratory tract infection
    B)   Examination under natural light
    C)   Pupillary exam
    D)   Examination of conjunctiva under slit lamp

130. The dilated vessels in Figure 10-52 were salmon-pink, moved freely with the conjunctiva, and blanched with the application of topical epinephrine. Which one of the following would be LEAST appropriate therapy?

    A)   Observation
    B)   Topical steroids
    C)   Topical antibiotics
    D)   Oral nonsteroidal agents

131. Which one of the following is the MOST destructive form of scleritis?

    A)   Diffuse anterior scleritis
    B)   Necrotizing scleritis with inflammation
    C)   Nodular anterior scleritis
    D)   Scleromalacia perforans

132. All of the following have been associated with scleritis EXCEPT:

    A)   gout
    B)   tuberculosis
    C)   leprosy
    D)   Behçet's disease

133. All of the following are acceptable therapies for scleritis EXCEPT:

   A) posterior sub-Tenon's steroid injection
   B) oral nonsteroidal anti-inflammatory agents (NSAIDs)
   C) topical cyclosporine
   D) systemic steroids

134. Which of the following is not associated with an abnormality of limbal stem cell proliferation?

   A) Shield ulcer
   B) Stevens-Johnson Syndrome
   C) Aniridia
   D) Chemical injury

135. Reduction of positive vitreous pressure during ocular surgery may be accomplished by all of the following EXCEPT:

   A) aspiration of liquid vitreous through the pars plana
   B) adjustment of a poorly fitting lid speculum
   C) IV mannitol
   D) hypoventilation during general anesthesia

136. You obtain a cornea for an elective penetrating keratoplasty and you notice that the color of the storage medium is yellow-orange instead of the usual pink. What does this indicate?

   A) Decrease in antibiotic levels
   B) Loss of epithelium
   C) A cornea over 3 days old
   D) Possible microbial contamination

137. Of the following, what is currently the MOST common indication for penetrating keratoplasty in adults?

   A) Fuchs' dystrophy
   B) Aphakic bullous keratopathy
   C) Pseudophakic bullous keratopathy
   D) Herpes simplex keratitis

138. Of the following, which is the MOST frequent indication for penetrating keratoplasty in children?

   A) Sclerocornea
   B) Interstitial keratitis
   C) Peters' anomaly
   D) Bacterial keratitis

139. Special considerations when performing penetrating keratoplasty in children include all of the following EXCEPT:

A) oversized grafts
B) scleral support during surgery
C) early removal of sutures postoperatively
D) frequent postoperative follow-up

140. Postoperative complications in pediatric penetrating keratoplasty include all of the following EXCEPT:

A) glaucoma
B) amblyopia
C) slow or delayed healing
D) graft rejection

141. Overall, approximately what percentage of corneal grafts are clear greater than 1 year postoperatively?

A) 90%
B) 65%
C) 50%
D) 40%

142. Approximately what percentage of corneal grafts performed for HSV keratitis remains clear greater than 1 year postoperatively?

A) 90%
B) 65%
C) 50%
D) 40%

143. Overall, the risk of an endothelial graft rejection episode is:

A) 1%
B) 5%
C) 20%
D) 40%

144. According to the Collaborative Corneal Transplant Study:

A) human leukocyte antigens (HLA) tissue matching was clearly advantageous
B) HLA tissue matching was considered cost-effective
C) ABO blood type incompatibility was shown to be a possible risk factor
D) Peripheral corneal vascularization was not a significant risk factor

145. Poor candidates for refractive surgery may include:

A) pathologic (posterior segment) myopia
B) keratoconus
C) history of HSV keratitis
D) all of the above

146. Most rigid gas permeable contact lens wearers should discontinue use of their lenses at least how many days before a refractive surgery evaluation?

A) 7 days
B) 21 days
C) 30 days
D) 60 days

147. Concerning radial keratotomy, after what number of incisions does the dioptric effect per incision decrease significantly?

A) 4 incisions
B) 8 incisions
C) 16 incisions
D) 32 incisions

148. Concerning astigmatic keratotomy for naturally occurring astigmatism, arcuate incisions greater than how many degrees are relatively contraindicated?

A) 60°
B) 90°
C) 120°
D) 130°

149. Which of the following was a conclusion of the Collaborative Corneal Transplant Study?

A) HLA-A, HLA-B, and HLA-DR matching the donor and recipient had no effect on overall graft survival.
B) Grafts with running sutures had earlier improvement of vision compared to grafts with interrupted sutures.
C) Matching donor and recipient age is beneficial to long-term graft survival.
D) ABO blood type matching does not reduce the risk of graft rejection.

150. Which of these quadrants of the paracentral cornea is most often the thinnest, based on intraoperative pachymetry in radial keratotomy patients?

A) Nasal
B) Inferior
C) Superior
D) Temporal

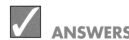 **ANSWERS**

1. D)   Stevens-Johnson syndrome

    This patient has a follicular conjunctivitis. Follicles are small avascular mounds of lymphocytes and plasma cells. Papillae are formed by edema and leakage of fluid from telangiectatic vessels. The differential diagnosis of a follicular conjunctivitis includes epidemic keratoconjunctivits (EKC), HSV, chlamydia, molluscum contagiosum, as well as topical drug reactions (type IV hypersensitivity to medications such as brimonidine or neomycin).

    Stevens-Johnson syndrome is a systemic autoimmune disease that causes sloughing of the mucous membranes (including the conjunctiva). This can be a reaction to medication from sulfonamides, Dilantin, and others. In milder cases, patients may present with a papillary conjunctivitis.

2. A)   Ligneous conjunctivitis

    Chlamydia trachomatis causes a variety of ocular and systemic diseases. Trachoma caused by *C. trachomatis* serotypes A, B, Ba, and C is considered to be the leading cause of blindness worldwide. In its early stages, trachoma presents as a follicular conjunctivitis. Severe inflammation can lead to tarsal scarring (which may lead to trichiasis and entropion), corneal scarring, and blindness. *Chlamydia trachomatis* serotypes D-K are associated with adult inclusion conjunctivitis, which can manifest as a chronic follicular conjunctivitis. Lymphogranuloma venereum is a result of infection by serotypes L1, L2, or L3. This disease does not usually affect the eyes.

    Ligneous conjunctivitis can result from any ocular infection that produces such a vigorous response that there is exudation of fibrin and formation of a hard, woody membrane. The etiology of ligneous is not known, but an inherited plasminogen deficiency has been suggested.

3. D)   Wegener's granulomatosis

    VDRL and RPR tests detect antilipoidal antibodies produced by the host during treponemal infection. Autoimmune diseases, such as rheumatoid arthritis and lupus erythematosus, have similar antibodies that may give a false-positive reading. Wegener's granulomatosis is associated with the antineutrophil cytoplasmic antibody.

4. C)   Löwenstein-Jensen agar

    This is a typical presentation of a fungal keratitis. Löwenstein-Jensen agar is used to help identify mycobacteria. Sabouraud's agar is used to help identify fungi. Calcofluor white binds to the cell walls of fungi and Acanthamoeba, enhancing their visibility under a fluorescent microscope. Giemsa stains are useful for identifying fungi, bacteria, and intracytoplasmic inclusions in Chlamydial infections by light microscopy.

5. A) Moraxella—blood agar in 5% to 10% carbon dioxide

Moraxella is a slow-growing, aerobic bacterium that grows best in the conditions described at 37°C. It is classically known for causing angular blepharitis, although less commonly than does Staphylococcus. Moraxella can also cause conjunctivitis and keratitis.

Cultures for ocular fungi should be plated onto Sabouraud's dextrose agar without cycloheximide, which, if present, will inhibit growth of saprophytic fungi. Loeffler's serum medium is used to speciate Moraxella based on growth characteristics. Löwenstein-Jensen medium is used for isolation of *Mycobacterium tuberculosis* while atypical mycobacteria will grow on blood agar. Haemophilus requires hemin and nicotinamide adenine dinucleotide (NAD) for growth and will not grow unless they are present, as in chocolate agar.

6. B) Natamycin

Natamycin is a polyene antifungal that is the drug of choice for filamentous fungi. Topical miconazole is the drug of choice for *Paecilomyces lilacinus*. Topical amphotericin is used to combat infections caused by *Aspergillus* and *Candida* spp. Flucytosine is used as an adjunctive agent for treatment of *Candida* spp.

7. B) acyclovir 800 mg five times daily

Options for managing primary HSV keratitis include trifluridine (Viroptic) nine times/day, vidarabine 3% ophthalmic ointment five times/day, or acyclovir 3% ophthalmic ointment five times/day. Débridement of the corneal lesions in primary herpes may expedite recovery. Débridement may also be necessary for resistant virus strains. In severe or recalcitrant cases, oral acyclovir may be beneficial as adjunctive therapy. Famciclovir 500 mg twice daily or valacyclovir 500 to 1000 mg twice daily for 5 days are the treatments of choice. Acyclovir 800 mg five times daily is the dosing for herpes zoster ophthalmicus.

8. D) Associated with Down syndrome

Megalocornea is usually an X-linked, isolated, nonprogressive congenital corneal enlargement with a horizontal corneal diameter of greater than 13 mm. It has been associated with systemic conditions such as Down, Marfan's, and Alport's syndromes, craniosynostosis, and facial hemiatrophy.

9. A) Peters' anomaly

10. A) Peters' anomaly

11. C) both

Condition	Inheritance	Anterior segment findings	Other findings
Posterior embryotoxon	autosomal dominant	Anteriorly displaced Schwalbe's line	
Axenfeld's anomaly	autosomal dominant	Posterior embryotoxon AND prominent iris processes attaching to Schwalbe's line	
Axenfeld's syndrome	autosomal dominant	Axenfeld's anomaly	Glaucoma, skeletal abnormalities, hypertelorism, hypoplastic shoulder
Rieger's anomaly	autosomal dominant	Axenfeld's anomaly AND anterior iris stromal hypoplasia	Glaucoma in 60%
Rieger's syndrome	autosomal dominant	Rieger's anomaly	Maxillary hypoplasia, microdontia, bony malformations
Peter's anomaly	sporadic	Absence of posterior corneal tissue and leukoma, ±iris adhesions to leukoma, ±lens–corneal adhesions	

12. D)   Marfan's syndrome

Hurler's syndrome, or mucopolysaccharidosis type 1, is associated with cloudy corneas, mental retardation, and skeletal defects. Turner's syndrome has an XO chromosomal abnormality and is associated with ptosis, cataract, blue sclera, and nystagmus. Although Marfan's disease is a disorder of collagen synthesis, blue sclera are not seen in this condition.

13. D)   superior limbic keratoconjunctivitis

Stevens-Johnson syndrome, ocular cicatricial pemphigoid, and atopic keratoconjunctivitis are associated with conjunctival cicatrization. Other etiologies include, but are not limited to, chemical burns, trachoma, squamous cell carcinoma, infectious conjunctivitis, and scleroderma. Superior limbic keratoconjunctivitis does not cause conjunctival scarring, but it does cause a papillary reaction on the superior tarsus and keratinization and redundancy of the superior bulbar conjunctiva.

14. D)   This process is nonprogressive.

Sclerocornea is a nonprogressive, noninflammatory scleralization of the cornea. Ninety percent of cases are bilateral with no gender predilection. Half are sporadic. The remaining may be either dominant or recessive.

15. D)   posterior embryotoxon

The ICE syndrome is a spectrum of diseases including progressive (essential) iris atrophy, Chandler's syndrome, and Cogan-Reese syndrome (iris-nevus syndrome). All are characterized by a "hammered silver" appearance to the corneal endothelium and varying degrees of iris changes, such as corectopia, holes, and atrophy. Chandler's syndrome typically has more severe corneal edema than the others. Essential iris atrophy is associated with polycoria and iris stretch holes. Cogan-Reese syndrome is characterized by numerous small pigmented nodules, iris atrophy, and pupillary distortion. Posterior polymorphous dystrophy of the cornea is considered by some to be related to the ICE syndrome. Posterior embryotoxon is anterior displacement of Schwalbe's line and is not related to this syndrome.

16. D) sclerocornea

Fetal alcohol syndrome is associated with multiple systemic and ocular abnormalities, including epicanthal folds, strabismus, blepharophimosis, long eyelashes, microphthalmia, telecanthus, anterior segment dysgenesis, and a persistent hyaloid vessel. In mothers who abuse alcohol, 30% of infants are affected. Disulfiram (Antabuse) is given to mothers in an effort to prevent them from drinking.

17. A) Autosomal dominant inheritance

The other findings are part of the Rieger's syndrome, which includes Rieger's anomaly (posterior embryotoxon, iris processes, iris atrophy) in addition to skeletal abnormalities.

18. D) Iridocorneal endothelial syndrome

Each one of the conditions listed in this question is characterized by corneal clouding noted soon after birth. Congenital hereditary stromal dystrophy is associated with normal eye pressures, normal stromal thickness, and normal corneal diameter. Peters' anomaly is part of the spectrum of anterior segment dysgenesis and is associated with absence of corneal endothelium and Descemet's membrane in the opacified area of the corneal leukoma. Congenital glaucoma is characterized by photophobia, tearing, enlarged corneal diameters, and increased eye pressures. ICE may have abnormalities of the endothelium; however, it does not usually have corneal edema or opacification as shown.

19. A) Dermolipoma

Choristomas represent normal tissue in an abnormal location, whereas *hamartomas* represent abnormal growth of tissue in its normal location. Choristomas include dermolipomas and dermoids. Hemangiomas and lymphangiomas represent hamartomas.

20. B) These are benign with no malignant potential.

Limbal dermoids are well-circumscribed, white-pale yellow, round lesions that are choristomas (heterotopic congenital lesion that results from normal tissue residing in an abnormal location). The flattest meridian of the cornea is adjacent to the dermoid. They have no malignant potential. They tend to grow as the child grows but usually very slowly. They can be associated with Goldenhar's syndrome, a triad of epibulbar dermoids, facial anomalies, and skeletal anomalies.

21. B) Muscle

Dermoids are choristomas containing ectodermal elements (skin, hair, fat, and sebaceous glands). Muscle tissue is not expected to be found in such a lesion.

22.   A)   iris colobomas may be present

Goldenhar's syndrome is a sporadic or autosomal dominant inherited syndrome of the first branchial arch. It consists of a triad: epibulbar dermoids; facial anomalies including upper eyelid colobomas, preauricular skin tags, and aural fistulas; and skeletal anomalies.

23.   D)   All of the above

Numerous medications are associated with the Stevens-Johnson syndrome. Some of these include penicillin, barbiturates, and sulfonamides, as well as some topical medications (sulfonamides, cycloplegics). Many infectious etiologies have also been implicated in precipitating a Stevens-Johnson syndrome. These include mycoplasma pneumonia, coxsackievirus, echovirus, and influenza virus.

24.   D)   Multiple endocrine neoplasia (MEN), type I

Multiple endocrine neoplasia, type IIb (Sipple-Gorlin syndrome), is associated with enlarged corneal nerves, medullary carcinoma of the thyroid gland, pheochromocytoma, and mucosal neuromas. Enlarged nerves may be found in Refsum's disease, ichthyosis, congenital glaucoma, and other diseases.

25.   C)   Figure 10-5C

26.   C)   Incision

27.   A)   rheumatoid arthritis

Figure 10-5A is a patient with atopy. Atopic patients have hyperactive immune systems that react to many environmental allergens. They can also have other allergic conditions including asthma, eczema, or seasonal allergies.
   Figure 10-5B is a chalazion. This is due to blockage of a meibomian gland orifice. The gland secretions collect, causing the nodular swelling of the lid. Incision and drainage is the definitive treatment.
   Figure 10-5C is due to HSV. The vesicular lesions on the upper lid can ulcerate and crust. Superinfection with bacteria is possible. Patients should be monitored for development of corneal dendrites.
   Figure 10-5D is a molluscum contagiosum lid lesion. The patients may have an associated follicular conjunctivitis. Treatment options include observation, chemical or thermal cautery, and excision. Incision of these lesions has also resulted in spontaneous involution of these lesions.

28.   B)   *Haemophilus influenzae*

A number of bacteria are found commonly in the environment. These can be recovered from the eyelashes, and most of the time they do not cause ocular disease. *Corynebacterium* spp, *Staphylococcus epidermidis, Moraxella catarrhalis,* and *Streptococcus viridans* are frequently found. Gram-negative organisms are not usually found on the ocular surface. Pathogenic bacteria include *Haemophilus influenzae, Pseudomonas aeruginosa, Streptococcus pneumoniae, Staphylococcus aureus, Bacillus subtilis,* and *Neisseria gonorrhoeae.*

29. C)   Physostigmine acts as a respiratory poison to Phthirus pubis.

Phthirus pubis (crab louse) infests pubic hair and eyelashes (Fig. 10-6) and is transmitted by sexual contact. Treatment is by mechanical removal or with bland ointments applied to the lids to suffocate adult lice. Physostigmine is effective as a respiratory poison against the lice but has many ocular side effects, limiting its effectiveness. Demodex is a normal commensal in adults living in meibomian glands. Classically, "sleeves" are found at the base of lashes, indicating Demodex infestation. Treatment is through lid scrubs. Collarettes are found more commonly with staphylococcal blepharitis.

30. C)   ketorolac

Figure 10-7 shows a case of contact dermatitis associated with allergy to a topical medication. Patients often have an accompanying follicular conjunctivitis. Allergies occur with topical ophthalmic medications, including atropine, neomycin, apraclonidine, and dipivefrin (Propine).

31. C)   Nocardia

Figure 10-8 shows dacryocystitis. Swelling and tenderness in the area of the lacrimal sac is evident. Streptococci and Staphylococci are known etiologies. Haemophilus is a common cause of dacryocystitis in children. Nocardia, a filamentous bacterium, is not a common cause of dacryocystitis but rather causes canaliculitis (less so than Actinomyces) and, rarely, keratitis or scleritis after trauma.

32. B)   Topical prednisolone drops

33. D)   can produce keratin

Squamous cell carcinoma of the limbus is rare. These lesions tend to be gelatinous, leukoplakic, or, occasionally, papilliform in appearance. Histologically, epidermoid and spindle-shaped cells replace the normal conjunctival epithelium. They can produce a whitish keratin plaque as they grow. Squamous cell carcinoma can primarily invade the cornea without conjunctival involvement. It can also invade intraocular structures. Most lesions may be treated with local excision with wide margins followed by cryotherapy. During larger resections, Mohs' technique is valuable. Local radiotherapy with a ruthenium 106 plaque after excision may also be employed. Adjunctive therapy with mitomycin C has been used in several case reports. Topical steroids would not be expected to affect this lesion.

34. D)   A salmon-colored lesion on the bulbar conjunctiva is characteristic.

Conjunctival lymphoma usually presents as a painless, salmon-colored lesion on the bulbar conjunctiva. It may be an isolated finding or may be associated with systemic disease. Histopathologic finding of monoclonal B-lymphocytes is associated with malignancy, so the finding of cellular atypia is not a criteria for malignant potential. Treatment may consist of surgery, local chemotherapy, or radiation.

35.   B)   it represents a more aggressive variant of basal cell carcinoma

Mucoepidermoid carcinoma of the conjunctiva is a more aggressive variant of squamous cell carcinoma. It should be suspected in cases involving recurrence after primary excision or in which no invasion into the globe occurs. It typically occurs in patients over age 60 and involves cells that are able to produce malignant mucus-secreting cells (goblet cells).

36.   A)   have immunoglobulins bound to the conjunctival basement membrane

Cicatricial pemphigoid is a chronic disease that affects mucosal surfaces typically in the elderly population. Immunoglobulins at the level of the basement membrane can be seen with immunofluorescent stains. Ocular cicatricial pemphigoid is usually bilateral (but may be very asymmetric) and associated with a chronic conjunctivitis. This leads to subconjunctival fibrosis and a drop in the number of goblet cells. The subconjunctival fibrosis also may lead to obstruction of the ducts of the lacrimal and accessory lacrimal glands. Progression usually results in symblepharon, foreshortening of the fornices, and ankyloblepharon. Keratinization of the conjunctival epithelium as well as corneal neovascularization and scarring are characteristic of end-stage ocular cicatricial pemphigoid.

37.   B)   Acanthotic epithelium over fibrovascular cores

Figure 10-10 shows a conjunctival papilloma. In children and young adults, lesions may be multiple and are usually found on the palpebral conjunctiva. They are of viral origin, and spontaneous resolution is common. These lesions contrast with noninfectious papillomas, which occur in older adults and are almost always single in occurrence, often at the limbus. Atypical cells with dark nuclei may be found histopathologically. Small caliber vascular channels in a collagenase stroma are found in pyogenic granuloma, and lined nonkeratinizing stratified squamous epithelia are found in epithelial inclusion cysts.

38.   A)   Observation

Past episodes with spontaneous resolution suggests viral origin. Incomplete excision or bleeding during excision may lead to seeding of other sites and multiple papillomas. Cryotherapy alone or in conjunction with excision with 2- to 3-mm margins is the preferred surgical treatment. Photocoagulation is not indicated.

39.   B)   Human papillomavirus

Human papillomavirus DNA has been found in papillomatous lesions of the conjunctiva. This virus has also been implicated in cases of squamous cell carcinoma of the conjunctiva.

40.   B)   Squamous cell carcinoma

Basal cell carcinoma is the most common malignant tumor of the eyelid skin, but squamous cell carcinoma is the most frequently occurring malignancy of the conjunctiva. Squamous papillomas are benign lesions that can, on rare occasions, undergo malignant transformation.

41. D)   The entire thickness of the epithelium may be involved.

Conjunctival intraepithelial neoplasia is the preinvasive stage of squamous cell carcinoma. By definition, there is no invasion of the basement membrane, but the entire thickness of the epithelium may be involved in conjunctival intraepithelial neoplasia (at which point it is called *carcinoma in-situ*). It invariably occurs in the interpalpebral area and is characterized by leukoplakia, thickening of the epithelium, and abnormal vascularization. Treatment is by excisional biopsy with or without supplemental cryotherapy to the base.

42. D)   Scleritis

Causes of secondary acquired conjunctival melanosis include Addison's disease, radiation, and pregnancy. Black conjunctival adrenochrome deposits result from the oxidative byproducts of epinephrine compounds.

43. C)   Figure 10-13

44. C)   Figure 10-13

45. B)   Figure 10-12

46. A)   Figure 10-11

Conjunctival malignant melanoma (Fig. 10-11) is a pigmented elevated lesion that enlarges progressively with time. It occurs most commonly on the bulbar conjunctiva. These tumors are very vascular, and dilated vessels may be seen feeding the tumor. The prognosis is generally better than cutaneous melanomas. A systemic metastatic work-up is necessary to direct treatment. Conjunctival melanomas can arise de novo (30%), from nevi (40%), or from primary acquired melanosis (30%).

A conjunctival nevus (Fig. 10-12) is a flat or slightly elevated pigmented lesion of the bulbar conjunctiva. It may have epithelial inclusion cysts within its substance. These lesions can grow or enlarge during adolescence or with pregnancy. Suspicious lesions should be biopsied to rule out melanoma.

Primary acquired melanosis (Fig. 10-14) is a unilateral condition found in middle-aged white people. These multiple, superficial, flat patches of pigmentation develop into malignant melanoma in 20% to 30% of these patients. Excisional biopsy should be performed on any suspicious nodular lesions.

Racial or ocular melanosis (Fig. 10-13) is found most commonly in pigmented individuals and represents benign collections of melanin in the conjunctiva. It appears as a perilimbal dusting of light brown pigment. No malignant potential exists.

47. D)   distant metastasis

48. A)   simple excision, leaving bare sclera

49. C)   Prolonged actinic exposure is a risk factor.

Figure 10-15 shows a pterygium of the right eye. Pterygia are wing-shaped folds of conjunctiva and fibrovascular tissue that invade the superficial cornea. The exact etiology is not known, but a strong causal relationship has been documented with ultraviolet light exposure. Destruction of Bowman's layer and changes in corneal astigmatism often occur. If inflamed, they may become hypertrophic with localized changes of the adjacent cornea, which may include punctate keratopathy and even dellen formation. Iron deposition at the leading edge of the pterygium is known as a Stocker's line. They may be observed, but excision is often indicated if the visual axis is threatened or if extreme irritation exists. The recurrence rate is significant, with approximately 40% recurring by simple excision. Conjunctival autograft and amniotic membrane graft may lower recurrence rate according to some studies. Application of mitomycin C may also prevent recurrence. These lesions are rarely malignant, and metastasis would be extremely uncommon.

50.   B)   Resection of the adjacent conjunctiva may be indicated

Figure 10-16 shows superior limbal hyperemia and mild keratitis consistent with superior limbal keratoconjunctivitis. Superior palpebral conjunctival papillary reaction, micropannus, and filaments may also be present. Rose bengal or lissamine green (Fig. 10-53) are vital dyes that highlight the affected conjunctiva. Treatment may include 0.5% to 1.0% silver nitrate solution (not a silver nitrate stick), pressure patching, mechanical scraping, conjunctival resection, or bandage contact lens. Thyroid dysfunction must be considered and thyroid function tests performed.

Reduced corneal sensation is a common finding in herpetic disease and is not associated with superior limbic keratoconjunctivitis. Floppy eyelid syndrome, which is most common in obese individuals and is characterized by easy eversion of superior tarsus and papillary response, responds well to sleeping with a protective eye shield.

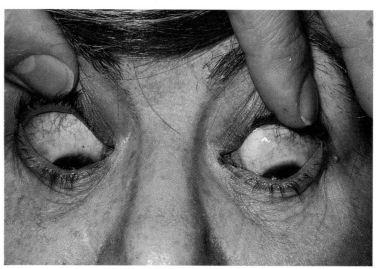

FIGURE 10-53

51.   D)   Decreased thyroid stimulating hormone

Thyroid abnormalities have been associated with superior limbic keratoconjunctivitis. A skin rash may be found in herpes simplex or zoster infections.

52. D)   Topical mast cell stabilizers or corticosteroid drops

Although *giant papillary conjunctivitis* (GPC) is historically classified as an ocular allergy, it is likely secondary to mechanical irritation. GPC does not signify a systemic allergic predisposition. It is usually associated with soft contact lenses (rarely caused by rigid gas permeable lenses), ocular prostheses, or exposed sutures. Large follicles (>1.0 mm in diameter, typically confined to the upper palpebral conjunctiva), conjunctival hyperemia, and a mucus discharge are signs associated with GPC. Limbal follicles (typically associated with vernal conjunctivitis) have also been reported. Treatment includes mast cell stabilizers, corticosteroids, improving lens hygiene, or changing contact lenses to a better-tolerated lens. If contact lens wear is discontinued, GPC generally resolves. Moxifloxacin is a fourth generation fluoroquinolone. This is not necessary because this is not an infectious condition.

53. A)   Figure 10-18M

54. C)   Figure 10-18N

55. A)   Superior limbic keratitis

The staining patterns correspond to the conditions listed:

    B = keratoconjunctivitis sicca
    D = contact lens-induced keratoconjunctivitis
    E = soft contact lens wearer
    J = superior limbic keratoconjunctivitis
    K = vernal catarrh, "floppy eyelid" syndrome
    M = lagophthalmos
    N = focal epithelial keratitis (Thygeson's, EKC, molluscum)

56. B)   lithium

Cornea verticillata is a whorl-like deposition of material in the corneal epithelium. Drugs that may cause this include amiodarone, chlorpromazine, chloroquine, indomethacin, meperidine, and tamoxifen.

57. A)   Fabry's disease

Fabry's disease is a glycolipidosis. Findings include cornea verticillata; cataracts; angiokeratomas; vascular anomalies of the heart, kidney, and brain; and burning pain in the hands and feet.

58. D)   The cystine deposits begin centrally within the anterior stroma and progress to involve the entire cornea.

In cystinosis, corneal crystals are evident in the anterior stroma and are often found on routine examination. Three forms of cystinosis are known, the infantile form being most severe with dwarfism, rickets, and renal failure. Most die before puberty, but some reach adulthood through dialysis or renal transplantation. The adolescent form is similar to, but less severe than, the infantile form, and both are autosomal recessive. Those with the adult form are usually asymptomatic and do not have the systemic findings indicated earlier. Mode of inheritance is uncertain and life expectancy is normal. All forms have in common the deposition of cystine crystals in the cornea and conjunctiva (as well as in the uveal tract).

59. D) Descemet's membrane

60. B) The corneal findings can be used to monitor therapy.

Figure 10-20 shows a Kayser-Fleischer ring in the cornea, which represents deposition of copper in the posterior lamella of Descemet's membrane. Such a ring may be seen in Wilson's disease, primary biliary cirrhosis, chronic hepatitis, or progressive intrahepatic cholestasis of childhood, but only patients with Wilson's disease will show neurologic findings. Treatment of Wilson's disease is with penicillamine, and the Kayser-Fleischer ring will disappear with appropriate treatment, thereby providing a means to monitor therapy. The defect in Wilson's disease is a decreased production of ceruloplasmin by the liver.

61. C) Trachoma

Figure 10-21 shows Herbert's pits found in trachoma. They are the scarred remnants of inflammatory nodules on the limbus. Horner-Trantas dots, seen in vernal keratoconjunctivitis, are focal limbal infiltrates of eosinophils. Staphylococcal marginal keratitis has corneal infiltrates characteristically with clear cornea between it and the limbus.

62. D) leukoplakia

Manifestations of trachoma include superior corneal pannus, conjunctival scarring, and superior conjunctival follicles. Leukoplakia is suspicious for squamous cell carcinoma of the conjunctiva.

63. B) This patient may have deposition of copper in the liver, kidneys, and brain.

Figure 10-22 shows calcific band keratopathy with a degeneration of the superficial cornea involving deposition of calcium hydroxyapatite, mainly in Bowman's layer. *Hepatolenticular degeneration,* or Wilson's disease, is associated with a Kayser-Fleischer ring in the peripheral cornea. Band keratopathy may be a hereditary condition or may be associated with chronic mercurial exposure. Other causes include chronic ocular disease, inflammation, hypercalcemia, or hyperphosphatemia.

64. A) Ethylenediaminetetraacetic acid (EDTA)

EDTA is able to chelate the calcium found in band keratopathy. It is necessary to scrape to epithelium to expose the calcium to the EDTA. Penicillamine binds heavy metal ions, such as iron, copper, and lead and may be helpful in Wilson's disease and hemochromatosis. Acetylcysteine is an anticollagenolytic agent.

65. B) Pathologically, it appears as lipid deposition in the cornea.

Spheroidal degeneration involves proteinaceous deposits in the superficial stroma that are thought to be caused, in part, by sunlight exposure. It is usually bilateral and is more common in men.

66. D) Epithelium remains intact.

Figure 10-23 shows a case of Terrien's marginal degeneration. Peripheral thinning occurs superiorly first, then circumferentially. Unlike Mooren's ulcer or peripheral ulcerative keratitis of autoimmune disease, thinning occurs with an intact epithelium in an essentially quiet eye. Thinning to perforation is rare. Against-the-rule astigmatism is often induced. Thinning that is more apparent than real is a characteristic of furrow degeneration, a benign condition that does not affect vision.

67. A)   Biopsy of the adjacent conjunctiva may show increased plasma cells.

Figure 10-24 shows a case of Mooren's ulcer. Note the conjunctival injection, ulceration of the peripheral cornea, and undermined leading edge. Pain may be severe and accompanied by photophobia. An autoimmune process likely plays a role as immunoglobulin, complement, and plasma cells are found in the adjacent conjunctiva. Two clinical types have been described. The type found in older adults is usually unilateral accompanied by mild pain, and it is more responsive to therapy such as topical steroids. Corneal perforation is rare. The other type is bilateral, often found in younger black males, and rapidly progressive. These lesions respond poorly to therapy, and systemic immunosuppressives are often necessary.

68. C)   This is a bilateral condition.

Pellucid marginal degeneration is a bilateral, nonhereditary condition. There is protrusion of the cornea above the area of maximal thinning inferiorly in the cornea, whereas in keratoconus, corneal protrusion is at the point of maximal thinning. It affects both men and women equally, and is frequently diagnosed between 20 and 40 years of age. No vascularization or lipid occurs, and vision is decreased secondary to high irregular astigmatism.

69. C)   Spontaneous perforation

The corneal topography shown is characteristic of keratoconus. Steepening inferotemporally is evident in this particular case (Fig. 10-54), but it may be inferior, inferonasal, or even central on corneal topography depending on the site of thinning and cone formation. Almost all cases are bilateral, but they may be very asymmetric with perhaps only mild astigmatism in one eye. Scissoring of the red reflex on retinoscopy is often an early sign. Deposits of iron around the base of the cone (Fleischer ring) and deep vertical stromal lines (Vogt striae) (Fig. 10-55) are also characteristic of keratoconus. Acute ruptures of Descemet's membrane or acute hydrops may occur, leading to corneal edema that often resolves spontaneously, leaving stromal scarring. Corneal perforation is rare unless associated with trauma.

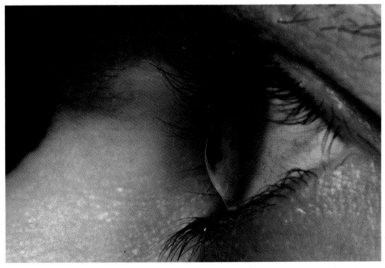

FIGURE 10-54

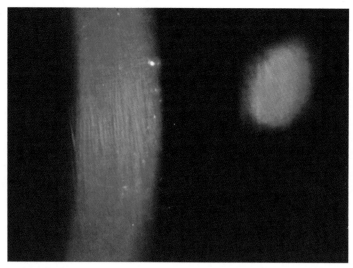

FIGURE 10-55

70.   D)   photorefractive keratectomy

Spectacle correction may be adequate in early or mild cases of keratoconus if acceptable visual acuity can be achieved. A hard contact lens will neutralize irregular astigmatism, although fitting may be difficult, especially in advanced cases with pronounced cones. If vision is unacceptable with hard contact lenses, proper fitting cannot be performed, or, if contact lens intolerance arises, penetrating keratoplasty should be considered. Prognosis for corneal transplant in these patients is excellent. Photorefractive keratectomy using the excimer laser is contraindicated in keratoconus as a result of corneal thinning and potential progression of the disease.

71.   A)   Hypertonic saline

This keratoconus patient has developed hydrops from a rupture of Descemet's membrane. Fluid from the anterior chamber can flow into the corneal stroma, causing edema and opacification. The initial therapy includes topical steroids, cycloplegics, and hypertonic saline drops.

72.   C)   It is unilateral with sporadic occurrence.

Circumscribed posterior keratoconus is seen mostly in women and is characterized by a localized central indentation of the posterior cornea with variable amounts of stromal haze. Loss of stromal substance occurs, but Descemet's membrane and endothelium are intact. Occurrence is sporadic, usually unilateral and nonprogressive. Amblyopia may occur.

73.   A)   it typically occurs in patients over age 60 years

Pellucid marginal degeneration is a noninflammatory degeneration of the peripheral cornea that usually affects the inferior cornea. It occurs most commonly in patients between the ages of 20 and 40 years and is more common in patients of European or Japanese descent. There is no gender predilection. It is a bilateral process that results in irregular, against-the-rule astigmatism. Treatment may consist of contact lenses and, eventually, penetrating keratoplasty.

74. C) The recessive form is nonprogressive, whereas the dominantly inherited form is slowly progressive.

Nystagmus is associated with the recessive, but not the dominant, form of the disease. There are no known associated ocular or systemic diseases. Corneal edema is present at birth in the recessive form, whereas corneal decompensation usually does not occur until the first or second year of life in the dominant form of the disease.

75. B) Pain, tearing, photophobia

Congenital hereditary stromal dystrophy is a rare, autosomal dominant condition presenting at birth as a central, anterior stromal feathery opacity that may cause reduced visual acuity. The corneal periphery is clear. There is no pain, photophobia, or tearing because IOP is normal.

76. A) Lattice stromal dystrophy

The most common stromal dystrophy is lattice, followed by granular. Meesmann dystrophy is a very rare epithelial dystrophy.

77. C) Acid mucopolysaccharides

78. B) The disease is caused by a defect in the synthesis of keratan sulfate.

Figure 10-27 shows *macular corneal dystrophy,* the least common of the classic stromal dystrophies. It usually leads to symptoms at an earlier age than either lattice or granular dystrophy and is caused by an error in the synthesis of keratan sulfate, leading to unsulfated keratan that is not degraded effectively. These mucopolysaccharide deposits accumulate throughout the cornea (including the periphery) and stain with colloidal iron and alcian blue.

79. D) Skin findings and nerve palsies are manifestations of systemic involvement.

80. C) alcian blue

Lattice corneal dystrophy, shown in Figure 10-28, is an autosomal dominantly inherited corneal dystrophy that consists of amyloid deposition into the anterior corneal stroma, which is best seen by retroillumination. There are two recognized forms of the disease: type I is localized to the cornea, and type II (Meretoja syndrome) involves widespread deposition of amyloid and results in systemic findings such as dry, lax skin; cranial nerve palsies; abnormal ears; and a mask facies. Lattice dystrophy is a frequent cause of recurrent erosion because the amyloid deposition in the anterior stroma leads to weak adherence of the epithelium to Bowman's layer. Amyloid stains with Congo red, metachromatically with crystal violet, and also with thioflavin T. It also exhibits birefringence and dichroism under the polarized microscope.

81. C) recurrent erosions are common

Recurrent erosions are uncommon in granular dystrophy as opposed to lattice dystrophy, in which they occur much more frequently. *Granular dystrophy* is an autosomal dominant inherited disease that occurs early in life, although symptoms do not usually occur until years later. In macular corneal dystrophy, the intervening cornea is cloudy, whereas in granular dystrophy, it remains clear. Masson trichrome stains the hyaline deposits vividly.

82.   C)   Both

83.   C)   Both

84.   D)   Neither

85.   A)   Figure 10-29

86.   D)   Neither

	Lattice	Granular	Macular
Inheritance	Autosomal dominant	Autosomal dominant	Autosomal recessive
Symptoms	Recurrent epithelial erosions	Mild irritation	Severely decreased vision
Appearance	Lattice lines, dots and flakes, clear between opacities	Dusting of "bread crumbs," clear stroma between opacities	Indistinct grey opacities, cloudy intervening stroma
Material	Amyloid deposition	Hyaline	Mucopolysaccharide
Typical stain	Congo red	Masson trichrome	Alcian blue
Recurrence in grafts	Yes	Yes	Yes

87.   B)   The lesions are among the most common to recur after penetrating keratoplasty.

This is a case of *Reis-Bucklers' dystrophy,* an autosomal dominant, progressive dystrophy. Symptoms often develop in adulthood and include painful recurrent erosions and decreased visual acuity. Lesions occur at the level of Bowman's layer. Treatment may include superficial keratectomy, excimer laser phototherapeutic keratectomy, or penetrating keratoplasty. Recurrence in the graft is common in both Reis-Bucklers' dystrophy and lattice dystrophy.

88.   A)   disruption and absence of Bowman's layer

Histopathology shows replacement of Bowman's layer by a fibrocellular tissue. "Peculiar substance" is found in epithelial cells in Meesmann dystrophy. Amyloid exhibits birefringence and dichroism when viewed under a polarizing microscope. Oil red O stain is used to stain the stromal opacities made of cholesterol in Schnyder's crystalline dystrophy.

89. C)   it occurs as a unilateral disease

Anterior membrane (map-dot-fingerprint) dystrophy of the cornea occurs bilaterally but may be asymmetric. It may be dominantly inherited. Characteristic clinical findings consist of cystic, geographic, or fingerprint formations that may be seen with sclerotic scatter or retroillumination. Pathologic findings consist of thickened basement membrane, abnormal epithelial cells with microcysts, and fibrillar material between the basement membrane and Bowman's layer. Symptoms typically occur between the fourth and sixth decades of life. Treatment options include topical lubricants, 5% sodium chloride, scraping, patching, anterior stromal puncture, or possibly phototherapeutic keratectomy.

90. A)   Multilaminar Descemet's membrane studded with excrescences

Patients with Fuchs' endothelial dystrophy have malfunctioning Na-K ATPase pumps in the lateral cell wall of the endothelial cells. This diminished pump function results in swelling of the corneal stroma. Cytochrome oxidase is also reduced, which may indicate a decrease in the metabolic activity of the endothelial mitochondria. Histologic examination would reveal a multilaminar Descemet's membrane studded with excrescences (Fig. 10-56). This abnormal tissue is a nonspecific response. As the disease progresses, specular microscopy may demonstrate a more pleomorphic endothelium with a reduction of endothelial cell density.

   Pigment deposition in the trabecular meshwork could result in elevated IOP and corneal edema. Descemet's breaks with keratoconus or birth trauma would be apparent as discrete lines visible on retroillumination.

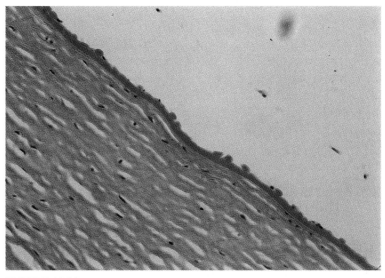

FIGURE 10-56

91. C)   Specular microscopy

Fuchs' endothelial dystrophy is an autosomal dominant (variable) corneal dystrophy that usually affects postmenopausal women. Clinical findings may include corneal guttae and Descemet's folds. In more advanced disease with endothelial decompensation, stromal, epithelial edema, and epithelial bullae may be present.

There is polymegathism and pleomorphism of the corneal endothelial cells with excrescences and thickening of Descemet's membrane best evaluated using specular microscopy. Symptoms are usually worse in the morning as a result of decreased surface evaporation during sleep. Similar findings can be duplicated by having the patient patch his or her affected eye for several hours. Pachymetry demonstrates thickening of the central cornea but does not indicate the etiology.

92. A)   Bandage contact lens may be used to treat ruptured bullae.

Treatment measures are aimed at limiting visual dysfunction and discomfort due to epithelial breakdown and ruptured bullae. Hypertonic solutions and ointments may provide some relief, but they do little when the edema is advanced. Some feel that lowering IOP may help control edema. Both hypertonic solutions and IOP-lowering agents, however, are only temporizing measures and are not long-term solutions. Ruptured bullae may be treated with patching or bandage contact lens. Penetrating keratoplasty carries a good prognosis in these patients. Anterior stromal puncture is not indicated in Fuchs' dystrophy, but it may be helpful in treating cases of recurrent erosion.

93. A)   retained viscoelastic material within the anterior chamber

Corneal edema following cataract surgery can be due to a number of factors. In Figure 10-34, there are prominent Descemet's and deep stromal folds rather than microcystic corneal edema. Injury to the endothelial cells or to Descemet's membrane are to be implicated. Retained viscoelastic would cause an elevation in IOP and the development of corneal bullae and microcystic edema on the epithelial surface.

94. A)   Meesmann dystrophy

All of these autosomal dominant dystrophies, except Meesmann dystrophy, have been linked to chromosome 5q31. *Meesmann dystrophy* involves thickened epithelium and basement membrane, with epithelial cells containing an electron-dense accumulation of "peculiar substance." *Reis-Buckler dystrophy* is a progressive dystrophy that affects Bowman's layer. *Avellino* (granular-lattice) dystrophy has hyaline deposits typical of granular dystrophy and amyloid deposits typical of lattice dystrophy seen.

95. D)   best treated by excimer laser phototherapeutic keratectomy

Salzmann's nodular degeneration is associated with many conditions, including trachoma, keratitis associated with rosacea, map-dot-fingerprint dystrophy, and vernal keratoconjunctivitis. These midperipheral, gray–blue subepithelial nodules gradually appear with chronic inflammation. After the inflammation subsides, these nodules persist. Histologically, there may be a nodular collagenous material between the epithelium and the intact Bowman's layer. This may allow for a cleavage plane during removal. Treatments include superficial keratectomy and lamellar keratoplasty. Excimer laser phototherapeutic keratectomy can be performed, but it is not first-line treatment.

96. C)   Discontinue her fluoroquinolone drop.

Figure 10-36 shows the precipitation of ciprofloxacin onto the corneal surface after cataract surgery. Corneal deposits do not result from the use of other fluoroquinolones. Disruption of the epithelial surface may permit the deposits to accumulate more easily. Discontinuation of the ciprofloxacin drops will allow the deposits to slowly resolve.

A bacterial or fungal infection would be very unusual in such a quiet eye. This may be confused with a shield ulcer from limbal-vernal keratoconjunctivitis, but the shield ulcer has a grayish stromal base with an overlying epithelial defect.

97. A) corneal sensation is reduced

Thygeson's superficial punctate keratitis is a bilateral (although it may be asymmetrical) disease consisting of a course punctate keratitis without an accompanying conjunctivitis. These lesions may or may not stain with fluorescein. Corneal sensation is normal. It is very responsive to topical corticosteroids, but this may increase the rate of recurrence. Topical cyclosporine may be beneficial. No clear etiology has been established, but a viral etiology has been postulated (although antiviral medications have not proven beneficial). People possessing the histocompatibility antigen HLA-DR3 have a 5.65 greater relative risk of having Thygeson's superficial punctate keratitis.

98. C) débridement

This is a typical photograph of adenovirus keratoconjunctivitis; serotypes 8, 11, and 19 are the most common causative agents. Therapy is mainly supportive. Cool compresses and lubrication can be recommended as can topical vasoconstrictors. There is little evidence to support the use of topical antibiotics. The use of topical steroids is controversial and is only indicated for the presence of a conjunctival membrane or pseudomembrane, marked foreign body sensation and chemosis, and reduced vision due to the epithelial and subepithelial keratitis. Débridement is not necessary for this condition.

99. C) *Staphylococcus aureus*

100. A) Blepharitis

101. A) Prednisolone acetate

Figure 10-39 shows a staphylococcal marginal infiltrate, which is thought to be caused by a hypersensitivity to staphylococcal exotoxins. The subepithelial infiltrate typically has a lucent area separating it from the limbus. The epithelium overlying the infiltrate may break down, causing many of the patient's symptoms. Patients commonly have blepharitis and meibomitis. Mild steroid drops (prednisolone 0.125%) effect quick resolution. A combination antibiotic and steroid drop is often an excellent choice. Slight corneal thinning and vascularization may be the only remnants of a previous episode.

102. D) *Haemophilus influenzae*

Figure 10-40 shows severe infectious keratitis; this clinical picture may be caused by many bacteria, such as *S. aureus, S. epidermidis,* and *P. aeruginosa*. Most bacteria require a break or disruption of the corneal epithelium to gain access and subsequent adherence to the underlying cornea. Hemophilus is one organism that can invade intact epithelium and establish infection. Other bacteria that do not require epithelial disruption include *Neisseria* spp., *Corynebacterium* spp., and *Listeria* spp.

103. D)   Disciform keratitis

Conjunctival injection, a large epithelial defect, and corneal infiltrate are present in Figure 10-41. Infectious keratitis, bacterial infection, and fungal infection should be considered. A noninfectious or sterile keratitis, such as that from topical anesthetic abuse, should also be considered. Disciform keratitis clinically shows corneal stromal edema, underlying keratic precipitates, and mild to moderate iridocyclitis. It is classically described in cases of herpes simplex, but it may also be seen in herpes zoster, mumps, varicella, and possibly chemical injury.

104. C)   corneal biopsy

Corneal smears and cultures would help identify an infectious etiology. However, a negative culture would not rule out an infectious cause. The patient should be questioned about the use of any topical medication other than those prescribed. In this case, the patient admitted to the use of topical proparacaine every 30 minutes. Topical anesthetics are known to be toxic to the corneal epithelium and can cause a nonhealing epithelial defect, stromal infiltrate, hypopyon, and corneal perforation with loss of the eye. Clinical suspicion is critical in making this diagnosis. Testing corneal sensation may be helpful in a significantly abnormal case. Corneal biopsy is not indicated at this time, but it may be needed if the other diagnostic tests are unrevealing.

105. C)   Both

106. C)   Both

107. B)   Herpes zoster keratitis

108. A)   Herpes simplex keratitis

109. C)   Both

A number of features are shared between dendritic infection from HSV and herpes zoster virus (HZV). Both may have an accompanying skin rash (along a dermatome in HZV) and corneal anesthesia. The active viral replication causes sloughing of epithelial cells in HSV, whereas in HZV, the epithelial cells are swollen and heaped up. Both conditions may recur. Iritis and elevation in IOP can be found with both viral infections; however, iris atrophy is more common with HZV.

110. D)   It is an indicator of elevation of systemic lipid levels.

Cholesterol and neutral fats accumulate in crystalline flecks in the corneal stroma in Schnyder's crystalline corneal dystrophy. The patients have excellent acuity despite a dense collection crystals in the visual axis. Recurrence in penetrating keratoplasties is possible. Although some patients have elevated lipid levels in association with this condition, the crystals are not indicative of a particular lipid level. Schnyder's can be found in patients with normal lipid profiles as well.

111. B)   Edges of these lesions stain with rose bengal.

Pictured is dendritic keratitis caused by HSV. The previous episode of redness may have represented primary ocular herpes, which usually lasts only a few days. The duration of dendritic keratitis is approximately 3 weeks, followed by resolution. Topical antiviral therapy is most commonly used for treatment to speed recovery, but simple débridement may be effective. Histopathology shows intranuclear inclusion bodies (Lipschütz bodies or Cowdry type A inclusions). Intracytoplasmic inclusions are present in Chlamydia.

Epithelial cells bordering dendritic lesions are devitalized and laden with virus, staining well with rose bengal; this is in contrast to pseudodendritic lesions of herpes zoster, which stain poorly.

112. A)   oral acyclovir will expedite recovery

Figure 10-43 shows disciform keratitis, in this case, secondary to HSV infection. Topical steroid therapy decreases the inflammatory response but may prolong disease activity, and tapering off steroids may be difficult. For this reason, peripheral lesions without significant neovascularization and central lesions that allow good visual acuity may be best untreated. When treatment is necessary, the lowest effective topical steroid dose is used, and most agree that a dose of prednisolone acetate 1% used more than once a day should be accompanied by a topical antiviral agent drop for drop. The Herpetic Eye Disease Study showed that no statistical or clinically significant benefit resulted from systemic acyclovir in patients receiving concomitant topical corticosteroids and antivirals with regard to treatment failure, resolution of keratitis, time to resolution, or 6-month best-corrected visual acuity. However, more patients in the acyclovir group had improvement in visual acuity after 6 months.

113. D)   Simple mechanical débridement may be curative when confined to the corneal epithelium.

The history described is classic for acanthamoeba keratitis. Patients often are contact lens wearers who clean their lenses with homemade solutions or tap water. Other risk factors include corneal trauma, direct exposure to soil, and exposure to standing water (well water, ponds, lakes). Pain commonly accompanies acanthamoeba keratitis but is often out of proportion to the clinical exam. Figure 10-41 shows a ring infiltrate corneal ulcer, a characteristic but late finding. Early stages may show small epithelial cysts, whereas late stages may show suppurative ulceration with hypopyon. More prominent corneal nerves, because of perineural infiltration, are a feature of this infection but are not pathognomonic. These free-living protozoans may grow well on standard media (blood and chocolate agar); however, they grow best on nonnutrient agar overlaid with *Escherichia coli* or *Enterococcus*. Various stains may allow identification with light microscopy, and confocal microscopy can be used to visualize the organisms in vivo. Figure 10-57 shows the appearance of cysts on a wet mount prep. Treatment includes simple débridement if infection is limited to the epithelium. Topical agents, including neomycin, propamidine, miconazole, polyhexamethylene biguanide, chlorhexidine, and oral ketoconazole, may be of benefit. More severe infections may require corneal transplantation but may be complicated by recurrences in the graft.

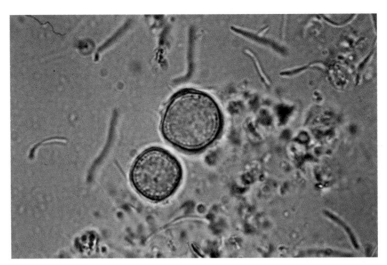

FIGURE 10-57

114. B)   double-walled cysts

Corneal ulceration in a contact lens wearer is most commonly caused by Gram-negative rods, especially *Pseudomonas* spp. In this case, however, acanthamoeba is the infectious agent, and the double-walled cyst form or the trophozoite is seen in corneal biopsy. Acid-fast pleomorphic rods may be *Mycobacterium* spp., which rarely cause keratitis. Branching hyphae are seen in fungal infections, and branching filaments may be found in infections caused by *Nocardia* spp. and *Actinomyces* spp.

115. B)   topical cefazolin

Pictured is a *Pseudomonas aeruginosa* corneal ulcer in a contact lens wearer. Initial antimicrobial therapy should provide broad-spectrum coverage for both Gram-positive and Gram-negative microbes. Combination therapy with a cephalosporin or vancomycin for Gram-positive coverage and an aminogylcoside (tobramycin or gentamicin) provide excellent coverage. Monotherapy with fourth generation fluoroquinolones (moxifloxacin and gatifloxacin) is also used. They have shown to provide coverage against both Gram-positive and Gram-negative microbes. Monotherapy with a cephalosporin (cefazolin) does not provide adequate Gram-negative coverage.

116. A)   Congenital syphilis

Tuberculosis, herpes simplex, and acquired syphilis would more likely cause a unilateral interstitial keratitis. Congenital syphilis causes a bilateral interstitial keratitis that may not become manifest until the patient is 10–20 years of age. Cogan's syndrome affects middle-aged adults with hearing loss, vertigo, and interstitial keratitis.

117. D)   Bell's palsy

Figure 10-46 shows a cornea with severe punctate epithelial erosions in the exposed interpalpebral area, such as that seen with exposure keratopathy. Causes for this include lagophthalmos, Bell's palsy, proptosis with incomplete closure of the lids, ectropion. The incomplete blink leaves the inferior third of the cornea exposed and dry. *Sjögren's syndrome* is a global dry eye state with decreased mucin production by the goblet cells and decreased tear production. It would appear as drying of the whole cornea. A chemical splash also would affect more of the cornea than is pictured here.

118. A)   Tarsorrhaphy

A tarsorrhaphy would be an excellent treatment to help close the lids and reduce the area that remains exposed. A contact lens would not be tolerated in this dry eye. Penetrating keratoplasties in dry eyes such as this have high rates of failure. Anterior stromal micropuncture may be useful for patients with recurrent erosions.

119. C)   corneal scarring and vascularization are successfully treated with penetrating keratoplasty

120. A)   Dapsone

Pictured in Figure 10-47 are conjunctival scarring and symblepharon formation caused by ocular cicatricial pemphigoid. Patients often present with symptoms of dry eyes and nonspecific erythema. Extraocular mucosal and skin lesions are common. Subconjunctival fibrosis and symblepharon formation are important findings. Severe dry eyes, corneal scarring, and vascularization develop. Conjunctival scrapings show lymphocytes, plasma cells, and eosinophils. Immunopathology from conjunctival biopsy specimens show deposits of IgA along the basement membrane zone. It is imperative to question the use of topical ocular preparations when encountering this clinical picture. Other causes of cicatrizing conjunctivitis or pemphigoid-like presentation include the use of antivirals, miotics (both direct and indirect), epinephrine, and timolol. Differential diagnosis also includes chemical burns, radiation treatment, ocular rosacea, and the Stevens-Johnson syndrome. Strictly monocular findings may be postsurgical, but they should also raise suspicion of conjunctival carcinoma. Treatment includes oral dapsone therapy with systemic prednisone for acute exacerbations. Cyclophosphamide may be beneficial when treatment failure or intolerance develops with dapsone. Because this is due to a systemic autoimmune disease, topical cyclosporine will be of limited benefit.

121. D)   Staphylococcal hypersensitivity

Staphylococcal hypersensitivity may cause irritation, corneal infiltrates, and a localized conjunctivitis. It does not result in conjunctival scarring.

122. D)   floppy eyelid syndrome

Filaments are strands of mucus and epithelial cells that have not been sloughed by the blinking action of the lids. They can be found in many dry eye states, with prolonged patching, and in conditions such as superior limbic keratoconjunctivitis. Floppy eyelid syndrome would have a papillary conjunctival reaction. Filaments are not associated with this condition.

123. B)   Long-term steroids are helpful.

Figure 10-49 shows a corneal epithelial defect. In a cornea with markedly abnormal sensation without trauma, this defect most likely represents neurotrophic keratitis.

This condition is caused by trigeminal nerve palsy or inflammation, especially the ophthalmic division. Causes include herpes simplex or zoster, surgery, strokes, and tumors. Evidence of herpetic etiology includes a previous history of a red eye with or without pain, shingles, lid and/or conjunctival scarring, corneal stromal haze or scarring, endothelial keratic precipitates, iritis, and sectoral iris atrophy.

An oval epithelial defect is usually present in the inferior half of the cornea with rolled, thickened edges. Chronic defects may be accompanied by stromal loss. Treatment includes lubricants, antibiotic prophylaxis, patching, or lid taping. Bandage contact lenses may be considered but must be used with caution. Punctal occlusion may be beneficial. Chronic inflammation at the level of the epithelial basement membrane may inhibit complete healing of the epithelial defect; therefore, low-dose topical steroids may promote healing in some cases. However, steroids must be used with great caution as they may potentiate collagenase activity and corneal thinning. Therefore, they are generally not indicated. Tarsorrhaphy may be necessary in refractory cases, especially in those with markedly abnormal corneal sensation and lid disorders.

124. D)   All of the above

For a traumatic hyphema with normal IOP, observation is appropriate with the modalities to reduce the risk of a rebleed; this includes bed rest, elevation of the head, and patching of the eyes to reduce eye movement. Oral aminocaproic acid may also be helpful to prevent a rebleed. In black patients, a sickle cell prep is essential.

125. A)   Anterior chamber washout

If IOP is elevated in hyphema and there are no signs of corneal blood staining, medical management of the IOP is appropriate. A carbonic anhydrase inhibitor may not be the best agent to lower IOP with the possibility of sickle cell in a black patient. If the IOP still remains elevated and/or signs of corneal blood staining appear, then surgical intervention is necessary with an anterior chamber washout. Intracameral t-PA may be able to lyse the clot; however, the blood breakdown products will still remain in the anterior chamber, and the IOP will be unaffected.

126. D)   Fleck dystrophy

Superficial phototherapeutic keratectomy uses the excimer laser to ablate the superficial layers of the cornea (epithelium, Bowman's layer, or superficial stroma) to remove dystrophic or scarred tissue. Granular and Reis-Buckler dystrophies are associated with recurrent erosions, which are treated by superficial keratectomy or phototherapeutic keratectomy. Epithelial basement membrane dystrophy (also called *map-dot-fingerprint* or *Cogan microcystic dystrophy*) is an abnormality in epithelial maturation, turnover, and production of basement membrane. Removal of damaged epithelium and anterior basement membrane is effective and can be done with phototherapeutic keratectomy. Fleck dystrophy is a nonprogressive, usually asymptomatic stromal dystrophy with gray-white opacities in the stroma. The epithelium, Bowman's layer, Descemet's membrane, and endothelium are not affected.

127. D)   Severe uveitis and glaucoma may occur.

Chemical injury with acid substances causes denaturation and precipitation of proteins, which limits ocular penetration. Alkali burns, in contrast, penetrate the globe rapidly with progressive damage. Symblepharon formation, severe uveitis, anterior segment neovascularization, glaucoma, and cataract are all later complications. Burns at the limbus carry a particularly poor prognosis because of potential ischemia and growth of neovascular tissue.

128. C) topical steroids are used long-term to decrease the inflammatory response

Copious irrigation should be started immediately. Débridement of necrotic conjunctiva and particulate matter should be performed as they may harbor more chemical. pH testing of the conjunctival fornices is helpful during and after irrigation. Patching or bandage contact lens may be used to aid in healing epithelium with antibiotic prophylaxis. Topical steroids are useful to suppress the inflammatory response; however, their use should be limited to the first 7 days after injury as they may potentiate the action of collagenases leading to continued stromal loss. Cicatricial lid changes should be repaired before penetrating keratoplasty.

129. C) Pupillary exam

Although an integral part of any eye exam, the pupillary exam would add little clinical information. The most likely diagnoses include episcleritis, conjunctivitis (allergic and viral), scleritis, anterior uveitis, and trauma.

130. C) Topical antibiotics

The clinical entity pictured in Figure 10-52 is episcleritis. Although it is usually self-limited, if symptoms warrant, topical steroids, lubricants, or oral nonsteroidals are reasonable therapies. Topical antibiotics are not necessary or helpful given the noninfectious nature of the process. If purulent drainage or other signs of infection are present, culture and then appropriate coverage with antimicrobial agents are necessary.

131. B) Necrotizing scleritis with inflammation

The most benign form of scleritis is diffuse anterior. In necrotizing scleritis with inflammation, 60% develop complications such as keratitis, cataract, uveitis, and scleral thinning, and 40% suffer visual loss. Many patients with this process die within a few years of diagnosis secondary to severe systemic autoimmune diseases, such as rheumatoid arthritis, polyarteritis nodosa, and Wegener's granulomatosis.

132. D) Behçet's disease

Scleritis has been associated with infectious diseases (syphilis, tuberculosis, herpes zoster, and leprosy), autoimmune diseases (rheumatoid arthritis, Wegener's granulomatosis, systemic lupus erythematosus, and polyarteritis nodosa), and metabolic diseases (gout).

133. A) Posterior sub-Tenon's steroid injection

Injection of steroids into sub-Tenon's space is contraindicated because it may increase the risk of scleral thinning and melting. Initial management is usually with an oral NSAID agent followed by systemic steroids and topical cyclosporine. Eventually, systemic immunosuppressives with azathioprine or methotrexate may be necessary.

134. A)   Shield ulcer

Several ocular surface disorders result from an abnormality of the limbal stem cells. Acquired disorders include injuries, both chemical and thermal, contact lens induced superior limbal keratoconjunctivitis, and Stevens-Johnson syndrome. Some hereditary etiologies include keratitis associated with multiple endocrine deficiencies and bilateral aniridia. Shield ulcers occur with limbal–vernal keratoconjunctivitis. No limbal stem cell deficiency is present with this condition.

135. D)   hypoventilation during general anesthesia

Reduction of positive vitreous pressure is important during most intraocular surgeries, especially "open sky" procedures such as penetrating keratoplasty. Intraoperative maneuvers to reduce vitreous pressure include reducing vitreous volume by aspiration or dehydration (IV mannitol) and removing pressure on the globe. Hyperventilation, rather than hypoventilation, also can be used during cases under general anesthesia to decrease vitreous pressure.

136. D)   Possible microbial contamination

Corneal storage medium often contains colorimetric pH indicators. Such a color change indicates a change in pH, which may be consistent with microbial contamination.

137. C)   Pseudophakic bullous keratopathy

Pseudophakic bullous keratopathy is the most frequent indication for penetrating keratoplasty in adults. This condition may decline in the future because of improvements in the design of anterior chamber and iris-fixated IOLs and in phacoemulsification techniques. Regrafts and keratoconus are also frequent indications for keratoplasty.

138. C)   Peters' anomaly

Peters' anomaly is the most frequent indication for penetrating keratoplasty in children.

139. A)   oversized grafts

Penetrating keratoplasty in children can be very challenging. The eye wall is extremely flaccid, and scleral support is often crucial. Anterior bulging of the lens–iris diaphragm is common, and many surgeons prefer to use a small-sized graft to reduce this problem as well as to reduce the chance of peripheral synechiae formation. Frequent postoperative follow-up and early suture removal (as early as 2 to 4 weeks postoperatively in neonates) help reduce the incidence of neovascularization of the graft.

140. C)   slow or delayed healing

Corneal transplants in children and young adults heal very quickly with sutures becoming vascularized and loosening within the first several months. Glaucoma and graft rejection are possible just as in adult transplants. In very young children, amblyopia presents a very real and difficult challenge. Fitting these children with contact lenses may restore vision more quickly and lessen the degree of amblyopia that develops. In addition to the previous complications, self-induced trauma is a frequent problem.

141. A)   90%

Corneal graft survival is excellent with current techniques. The incidence is even higher for conditions such as keratoconus.

142. B)   65%

Graft clarity is often higher for noninflamed eyes. Therefore, penetrating keratoplasty should be delayed until the eye is quiet (if possible).

143. C)   20%

Overall, the chance of an endothelial graft rejection episode is 20% to 25% according to most studies. If the rejection is recognized early, intensive treatment may save the graft from failure.

144. C)   ABO blood type incompatibility was shown to be a possible risk factor

The most interesting conclusion of this study was that even for high-risk keratoplasties, HLA tissue matching was neither clearly advantageous nor cost-effective. The possibility also existed of a correlation of risk and ABO blood type incompatibility. Further study is needed to decide whether this is a necessary screening test.

145. D)   all of the above

Patients with connective tissue disorders, traumatic or hereditary epithelial surface disorders, poorly controlled blepharitis or keratoconjunctivitis sicca, and unrealistic expectations are also poor candidates.

146. B)   21 days

Most contact lens wearers are very reluctant to discontinue use of their lenses for any significant amount of time. Stability of refraction and topography are important when deciding on a surgical plan. Most surgeons require at least 2 to 3 weeks of a contact lens "holiday" to verify stability. Some individuals require a longer period before they show stability.

147. B)   8 incisions

The addition of 8 incisions to an 8-incision radial keratotomy will often add little more myopic effect and may lead to more problems with corneal destabilization, wound gape, and, potentially, an increased risk of progressive hyperopia. Also, it is technically difficult to make such incisions sufficiently deep and uniform after placing the first 8.

148. B)   90°

Most surgeons will rarely perform arcuate incisions greater than 90° because of decreased efficacy and increased instability of effect.

149. A) HLA-A, HLA-B, and HLA-DR matching the donor and recipient had no effect on overall graft survival.

The Collaborative Corneal Transplantation Studies are a set of multicenter trials that investigated the efficacy of matching the donor-recipient HLAs on the incidence of graft rejection and graft survival in high-risk recipients undergoing penetrating keratoplasty. Matching HLA-A, HLA-B, and HLA-DR had no effect on overall graft survival or on the incidence of irreversible graft rejection. It is uncertain whether ABO blood group matching may reduce the risk of graft rejection. Matching donor-recipient age was not evaluated. These are being further studied in the ongoing Cornea Donor Study. Suturing technique and visual outcomes were not evaluated in the Collaborative Corneal Transplant Study.

150. D) Temporal

The inferotemporal quadrant is the thinnest in most patients (38%). Of the provided choices, the thinnest quadrants (in descending order) are the temporal (28%), inferior (19%), nasal (11%), and superior (4%). Variation exists in individual patients; therefore, multiple paracentral measurements are important to determine the thinnest region. Determination of the thinnest paracentral corneal measurement is used to set the blade depth for radial keratotomy as well as to determine which quadrant to incise first.

Notes

Notes

11

Lens/Cataract

QUESTIONS

Questions 1–5 Pertain to Figures 11-1 to 11-6.

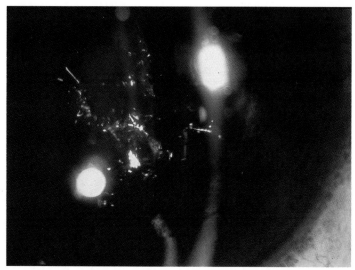

FIGURE 11-1

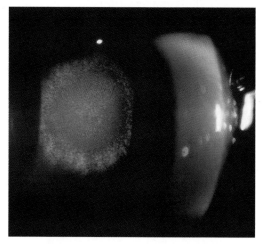

FIGURE 11-2

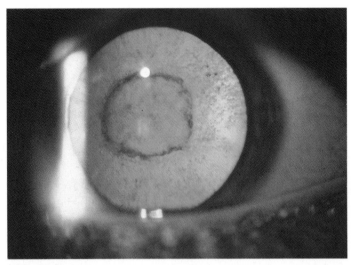

FIGURE 11-3

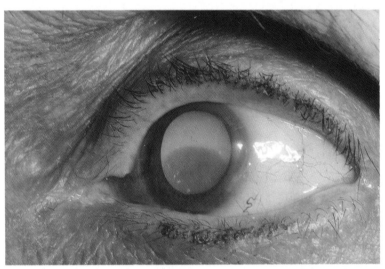

FIGURE 11-4

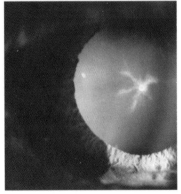

FIGURE 11-5

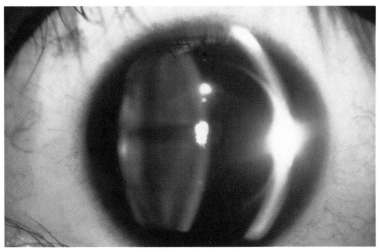

FIGURE 11-6. From Wright K. Textbook of ophthalmology. Baltimore: Williams & Wilkins, 1997.

1. Which cataract is associated with the long-term use of corticosteroids?

    A) Figure 11-3
    B) Figure 11-2
    C) Figure 11-6
    D) Figure 11-4

2. Which can be found in a patient with deafness and hemorrhagic nephritis?

    A) Figure 11-4
    B) Figure 11-2
    C) Figure 11-5
    D) Figure 11-6

3. A patient has the cataract pictured in Figure 11-2. Which is NOT a true statement about this patient?

    A) A Kayser-Fleischer ring can be found on the cornea.
    B) The cataract was caused by iron deposits in the anterior lens capsule.
    C) Patients may also have involvement of their liver and brain.
    D) The cataract is not usually visually significant.

4. What additional finding might be seen in the patient with the cataract displayed in Figure 11-1?

    A) Elevated blood sugar
    B) Muscle weakness
    C) Angle closure glaucoma
    D) Keratic precipitates

5. Which cataract might be found in a 1-month-old infant?

    A) Figure 11-5
    B) Figure 11-3
    C) Figure 11-6
    D) Figure 11-1

6. The lens finding shown in Figure 11-4 is due to

   A) traumatic injury
   B) systemic metabolic disease
   C) radiation damage
   D) advanced mature lens changes

7. Which of the following is NOT associated with retained lens nuclei?

   A) Trisomy 13
   B) Rubella
   C) Peters' anomaly
   D) Lowe's syndrome

8. Which of the following types of cataracts is classically associated with myotonic dystrophy?

   A) Nuclear cataract
   B) Polychromatic crystalline cataract
   C) Posterior subcapsular cataract
   D) Anterior polar cataract

9. A 5-year-old white boy presents with difficulty seeing the blackboard at school. Upon examination, he is found to be highly myopic. He is short of stature and has short stubby fingers with broad hands and tight joints. Which of the following is MOST likely?

   A) Prone to angle closure glaucoma aggravated by the administration of pilocarpine
   B) Prone to angle closure glaucoma aggravated by the administration of a cycloplegic
   C) Normal appearing parents
   D) Higher risk of lens dislocation with minor trauma

10. Which of the following test acuity by means of contrast sensitivity?

    A) Pelli-Robson chart
    B) Purkinje vascular phenomenon
    C) PAM (Potential Acuity Meter)
    D) Blue-field entoptic test

11. When did the cataract in Figure 11-7 develop?

    A) Between birth and 2 years of age
    B) During adolescence
    C) In utero
    D) Over age 40

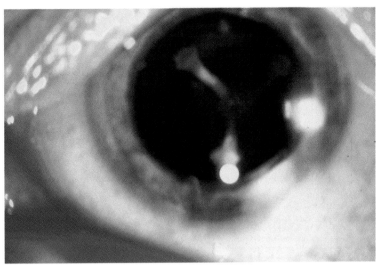

FIGURE 11-7

12. Which of the following is CORRECT concerning drug-induced cataracts?

   A) Amiodarone causes stellate anterior axial pigment deposition.
   B) Phenothiazine causes pigment deposition in the posterior lens capsule.
   C) Prolonged treatment of eyelid dermatitis with topical steroids does not cause cataracts.
   D) Echothiophate use in children causes progressive cataract formation.

Questions 13–14

13. Which of the following would LEAST likely be associated with the eyes shown in Figure 11-8?

   A) Long, spider-like fingers
   B) Nonprogressive lens subluxation
   C) Low risk of retinal detachment
   D) Abnormality in fibrillin

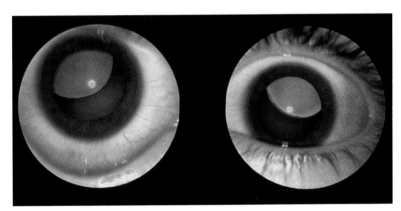

FIGURE 11-8

14. Which of the following would be the MOST appropriate initial management in the patient in Figure 11-8?

    A) Immediate surgical removal of the lens
    B) Spectacle or contact lens correction of the refractive error
    C) No treatment because there is only a low risk of amblyopia
    D) Pilocarpine to constrict the pupil

Questions 15–16

15. The following are characteristics of the condition shown in Figure 11-9 EXCEPT:

    A) prone to angle closure glaucoma
    B) progressive cataract formation
    C) unilateral process
    D) autosomal dominant inheritance

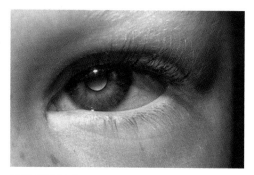

FIGURE 11-9. From Wright K. Textbook of ophthalmology. Baltimore: Williams & Wilkins, 1997.

16. Differential diagnosis of the patient in Figure 11-9 includes all of the following EXCEPT:

    A) retinoblastoma
    B) retinopathy of prematurity
    C) homocystinuria
    D) Coats' disease

17. A 6-month-old infant presents with unilateral, complete cataracts. There is no family history of eye disease. Which would be LEAST helpful in determining the etiology?

    A) TORCH (toxoplasmosis, other agents, rubella, cytomegalovirus, herpes simplex) titers and syphilis serology
    B) B-scan ultrasonography
    C) Chromosomal analysis
    D) Urine protein and reducing substances

18. Regarding age-related cataracts, which is CORRECT concerning the following histopathologic changes?

    A) Posterior subcapsular cataract—morgagnian globules
    B) Cortical cataracts—Wedl (bladder) cells
    C) Nuclear sclerotic cataracts—homogenous, loss of cellular laminations
    D) Elschnig pearls—proliferation of lens capsule

Questions 19–20

19. A 10-year-old boy presents with bilateral, symmetric findings. His left eye is pictured in Figure 11-10. He is tall with blond hair. Both of his parents appear normal. Which of the following is LEAST likely to be found in this patient?

    A) Mental retardation
    B) Osteoporosis
    C) Decreased serum levels of methionine
    D) Increased of thromboembolism with surgery and general anesthesia

20. Which would be appropriate therapy for this patient (Fig. 11-10)?

    A) Vitamin A
    B) Coenzyme Q
    C) Vitamin B_6
    D) Low phenylalanine diet

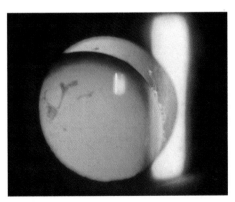

FIGURE 11-10

21. Which of the following concerning polar cataracts is CORRECT?

    A) Anterior polar cataracts usually cause more visual disturbance than posterior polar cataracts.
    B) Posterior polar cataracts have been associated with remnants of the tunica vasculosa lentis.
    C) Both anterior and posterior polar cataracts can be sporadic or recessively inherited.
    D) Posterior polar cataracts invariably progress to complete cataracts.

Questions 22–23

22. Complications during or after cataract surgery in the patient shown in Figure 11-11 will likely be due to:

    A) severe postoperative inflammation
    B) zonular dehiscence
    C) corneal decompensation
    D) retention of viscoelastic

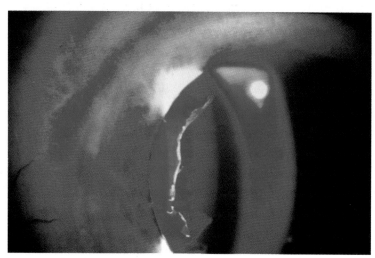

FIGURE 11-11

23. In which of the following individuals is this most typically found?

    A) Young, myopic males
    B) Men with type A personality
    C) Women with tall, thin stature
    D) Elderly, white women

24. A dispersive viscoelastic used in phacoemulsification has which of the following properties?

    A) Adheres to and protects endothelium from damage
    B) Easy to remove at end of case
    C) Retained viscoelastic does not cause increase in IOP postoperatively
    D) Prevents collapse of the anterior chamber during high vacuum

25. During a complicated cataract removal case, the lens and capsular bag were both removed and an anterior chamber lens was placed. The first day postoperatively, the IOP is 50 mmHg and the iris is bowed forward around the IOL. Which of the following measures would be most effective?

    A) Topical glaucoma medications and close observation
    B) Laser peripheral iridectomy
    C) Increased frequency of the topical steroid
    D) Paracentesis to release aqueous fluid

26. A patient has with-the-rule astigmatism. During uncomplicated cataract surgery, a toric posterior chamber intraocular lens (IOL) is placed into the capsular bag and aligned with the astigmatism. The day following surgery, the lens appears to have rotated 90°. Which of the following statements is most accurate?

    A) Lens explant is necessary because the lens is not stable.
    B) The measured astigmatism has increased.
    C) The lens should have been placed in the ciliary sulcus.
    D) Rotation of the lens can be done anytime during the first 3 months.

27. Which of the following is NOT associated with microspherophakia?

    A) Small stature, stubby fingers, reduced joint mobility
    B) Alport's syndrome
    C) Congenital rubella
    D) Hyperlysinemia

Questions 28–29

A 1-week-old baby is noted by the pediatrician to have an abnormal red reflex of both eyes. His right eye is shown in Figure 11-12. The left eye has a similar appearance. Both eyes are otherwise normal.

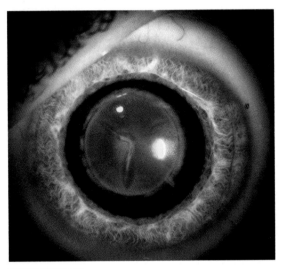

FIGURE 11-12

28. Which of the following may be the most appropriate therapy for this infant?

    A) Patch the eye that best fixes and follows and perform surgery on the other eye.
    B) Perform surgery on one eye as soon as possible and the other eye after 3 months of age.
    C) Perform surgery on one eye with immediate aphakic correction; perform surgery on the other eye before 3 months of age.
    D) Observe until 3 months of age and perform cataract surgery only if nystagmus develops.

29. Appropriate surgical methods or steps during cataract surgery on this infant include all of the following EXCEPT:

A) aspiration of the cataractous lens
B) implantation of posterior chamber IOL
C) posterior capsulectomy and limited anterior vitrectomy
D) extracapsular cataract extraction

30. What is the cause for posterior capsular opacification following phacoemulsification and implantation of an IOL?

A) Fibrovascular ingrowth stimulated by the lens
B) Bacterial sequestration and colonization
C) Proliferation of residual lens epithelium
D) Toxicity of the IOL

31. Which of the following is NOT a reported complication following yttrium-aluminum-garnet (YAG) capsulotomy?

A) Iritis
B) Retinal detachment
C) Corneal edema
D) Subluxation of the lens

32. Which of the following is true concerning the different designs of phacoemulsification machines?

A) The peristaltic pump requires a slow building of vacuum for aspiration.
B) The diaphragm pump allows instantaneous vacuum.
C) The Venturi pump has stepwise increases in vacuum.
D) The speed of rollers in the peristaltic pump allows linear control of vacuum.

33. Excessive iris prolapse during extracapsular cataract extraction via phacoemulsification may be caused by all of the following EXCEPT:

A) infusion bottle height too high
B) wound size too large for phacoemulsification tip
C) excessive phacoemulsification power
D) suprachoroidal hemorrhage

Questions 34–35

A 37-year-old woman is hit in the left eye with a metallic foreign body. On examination, you observe a corneal laceration, rupture of the lens capsule with lens opacification and subluxation, and vitreous present anterior to the lens. No foreign body is found and the posterior pole appears normal.

34. Following repair of the corneal laceration, which of the following is the best approach?

A) Pars plana vitrectomy, lensectomy
B) Extracapsular cataract extraction via nucleus expression, anterior vitrectomy
C) Extracapsular cataract extraction via phacoemulsification, anterior vitrectomy
D) Intracapsular cataract extraction, anterior vitrectomy

35. Following lens removal and vitrectomy, you notice an iridodialysis that extends from the 5 o'clock position to the 7 o'clock position. Which of the following is the most correct statement regarding secondary lens implantation in this patient?

A) A posterior chamber lens would likely have adequate support.

B) A sutured posterior chamber lens is appropriate.

C) Anterior chamber lens implantation would be technically easiest and most stable.

D) The patient is best left aphakic and should wear an aphakic contact lens.

36. Irrigation of polymethylmethacrylate (PMMA) IOLs just before insertion is intended to:

A) hydrate the lens to achieve the correct refractive power

B) facilitate insertion through a tight wound

C) remove static charges, which attract debris

D) wash off residual oils left from the manufacturing process

37. Which of the following is correct concerning cataract surgery in patients with nanophthalmos?

A) The chances for a poor visual outcome are similar to those in other cataract surgeries.

B) Extracapsular cataract extraction without IOL insertion is the recommended procedure.

C) Trabeculectomy is not recommended at the time of cataract extraction.

D) Anterior sclerotomies may be indicated at the time of surgery.

38. A 76-year-old man is scheduled for cataract surgery in his right eye as his visual acuity has dropped to 20/200 due to lens opacity. He previously underwent cataract surgery in the opposite eye, which resulted in an expulsive choroidal hemorrhage and no light perception vision. All of the following may be steps to prevent an expulsive hemorrhage in this eye EXCEPT:

A) clear corneal incision

B) use of a Honan balloon after retrobulbar anesthesia

C) closure of the wound with nylon sutures

D) blood pressure kept well controlled during surgery

39. Which of the following is correct regarding cataract surgery in patients with uveitis?

A) Placement of the IOL should be in the posterior chamber in patients with juvenile rheumatoid arthritis and iridocyclitis.

B) Ideally, uveitis should be quiet for 3 to 6 months before elective surgery.

C) Patients with Fuchs' heterochromic iridocyclitis have a poor prognosis.

D) The risk of complications is increased in patients with pars planitis.

40. The risk of complications during cataract extraction in an eye that has previously undergone pars plana vitrectomy is primarily due to:

A) collapse of the globe during surgery

B) positive pressure from the vitreous cavity

C) the excessive mobility of the posterior capsule

D) iridodonesis

41. A patient is sent to you for decreased visual acuity due to cataracts. On examination, you find significant nuclear sclerotic cataracts and a visual acuity of 20/80 in each eyes. Dilated fundus examination shows proliferative diabetic retinopathy and clinically significant macular edema. Regarding cataract surgery, you should tell the patient that:

    A) cataract surgery should be performed as soon as possible to better visualize the fundus
    B) an attempt should be made to perform photocoagulation before cataract surgery
    C) extracapsular cataract extraction without IOL implantation is the procedure of choice
    D) extracapsular cataract extraction with intact posterior capsule is associated with a greater chance of neovascular glaucoma postoperatively

42. A 72-year-old woman presents complaining of pain and redness in her left eye (Fig. 11-13). Moderate anterior chamber cell and flare are present as is minimal corneal edema. IOP is 38 mmHg, and the angle appears open although the view is poor. She has had very poor vision in this eye for at least 6 months. No relative afferent pupillary defect is noted. All of the following are acceptable management options at this time EXCEPT:

    A) IOP-lowering agents and topical steroids
    B) laser peripheral iridotomy and topical steroids
    C) extracapsular cataract extraction with posterior chamber IOL insertion
    D) intracapsular cataract extraction if significant zonular dehiscence is present

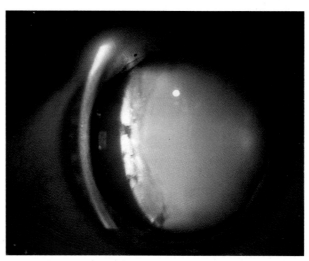

FIGURE 11-13

43. A 60-year-old man successfully undergoes phacoemulsification of the nuclear sclerotic cataract in his right eye. The surgeon accidentally leaves a moderate amount of viscoelastic in his eye. How long after completion of the case might the patient experience a significant spike in IOP?

    A) 30 minutes
    B) 4 hours
    C) 10 hours
    D) 24 hours

Questions 44–45

A 65-year-old man underwent cataract surgery with placement of a posterior chamber IOL. He presents 2 years later as shown in Figure 11-14. He has low-grade inflammation and 1+ anterior chamber cellular reaction.

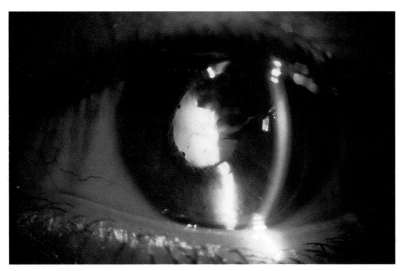

FIGURE 11-14

44. The cause for this condition is often attributed to:

A) infection with *P. acnes*
B) use of silicone IOLs
C) retained cortical material
D) a small capsulorrhexis

45. Treatment for this might be:

A) topical steroids
B) intraocular vancomycin
C) IOL exchange
D) use of the YAG laser to disrupt the whitish material

46. A patient with the preoperative refraction OD of − 3.00 + 2.00 × 90 has a visually significant cataract in this eye. Keratometry is 40.00 @ 180 and 42.00 @ 90. Which length and location of the cataract scleral tunnel might help decrease the amount of late postoperative astigmatism for the patient?

A) 3.5-mm scleral incision superiorly
B) 6.0-mm scleral incision superiorly
C) 3.5-mm scleral incision temporally
D) 6.0-mm scleral incision temporally

47. After removal of the anterior chamber IOL, you decide to place a scleral-sutured posterior chamber IOL. The needle should be passed approximately how far posterior to the limbus?

   A) 2.0 mm
   B) 1.5 mm
   C) 0.75 mm
   D) 0.25 mm

48. A 68-year-old man underwent cataract extraction with phacoemulsification and insertion of a posterior chamber IOL. The first day postoperatively, he comes back with moderate epithelial and stromal edema. One week later, the edema is still present. Which is NOT a cause for his persistent corneal edema?

   A) Elevated IOP
   B) Chemical toxicity
   C) Epithelial downgrowth
   D) Surgical trauma

49. A 70-year-old man underwent extracapsular cataract 2 years ago that was complicated by mild wound dehiscence. This was observed and he recovered good vision over the past month. His current IOP is 5 mmHg in that eye. Slit lamp examination reveals the finding shown in Figure 11-15. This most likely represents:

   A) localized bullous keratopathy
   B) limbal HSV infection
   C) conjunctival hyperplasia
   D) filtering bleb

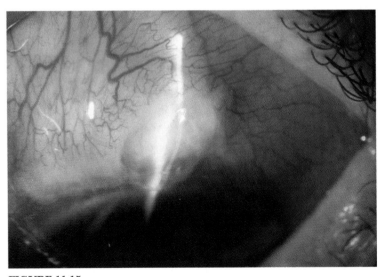

FIGURE 11-15

50. What is the incidence of clinical cystoid macular edema following uncomplicated extracapsular cataract extraction?

   A) less than 1%
   B) 1% to 2%
   C) 10%
   D) 20%

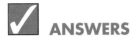

ANSWERS

1. A)   Figure 11-3

2. D)   Figure 11-6

3. B)   The cataract was caused by iron deposits in the anterior lens capsule.

4. B)   Muscle weakness

5. C)   Figure 11-6

6. D)   advanced mature lens changes

    The following figure numbers enumerate the pictured cataracts:
    Figure 11-1 = Christmas tree cataract, myotonic dystrophy
    Figure 11-2 = sunflower cataract, Wilson's disease
    Figure 11-3 = posterior subcapsular cataract
    Figure 11-4 = morgagnian cataract
    Figure 11-5 = phenothiazine cataract
    Figure 11-6 = anterior polar cataract

    The *multiple polychromatic crystalline cataract,* or "Christmas tree" cataract, is associated with myotonic dystrophy. These are not present at birth, but develop as the patient ages. Patients do not typically have symptoms from these crystals. Associated systemic findings with myotonic dystrophy include temporal bossing, muscular atrophy and weakness, mental retardation, and abnormalities in cardiac conduction.

    Wilson's disease is a multisystem disease as a result of abnormal copper metabolism. Copper accumulates in the anterior lens capsule producing the sunflower appearance. Copper deposition in Descemet's membrane produces the brownish Kayser-Fleischer ring as well. Systemic manifestations include cirrhosis, renal impairment, and degeneration of the basal ganglia. Treatment is directed toward lowering copper levels with penicillamine.

    The posterior subcapsular cataract can be found in many patients as a result of age-related changes; however, corticosteroid use has also been implicated in causing this opacity.

    Morgagnian cataracts are mature cataracts in which the peripheral cortical material becomes liquefied and the dense central nucleus can sink inferiorly.

    Phenothiazine and amiodarone can form deposits in the anterior lens capsule as shown in the cataract in Figure 11-5. These do not affect vision.

    Anterior polar cataracts are idiopathic (90%) remnants of the hyaloid system. These are typically present from birth, nonprogressive, and do not affect vision. They have been reported in association with anterior lenticonus as part of Alport's syndrome (deafness, glomerulonephritis).

7. C) Peters' anomaly

    Peters' anomaly falls into the spectrum of the anterior segment dysgeneses. It is characterized by lenticular-corneal adhesions and absence of Descemet's membrane in the region of the adhesion. The lens may be abnormal in these children; however, the lens nuclei are not retained.

8. B) Polychromatic crystalline cataract

    Cataracts occur in almost all adults with myotonic dystrophy. Iridescent crystals, usually red or green in color in the anterior and posterior subcapsular regions, make up the classic early lens changes.

9. A) Prone to angle closure glaucoma aggravated by the administration of pilocarpine

    The patient has a classic description of Weill-Marchesani syndrome, an autosomal recessively inherited disorder. Given the spherical shape of the lens, patients are prone to angle closure glaucoma, which is aggravated by miosis. Cycloplegia may decrease pupillary block by tightening zonules, decreasing anteroposterior lens diameter, and pulling the lens posteriorly.

10. A) Pelli-Robson chart

    The Pelli-Robson chart, Regan contrast sensitivity charts, and Vectorvision are contrast sensitivity tests. The Potential Acuity Meter uses the principle of the indirect ophthalmoscope to project an image of a letter chart on the macula of the patient. The Purkinje vascular phenomenon and the blue-field entopic test are visualizations of the vasculature of the eye itself when light is projected through the eyelids or sclera. These tests are highly subjective and variable.

11. C) In utero

    Pictured in Figure 11-7 is a sutural cataract demonstrating opacification of the fetal Y sutures. This is a congenital cataract with the formation occurring during development of the fetal lens nucleus.

12. A) Amiodarone causes stellate anterior axial pigment deposition.

    Amiodarone and phenothiazine cause stellate cataracts in the anterior lens capsule. All forms of steroids have been associated with cataract formation. Although echothiophate has been associated with progressive cataract formation in adults, this has not been reported in children.

13. C) Low risk of retinal detachment

    Marfan's syndrome is a genetic abnormality in fibrillin, a structural protein in collagen. Patients with Marfan's are tall; have long, thin fingers; have hyperextensible joints; and have aneurysms of the aorta. Ocular manifestations include subluxation of the lenses superotemporally and a high risk of retinal detachment.

14. B) Spectacle or contact lens correction of the refractive error

Given the high risk of retinal detachment, the increased risk of complications with routine cataract surgery, and the generally nonprogressive nature of the subluxation, spectacles or contact lenses should be tried first. Most cases are amenable to spectacles or contact lenses. Pupil dilation is sometimes helpful because it allows the patient to see around the subluxed lens. A reading add is needed secondary to poor accommodation of the lens due to zonular dehiscence.

15. D) autosomal dominant inheritance

Persistent hyperplastic primary vitreous (PHPV) is a congenital, nonhereditary ocular malformation. Associated findings include elongation of ciliary processes, prominent radial iris vessels, persistent hyaloid artery, microphthalmia, and ectopia lentis.

16. C) homocystinuria

PHPV is included in the differential diagnosis of leukocoria. Homocystinuria does not cause leukocoria but is associated with ectopia lentis along with PHPV.

17. D) Urine protein and reducing substances

With no family history and unilateral complete cataracts, screening labs are not warranted. Urine protein and reducing substance analysis are screens for Lowe's syndrome or galactosemia with bilateral cataracts. Bilateral cataracts are associated with chromosomal abnormalities such as trisomy 13 and Turner's syndrome. If no view to the fundus is possible, B-scan ultrasound of the eye is necessary to rule out secondary causes such as intraocular tumors.

18. C) Nuclear sclerotic cataracts – homogenous, loss of cellular laminations

In posterior subcapsular cataracts, there is posterior migration of lens epithelial cells, which swell along the posterior capsule. These swollen cells are called *Wedl* or *bladder cells*. In cortical cataracts, there is hydropic swelling of lens fibers. The eosinophilic, globular material between lens fibers is called *morgagnian globules*.

19. C) Decreased serum levels of methionine

The history and physical findings are consistent with a diagnosis of homocystinuria, in which serum levels of homocystine and methionine are elevated. Inheritance is autosomal recessive. Patients are normal at birth but develop seizures, osteoporosis, and mental retardation. Classic lens dislocation is bilateral, symmetric, usually inferonasal.

20. C) Vitamin B_6

In homocystinuria, there is a disorder in the metabolism of methionine. Deficient cysteine is thought to weaken zonules, which have a high concentration of cysteine. Vitamin B_6, a low methionine high cysteine diet, and vitamin supplementation have shown promise in treating these patients and in reducing ectopia lentis. Coenzyme Q has been touted for patients with Leber's hereditary optic neuropathy, and Vitamin A may be helpful in some cases of retinitis pigmentosa.

21. B)   Posterior polar cataracts have been associated with remnants of the tunica vasculosa lentis.

Anterior polar cataracts are usually small and nonprogressive, do not usually impair vision, and may be seen in association with microphthalmos, a persistent pupillary membrane, and anterior lenticonus. Posterior polar cataracts cause more visual impairment and tend to be larger than anterior polar cataracts. Both can be autosomal dominant or sporadic. Posterior polar cataracts may be associated with posterior lenticonus or a remnant of the tunica vasculosa lentis.

22. B)   zonular dehiscence

This is an example of pseudoexfoliation syndrome. Note the deposition of pseudoexfoliative debris on the anterior lens capsule and at the pupillary margin. This syndrome is associated with an approximately five times higher rate of vitreous loss during extracapsular cataract extraction. In some cases, phacodonesis or iridodonesis may be evident at the slit lamp, signaling lens subluxation. Other times, however, lens subluxation and zonular dehiscence may not be evident until during surgery. Severe postoperative inflammation and corneal decompensation are not necessarily more common in these patients. Retained viscoelastic may cause a temporary rise in IOP after surgery, which may complicate cases with pseudoexfoliative glaucoma.

23. D)   Elderly, white women

Pseudoexfoliation is typically found in people of Scandinavian descent, and the incidence increases with age. Young, myopic males may be predisposed to pigmentary dispersion syndrome. The central serous choroidopathy patient characteristically is a type A personality man. Tall, thin body habitus may be found with Marfan's syndrome.

24. A)   Adheres to and protects endothelium from damage

A dispersive viscoelastic has a low surface tension and when used in the eye has a higher retention than a cohesive viscoelastic. With high vacuum, the dispersive viscoelastic tends to fragment, making it harder to remove from the eye. A layer of this viscoelastic can protect the endothelium from lens fragments during phacoemulsification. All viscoelastics, if retained in the eye, can cause increases in IOP.

25. B)   Laser peripheral iridectomy

This case describes *iris bombé*, which can occur if the aqueous humor produced by the ciliary body is unable to move around the IOL to the trabecular meshwork. The iris is pushed forward peripherally and causes a secondary angle closure. A similar situation can occur in uveitis if synechiae form 360° around the pupillary border. A peripheral iridectomy is necessary to create an alternate location for the aqueous. A paracentesis would not be easy to perform with the forward position of the iris. Release of the aqueous may worsen the condition as well.

26. B)   The measured astigmatism has increased.

Toric lenses are designed to counteract the corneal astigmatism. When the lens rotates off axis, the amount of astigmatism correction decreases. When it rotates 90° off axis, the astigmatism measured will be greater than the corneal astigmatism. The lens should be rotated back to the correct position within the several weeks after surgery before the anterior and posterior capsule fuse together and make it more difficult to manipulate the lens. The lens should not be placed in the ciliary sulcus because it will not be stable in this location.

27. D) Hyperlysinemia

All of these conditions have been reported to be associated with microspherophakia, except hyperlysinemia, which has been related to ectopia lentis. Patients with Weill-Marchesani have small stature, stubby fingers with broad hands, and stiff joints. Weill-Marchesani is also associated with anterior dislocation of the lens.

28. C) Perform surgery on one eye with immediate aphakic correction; perform surgery on the other eye before 3 months of age.

Bilateral congenital cataracts of significant opacity, as in Figure 11-12, should be addressed surgically as soon as possible. Aphakic correction with an aphakic contact lens is performed immediately postoperatively. Surgery on the second eye should be done as soon as possible after the first eye. Vision may develop normally without surgery if the lens opacity is axial and the pupils are continuously dilated.

When indicated, surgery is ideally performed before the child is 3 months of age. Profound amblyopia is present by this age and nystagmus develops. Cataract surgery after the development of nystagmus often does not improve visual acuity and nystagmus persists.

29. B) implantation of posterior chamber IOL

Cataract surgery in infants differs from that in adults in several important ways. In infants, the nucleus, although opaque, is soft and gummy. Marked opacification and membrane formation occur on the posterior capsule and anterior hyaloid if the posterior capsule is left untouched. Additionally, significant adhesions exist between the lens and anterior hyaloid face. For these reasons, intracapsular cataract extraction is not considered because vitreous loss may occur. Extracapsular cataract extraction is performed by aspirating the nucleus and cortex with a phacoemulsification handpiece or vitrectomy instrument. A posterior capsulectomy is followed by a limited anterior vitrectomy. Postoperative aphakic correction via contact lens can be started immediately. Implantation of IOLs in children is controversial. In infants under 2 years of age, lenses are generally contraindicated because the eye undergoes a drastic change in refractive power as it grows. An implanted IOL would have to be removed or exchanged in later years.

30. C) Proliferation of residual lens epithelium

Opacification of the posterior capsule following extracapsular cataract extraction is not an uncommon problem. The main causes include proliferation of retained lens epithelium and capsular fibrosis and contraction. An opening in the capsule can be made with a YAG laser, providing a clear visual pathway.

31. C) Corneal edema

Complications of YAG capsulotomies result from the energy delivered to the eye. The YAG creates microexplosions that disrupt the posterior capsule. This may also put traction on the vitreous, causing a retinal break. Elevated IOP, iritis, and macular edema are also resulting complications. Corneal edema should not result if the laser is properly focused at the posterior capsule.

32. D)   The speed of rollers in the peristaltic pump allows linear control of vacuum.

Three kinds of aspiration systems exist in phacoemulsification machines. The *peristaltic pump* has rollers that move along tubing and create a relatively rapid rise in vacuum. The *diaphragm pump* has valves over both the inlet and outlet of a fluid chamber covered by a diaphragm. This system allows a slower build of vacuum. The *Venturi pump* produces the most rapid increase in vacuum. This, however, can be the most dangerous because it allows almost instantaneous engagement of unwanted tissues such as capsule or iris.

33. C)   excessive phacoemulsification power

Iris prolapse associated with an excessively deep anterior chamber suggests too high a bottle height, which can be remedied by simply lowering the bottle. If iris prolapse is associated with a normal or shallow anterior chamber depth, this may be caused by wound leak around the phacoemulsification tip or possibly suprachoroidal hemorrhage. If leak around the phaco tip is evident, a temporary suture may be placed. Peripheral iridectomy at the site of prolapse may also help reposit the iris. Excessive phacoemulsification power does not result in iris prolapse.

34. A)   Pars plana vitrectomy, lensectomy

When traumatic capsular rupture is present with lens subluxation and disruption of the anterior hyaloid face, the pars plana approach for lensectomy and vitrectomy is the most appropriate. The presence of a hard nucleus, if present, may make this technically difficult. Extracapsular cataract extraction would not be indicated with loss of zonular integrity and presence of free vitreous. Intracapsular cataract extraction is contraindicated when vitreous is present and the capsule is ruptured.

35. B)   A sutured posterior chamber lens is appropriate.

In this case, support for a posterior chamber lens, either in the sulcus or capsular bag, would very likely be inadequate. Anterior chamber lens placement should be considered, but the presence of a large iridodialysis may complicate placement. Other factors that are relative contraindications for anterior chamber lens placement, if present, include corneal endothelial dystrophy, abnormal angle vessels or structures, and peripheral anterior synechiae. Placement of an anterior chamber lens would, however, be technically easiest. Sulcus fixation via transscleral polypropylene (Prolene) sutures would be appropriate but is technically more difficult. Aphakic contact lens wear is an option but not the best one.

36. C)   remove static charges, which attract debris

PMMA lenses, when packaged, may pick up static charges that attract dust and debris when opened. Therefore, the lens may be rinsed with balanced salt solution before insertion. Silicone lenses do not require this and, in fact, may be more difficult to handle once they have gotten wet. Application of a viscoelastic, such as sodium hyaluronate, may facilitate insertion of a lens, especially a foldable one, through a small incision.

37. D)   Anterior sclerotomies may be indicated at the time of surgery.

The indications for cataract surgery in nanophthalmic patients are similar to those in other patients. However, the chances for complications and a poor visual outcome are significantly higher. These complications include retinal detachment, choroidal effusion, postoperative angle-closure glaucoma, flat anterior chamber, cystoid macular edema, corneal decompensation, and malignant glaucoma. Extracapsular cataract extraction with posterior chamber lens insertion is generally the procedure of choice, using the smallest incision possible. Some cases with refractory positive vitreous pressure and anterior segment crowding may do best without IOL implantation. In eyes with significant glaucoma, small incision cataract surgery may be combined with trabeculectomy. When the anterior chamber is shallow preoperatively and the choroid is thickened, anterior sclerotomies are indicated at the time of surgery.

38. A)   clear corneal incision

Risk factors for expulsive choroidal hemorrhage include myopia, glaucoma, atherosclerotic vascular disease, hypertension, and previous expulsive hemorrhage in the opposite eye. Using as small an incision as possible along with being ready to perform a sclerotomy is important. Decompression before opening the globe with digital pressure or other device may be helpful. Close the wound with nonabsorbable, preferably nylon, sutures to prevent delayed hemorrhage. It is also beneficial to keep blood pressure controlled and level of anesthesia deep (if general anesthesia is used) during surgery. Shelved or self-sealing incisions allow more rapid closure and repressurization of the globe should bleeding occur.

39. B)   Ideally, uveitis should be quiet for 3 to 6 months before elective surgery.

The indications for cataract surgery in patients with uveitis are similar to those in patients without uveitis. However, complications in the early or late postoperative period may arise in certain uveitides. Elective cataract surgery is best performed after inflammation is quiet for several months. Even minimal or baseline inflammation preoperatively may result in marked inflammation postoperatively. Prophylaxis or treatment may require hourly topical steroids or even systemic steroids.

IOL implantation is contraindicated in patients with juvenile rheumatoid arthritis–associated iridocyclitis. Development of cyclitic membranes and subsequent ciliary body detachment following extracapsular cataract extraction suggest the need for complete capsular removal. Therefore, combined lensectomy and subtotal vitrectomy is recommended either through the limbus or pars plana. Patients with Fuchs' heterochromic iridocyclitis are among the group that does best following cataract extraction and after IOLs have been safely implanted. A transient postoperative hyphema may develop but resolves without sequelae. Although those with pars planitis do not apparently have a significantly increased risk of complications associated with routine cataract surgery, pars plana lensectomy-vitrectomy may be indicated as postoperative vitreous opacities may limit visual acuity. Visual acuity may also be limited by cystoid macular edema.

40. C)   the excessive mobility of the posterior capsule

The posterior capsule is capable of moving more posterior than normal without support of the vitreous. Zonular dehiscence may result from attempted manual expression of the nucleus during extracapsular cataract extraction. The posterior capsule is also more likely to move forward with the lens during phacoemulsification and aspiration in extracapsular cataract extraction via phacoemulsification. As a result, capsular tears may be more likely. Collapse of the globe is usually not problematic with a well-formed phaco incision. Positive pressure from the posterior segment occurs more frequently when the vitreous cavity is occupied by the vitreous.

41.   B)   an attempt should be made to perform photocoagulation before cataract surgery

According to the Early Treatment of Diabetic Retinopathy Study (ETDRS), in diabetic retinopathy, argon laser photocoagulation should be attempted to the degree allowed by the lens opacity before cataract surgery. In this case, concomitant focal and panretinal photocoagulation or focal laser followed by panretinal photocoagulation should be performed. As many laser spots as possible to control neovascularization should be placed before surgery.

Although extracapsular cataract extraction with or without IOL implantation may be indicated following photocoagulation, maintenance of an intact posterior capsule appears to be important. The intact posterior capsule (or anterior hyaloid face) appears to act as a barrier, to some extent, to the proposed angiogenic factors that lead to development of neovascularization. Successful extracapsular cataract extraction with intact posterior capsule does not appear to increase the risk of anterior segment neovascularization leading to postoperative neovascular glaucoma.

42.   B)   laser peripheral iridotomy and topical steroids

This is a case of phacolytic glaucoma due to a hypermature cataract. A dense, white cataract along with anterior segment inflammation is noted. Lens proteins, which have liquefied, leak through an intact lens capsule and attract macrophages with resultant inflammation. The combination of lens proteins and macrophages then block the trabecular meshwork with elevation of the IOP.

Definitive treatment is cataract extraction. When possible, however, it may be beneficial to attempt control of inflammation and IOP medically before surgery. Most surgeons will perform extracapsular cataract extraction with IOL implantation, but intracapsular cataract extraction may be preferred if significant zonular dehiscence is discovered. Laser peripheral iridotomy is not indicated as glaucoma in this case is not due to angle closure.

43.   B)   4 hours

Lane and colleagues evaluated IOP elevation associated with three commonly used viscoelastic agents (sodium hyaluronate, chondroitin sulfate, and hydroxymethylcellulose) and all produced significant pressure elevations at 4 ± 1 hours postoperatively. Removing the viscoelastic did not eliminate significant postoperative IOP elevation, although when chondroitin sulfate was removed, the pressure elevation was slightly less.

44.   A)   infection with *P. acnes*

45. B)   intraocular vancomycin

Chronic postoperative endophthalmitis, as shown here, can occur months to years following cataract surgery. A number of bacterial organisms have been isolated from the whitish plaque, among them *Propionibacterium acnes*. The low-grade inflammation can wax and wane and responds to topical steroids. Treatment includes intracameral vancomycin and/or vitrectomy and excision of the plaque.

Retained cortical material can incite inflammation in the months following cataract surgery, but remote inflammation due to the cortical lens material is unusual. Proliferation of lens epithelium (Elschnig pearls and Soemmering's ring) is noninflammatory.

46. B)   6.0 mm scleral incision superiorly

The patient has with-the-rule astigmatism that has no obvious lenticular component. A 6.0-mm scleral incision placed superiorly may help decrease the patient's preoperative astigmatism 1.5 ± 0.5 D. A 3.5-mm incision would be more astigmatically neutral with 0.5 ± 0.3 D drift against-the-rule.

47. C)   0.75 mm

The ciliary sulcus is only 0.83-mm posterior to the limbus vertically and 0.46-mm posterior horizontally (Fig. 11-16). Avoid 3- to 9-o'clock alignment, if possible, because of the chance of damaging the long ciliary arteries and nerves. Figure 11-17 shows an example of a lens designed for transscleral suturing. Note the two eyelets for the sutures.

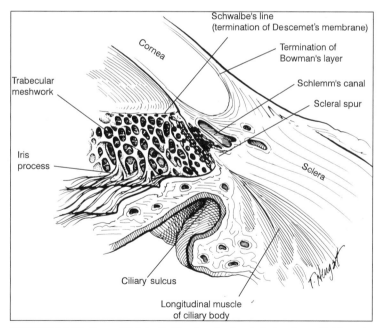

FIGURE 11-16. From Wright K. Textbook of ophthalmology. Baltimore: Williams & Wilkins, 1997.

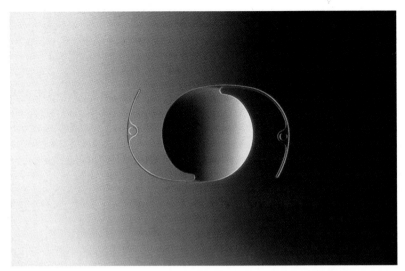

FIGURE 11-17. Photograph courtesy of Alcon Laboratories, Inc., Ft. Worth, TX.

48. C)   Epithelial downgrowth

Among the causes of corneal edema the day following cataract extraction are elevated IOP (from inflammation, glaucoma, debris clogging the trabecular meshwork), corneal decompensation (low endothelial counts as in Fuchs' dystrophy, endothelial chemical toxicity), or trauma to the endothelium. Epithelial downgrowth would not present immediately after surgery but would take weeks to develop. The corneal decompensation would overlie the area of the downgrowth, and a membrane may be seen on the endothelium and iris.

49. D)   filtering bleb

This is an inadvertent filtering bleb following cataract surgery.

50. A)   less than 1%

The incidence of clinical cystoid macular edema is less than 1% following uncomplicated cataract extraction. The incidence of angiographic evidence of cystoid macular edema is approximately 10 times this.

Notes

Notes

12

Retina and Vitreous

QUESTIONS

Questions 1–3

A 72-year-old man with a history of dizziness is examined for a chronic red eye and mildly decreased vision. Iris angiogram shows ipsilateral delayed filling. The posterior pole (Fig. 12-1A) and midperipheral hemorrhages (Fig. 12-1B) are shown.

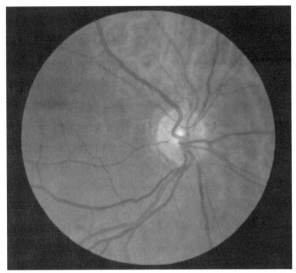

FIGURE 12-1A

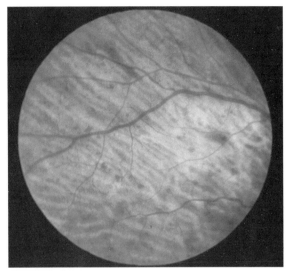

FIGURE 12-1B

1. Which condition is most likely responsible for his condition?

    A) Cardiac emboli
    B) Thrombosis of the central retinal vein
    C) Diabetes mellitus
    D) Carotid stenosis

2. What ocular finding would NOT be expected?

    A) Hypopyon
    B) Anterior chamber flare
    C) Hypotony
    D) Rubeosis

3. Which test would be most helpful in the diagnosis?

    A) Ophthalmodynamometry
    B) Electroretinogram (ERG)
    C) Color testing
    D) Glucose tolerance test

Questions 4–6

A 34-year-old white man reports that he has had floaters for 1 week. His fundus examination is shown in Figure 12-2.

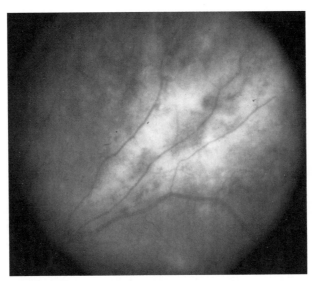

FIGURE 12-2

4. Which systemic condition is most relevant to the diagnosis?

    A) Insulin-dependent diabetes mellitus since age 11
    B) Uncontrolled hypertension
    C) Recurrent pneumonia, weight loss, and vascular skin lesions
    D) Sickle cell anemia

5. Which of the following would be seen histopathologically?

    A) Retinal necrosis
    B) Loss of pericytes
    C) Macroaneurysms
    D) Thickening and excrescences on Bruch's membrane

6. What ocular complication may be associated with this condition?

    A) Retinal detachment
    B) Neovascular glaucoma
    C) Neovascularization of the optic disc
    D) Siegrist streaks

Questions 7–8

A 60-year-old woman with diabetes mellitus and hypertension reports having difficulty reading for the past 4 months. Her visual acuity is 20/25. Her fundus photograph is shown in Figure 12-3.

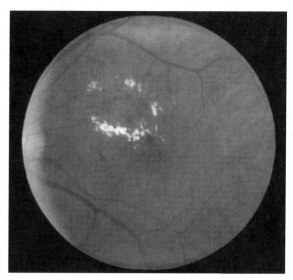

FIGURE 12-3

7. According to the Early Treatment of Diabetic Retinopathy Study (ETDRS), which one of the following is considered clinically significant diabetic macular edema?

   A) Hard exudates within 500 μm of the fovea
   B) Retinal thickening greater than 1 disc area in size and within 1 disc diameter of the center of the fovea
   C) Diffuse leakage on fluorescein angiography
   D) A circinate ring of exudates located 2 disc areas from the fovea

8. What treatment is indicated for the patient shown?

   A) No treatment, but re-evaluation in 2 months
   B) Focal laser photocoagulation if visual acuity is less than 20/40
   C) Panretinal laser photocoagulation
   D) Focal laser photocoagulation

Questions 9–11

A 7-year-old girl reports having poor vision for 2 weeks. She presents with a fundus as shown in Figure 12-4.

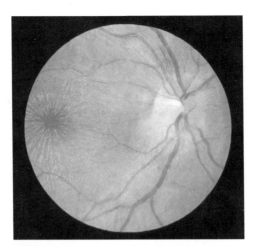

FIGURE 12-4. From Wright K. Textbook of ophthalmology. Baltimore: Williams & Wilkins, 1997.

9. What historical information might be helpful in the diagnosis?

   A) Prematurity with low birth weight
   B) Juvenile-onset diabetes mellitus
   C) Blunt trauma to orbit with a soccer ball
   D) A pet cat at home

10. What laboratory studies are appropriate?

   A) Urinalysis, stool for ova and parasites
   B) complete blood count (CBC), Venereal Disease Research Laboratories (VDRL) test, toxoplasma titer, viral titer screen
   C) Antinuclear antibodies, serum protein electrophoresis (SPEP)
   D) Lipoprotein, computed tomography (CT) of head and orbits

11. What treatment would you offer?

   A) Triple sulfa antibiotics
   B) Vitrectomy
   C) Observation
   D) Laser photocoagulation

12. Which one of the following about Coats' disease is TRUE?

    A) Usually bilateral
    B) Associated with microphthalmia
    C) Bimodal age distribution
    D) Equally common between males and females

13. In a nonperfused central retinal vein occlusion (CRVO), when is the MOST appropriate time to perform panretinal photocoagulation (PRP)?

    A) As soon as possible after the vein occlusion
    B) When there is development of neovascularization of any type
    C) If macular edema is present on IVFA
    D) After resolution of the retinal hemorrhages

14. Which one of the following is NOT a risk factor for CRVO?

    A) Hypertension
    B) Glaucoma
    C) Diabetes
    D) Prosthetic cardiac valves

15. Which one of the following conditions has been associated with foveal hypoplasia?

    A) Choroideremia
    B) Aniridia
    C) Juvenile X-linked retinoschisis
    D) Tay-Sachs disease

16. Which one of the following would NOT be associated with a viral prodrome?

    A) Acute posterior multifocal placoid pigment epitheliopathy
    B) Multiple evanescent white dot syndrome
    C) Diffuse unilateral subacute neuroretinopathy
    D) Leber's stellate neuroretinitis

17. Which retinal layer accounts for the petalloid cystic appearance of cystoid macular edema (CME)?

    A) Nerve fiber layer
    B) Inner plexiform layer
    C) Outer plexiform layer
    D) Outer nuclear layer

Questions 18–20

A 60-year-old white woman reports having poor vision in her left eye for 4 months. Her fundus is shown in Figure 12-5.

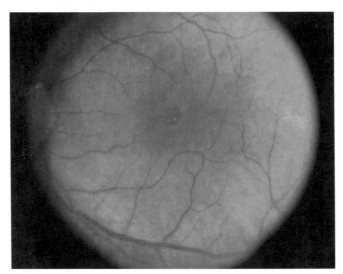

FIGURE 12-5

18.   What is her diagnosis?

   A)   Retinal detachment
   B)   Macular hole
   C)   CME
   D)   Epiretinal membrane

19.   What would fluorescein angiography show?

   A)   Central hypofluorescence due to blockage
   B)   Leakage in petalloid pattern
   C)   Central window defect
   D)   Pooling of fluorescein

20.   What treatment might be offered?

   A)   Vitrectomy with intraocular gas injection
   B)   Laser photocoagulation
   C)   Sub-Tenon's steroid injection
   D)   Scleral buckling procedure

21.   All of the following are associated with the clinical finding shown in Figure 12-6 EXCEPT:

   A)   vitreous hemorrhage
   B)   hypertension
   C)   renal cell carcinoma
   D)   macular edema

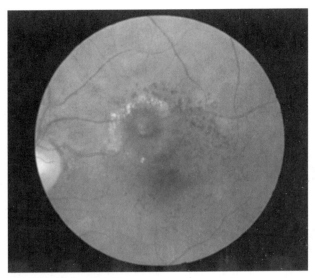

FIGURE 12-6

22. According to the Diabetic Retinopathy Study, all of the following meet the high-risk criteria for significant visual loss with proliferative diabetic retinopathy (PDR) EXCEPT:

   A) 1 DA isolated NVE
   B) 1/3 DA NVD
   C) 1/4 DA NVD with vitreous hemorrhage
   D) 1/2 DA NVE with preretinal hemorrhage

23. Which one of the following may be associated with the condition shown in Figure 12-7 and angiogram in Figure 12-8?

   A) Neovascularization of the disc
   B) Macular edema
   C) Cotton-wool spots
   D) Pigment epithelial detachment

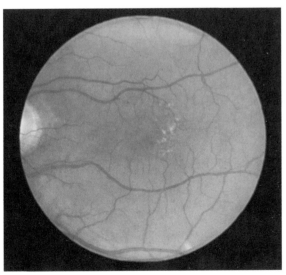

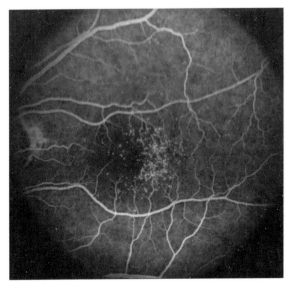

FIGURE 12-7   **FIGURE 12-8**

Questions 24–25

A 34-year-old lawyer presents with 2 days of painless blurring of vision in his right eye and the fundus shown in Figure 12-9. He had a similar episode 2 years ago.

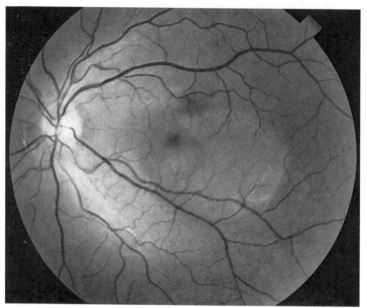

FIGURE 12-9. From Wright K. Textbook of ophthalmology. Baltimore: Williams & Wilkins, 1997.

24. What would the fluorescein angiogram most likely demonstrate?

    A) Diffuse choroidal oozing
    B) Focal leaking hot spot
    C) Lacy subfoveal choroidal neovascular membrane (CNVM)
    D) Leakage off optic nerve

25. Which therapy is MOST appropriate for this condition?

    A) Observation
    B) PRP
    C) Posterior sub-Tenon's injection of corticosteroids
    D) Scleral buckle and posterior drainage of fluid

Questions 26–28

A 27-year-old man presents with a 2-day history of blurred vision and metamorphopsia in his left eye. His fundus is shown in Figure 12-10, and fluorescein angiogram is pictured in Figure 12-11.

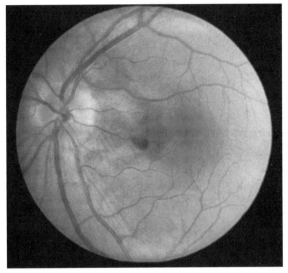

FIGURE 12-10

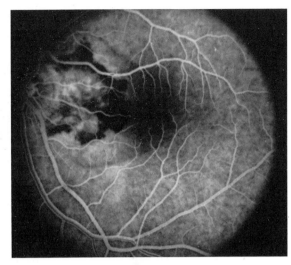

FIGURE 12-11

26. What peripheral retinal lesions might be expected?

  A) Bone spicules
  B) Sea fan neovascularization
  C) Snow banking exudates
  D) Punched-out chorioretinal scars

27. Where might this patient have lived?

  A) San Joaquin valley
  B) Ohio-Mississippi river valley
  C) Rocky Mountains
  D) North Carolina

28. What treatment is indicated?

  A) Submacular surgery
  B) Laser photocoagulation
  C) Oral steroids
  D) Triple sulfa antibiotics

29. You examine a patient with the fundus pictured in Figure 12-12. A yellowish refractile plaque can be seen in the retinal arteriole at the disc. Which one of the following symptoms is possible with this finding?

  A) Floaters
  B) Metamorphopsia
  C) Amaurosis
  D) Flashing lights

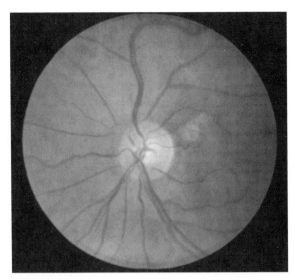

FIGURE 12-12

Questions 30–32

A 69-year-old patient reports not being able to see to write checks to manage his personal finances.

30. What does Figure 12-13 show?

    A)   CNVM
    B)   Pigment epithelial detachment
    C)   Retinal pigment epithelium (RPE) tear
    D)   Geographic atrophy (age-related macular degeneration [ARMD])

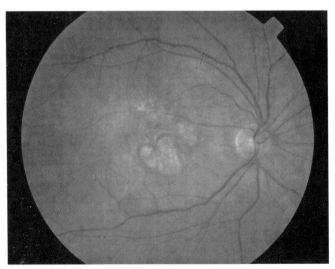

FIGURE 12-13

31. How would you treat this?

    A) Vitamin E therapy
    B) Counsel and monitor with an Amsler grid
    C) Immediate laser photocoagulation
    D) Subretinal surgery

32. Which finding in the fellow eye would be the most worrisome?

    A) Subretinal blood
    B) Geographic atrophy
    C) Soft drusen
    D) Photocoagulation scars

33. According to the Endophthalmitis Vitrectomy Study:

    A) All patients with acute endophthalmitis benefit from immediate vitrectomy.
    B) Systemic antibiotics are of benefit in the final visual outcome and should be instituted in addition to intravitreal antibiotics.
    C) Vitreous biopsy and injection of intravitreal antibiotics in patients with better than hand-motions vision did equally well as patients with immediate vitrectomy and injection of intravitreal antibiotics in final visual outcome.
    D) In patients with light-perception only vision, neither vitrectomy nor vitreous tap was of significant benefit in final visual outcome.

34. Which one of the following may present with peripheral retinal neovascularization?

    A) Incontinentia pigmenti
    B) Juxtafoveal telangiectasis
    C) Pathologic myopia
    D) Chorioretinitis sclopetaria

35. Which one of the following is the LEAST likely etiology of a central retinal artery occlusion (CRAO) in a 25-year-old woman?

    A) Cardiac emboli
    B) Oral contraceptives
    C) Migraine
    D) Atherosclerosis

36. All findings are associated with sickle cell disease EXCEPT:

    A) Dalen-Fuchs nodules
    B) sunbursts
    C) sea fan neovascularization
    D) salmon patch hemorrhages

37. Degeneration of which retinal cell is the principle cause of retinitis pigmentosa?

    A) retinal pigment epithelium (RPE)
    B) Rods
    C) Ganglion cells
    D) Cones

38. All of the following are true regarding sympathetic ophthalmia EXCEPT:

    A) It may occur 2 years following penetrating eye injury.
    B) The granulomatous uveitis occurs bilaterally.
    C) Histopathologically, it is a panuveitis with sparing of the choriocapillaris.
    D) The only effective treatment is enucleation of the traumatized eye.

39. All of the following may develop a similar complication leading to central visual loss EXCEPT:

    A) Presumed ocular histoplasmosis syndrome (POHS)
    B) angioid streaks
    C) pathologic myopia
    D) nanophthalmos

40. Which lesion might lead to development of a macular pucker (epiretinal membrane)?

    A) Cobblestone degeneration
    B) Retinal hole
    C) Choroidal nevus
    D) Bone spicule pigmentation

41. What percentage of the population will have a cilioretinal artery?

    A) 85%
    B) 65%
    C) 45%
    D) 25%

42. What ocular complication may result after a central retinal artery occulsion (CRAO)?

    A) Corneal edema
    B) Staphyloma
    C) Rubeosis iridis
    D) CNVM

43. The CME in which one of the following conditions would have leakage on fluorescein angiography?

    A) Goldmann-Favre
    B) Juvenile X-linked retinoschisis
    C) Nicotinic acid maculopathy
    D) Epiretinal membrane

44. All of the following may present with subretinal, intraretinal, and preretinal hemorrhage EXCEPT:

    A) choroidal neovascularization
    B) sickle cell retinopathy
    C) trauma
    D) macroaneurysm

45. A 35-year-old sickle cell patient comes in after being hit in the eye with a soccer ball as shown in Figure 12-14. He is in severe pain, with vision decreased to 20/50 and intraocular pressure (IOP) of 50 mmHg. Which one of the following is the MOST appropriate treatment?

A) Lowering the IOP with timolol and acetazolamide
B) Dilating the pupil with phenylephrine (Neo-Synephrine) and tropicamide
C) Anterior chamber washout
D) Cryopexy to reduce ischemic areas

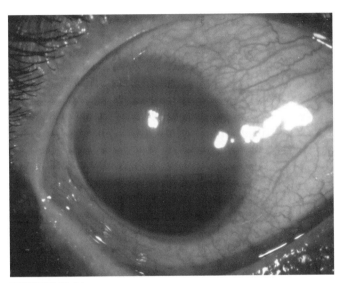

FIGURE 12-14

Questions 46–49

A 48-year-old African American man comes in for a routine eye examination, and the fluorescein angiogram pictured in Figure 12-15 is obtained.

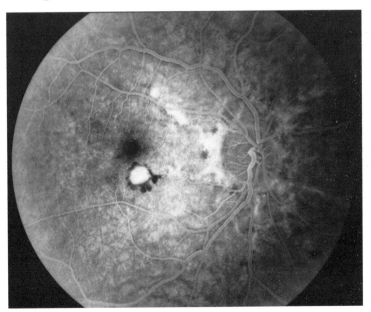

FIGURE 12-15. From Wright K. Textbook of ophthalmology. Baltimore: Williams & Wilkins, 1997.

46. Each of the following historical features would be helpful in confirming the etiology EXCEPT:

    A) hyperextensible joints
    B) fractures of both femurs
    C) recent splenectomy
    D) headaches and nausea

47. On further examination, this patient has areas of yellowish papular skin lesions and redundant and inelastic folds of skin on the neck and thighs. What ocular manifestation of this disease might be present?

    A) Optic nerve drusen
    B) Arterial macroaneurysms
    C) Salmon patches
    D) Blue sclera

48. Which systemic complication of this condition is possible?

    A) Peripheral neuropathy
    B) Gastrointestinal bleeding
    C) Carotid emboli and stroke
    D) Weight loss and anorexia

49. Which ocular complication may occur?

    A) Choroidal neovascularization
    B) RPE degeneration
    C) Retinal detachment
    D) Vitreous hemorrhage

50. Which laser would be best for PRP in a patient with proliferative diabetic retinopathy (PDR) and a mild vitreous hemorrhage?

    A) Xenon arc
    B) Krypton red
    C) Argon green
    D) Carbon dioxide laser

51. All of the following are true of pars plana cysts EXCEPT:

    A) they can occur in otherwise normal eyes
    B) they contain mucopolysaccharides
    C) they can occur in patients with multiple myeloma
    D) they occur in less than 1% of autopsy eyes

52. Which mucopolysaccharidosis does not cause RPE degeneration?

    A) Hunter's
    B) Hurler's
    C) Maroteaux-Lamy
    D) Scheie's

53. Retinal crystals may be seen with use of all of the following medications EXCEPT:

    A) tamoxifen
    B) canthaxanthine
    C) methoxyflurane
    D) chloroquine

54. Angiographically silent or black choroid can often be seen in:

    A) Hunter's disease
    B) APMPPE
    C) Stargardt's disease
    D) Giant cell arteritis

55. What method is used to repair retinal detachments due to cytomegalovirus (CMV)?

    A) Cryopexy and an intraocular gas bubble
    B) Vitrectomy and endolaser
    C) Scleral buckle with drainage of subretinal fluid
    D) Vitrectomy and silicone oil tamponade

56. Exudative detachments occur in all of the following conditions EXCEPT:

    A) Vogt-Koyanagi-Harada Syndrome (VKH)
    B) myopia
    C) toxemia of pregnancy
    D) CMV retinitis

57. A copper intraocular foreign body can cause all of the following EXCEPT:

    A) sunflower cataract
    B) Kayser-Fleischer rings
    C) suppurative endophthalmitis
    D) irreversibly flat ERG

58. A 67-year-old hypertensive white man awoke with acute, painless loss of vision. Examination reveals visual acuity of hand motions and an afferent pupillary defect. The fundus is shown in Figure 12-16. Which one of the following has NOT been advocated as a possible treatment for this condition?

    A) Hyperbaric oxygen
    B) Anterior chamber tap
    C) Acetazolamide and topical beta-blockers
    D) Coumadinization

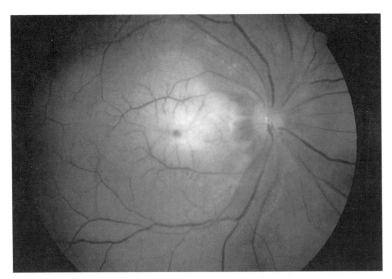

FIGURE 12-16

59. Which statement regarding uveal effusion syndrome is TRUE?

    A) It occurs in eyes with abnormally short axial length.
    B) It is effectively prevented by using a Flieringa ring.
    C) It is treated by vitrectomy to drain choroidals.
    D) Risk factors include hypertension and atherosclerosis.

60. What is the treatment for traumatic macular holes?

    A) Systemic corticosteroids
    B) Observation
    C) Scleral buckle and vitrectomy
    D) Vitrectomy and gas–fluid exchange

61. Which one of the following intraocular foreign bodies would be tolerated best?

    A) Sand
    B) Wood
    C) Brass
    D) Iron

62. Commotio retinae represents:

    A) retinal edema from contusion injury
    B) traumatic disruption of choroidal circulation resulting in retinal edema
    C) disruption of photoreceptor elements and damage to photoreceptor cells
    D) retinal edema from damage to retinal vasculature

63. What is, in order of frequency, the likelihood of traumatic retinal tears after blunt ocular injury?

    1. Tears around lattice
    2. Giant retinal tears

3. Inferotemporal dialysis
4. Superonasal dialysis
5. Flap tears

A) $3 > 2 > 4 > 5 > 1$
B) $4 > 3 > 2 > 1 > 5$
C) $3 > 4 > 2 > 5 > 1$
D) $4 > 2 > 3 > 5 > 1$

64. All of the following about retinopathy in shaken baby syndrome are true EXCEPT:

A) intra-retinal and pre-retinal hemorrhages are present
B) has a good visual prognosis with complete healing of retinal injuries
C) may also have vitreous hemorrhage
D) similar to CRVO, Purtscher's retinopathy, and Valsalva retinopathy

65. Terson's syndrome may have:

A) retinal hemorrhages in patients with spontaneous or traumatic subarachnoid hemorrhages
B) vitreous hemorrhage in patients with spontaneous or traumatic subarachnoid hemorrhages
C) both A and B
D) neither A nor B

66. Purtscher's retinopathy occurs in patients with all of the following EXCEPT:

A) severe chest compression trauma
B) acute pancreatitis
C) fat embolism syndrome
D) disseminated intravascular coagulation

67. Leakage is a common fluorescein angiographic finding in patients with:

A) solar maculopathy
B) photic injury
C) both A and B
D) neither A nor B

68. Persistent hyperplastic primary vitreous (PHPV):

A) is initially associated with a clear lens or minimal opacity that may later become densely cataractous
B) is often bilateral
C) always requires lensectomy and vitrectomy
D) is associated with buphthalmos

Questions 69–70

A 27-year-old had a ruptured right globe with uveal prolapse repaired 6 weeks before presenting with photophobia, blurry vision, and pain in the left eye.

69. Which one of the following statements regarding this patient is TRUE?

A) Granulomatous keratic precipitates are found in both eyes.
B) Enucleation of the right eye will be beneficial in this condition.
C) This is endogenous endophthalmitis and will benefit from IV antibiotics.
D) This condition occurs in 5% of cases of penetrating ocular trauma.

70. What treatment is indicated?

A) Posterior vitrectomy of left eye
B) Oral nonsteroidal anti-inflammatory medications
C) Topical and systemic corticosteroids
D) Intravitreal injection of antibiotics

71. Which one of the following is NOT a cause of white-centered retinal hemorrhages (Roth's spots)?

A) Subacute bacterial endocarditis
B) Leukemia
C) Measles
D) Collagen-vascular disease

72. All of the following are associated with punctate inner choroidopathy (PIC) EXCEPT:

A) myopia
B) female gender
C) viral prodrome
D) CNVMs

73. APMPPE is associated with:

A) female preponderance
B) severe irreversible vision loss
C) viral prodrome
D) onset in fifth and sixth decades

74. Typical fluorescein angiographic findings of APMPPE are:

A) early hyperfluorescence of lesions
B) late hyperfluorescence of lesions
C) late hypofluorescence of lesions
D) leakage from optic nerve

75. Fluorescein angiographic findings of multiple evanescent white dot syndrome (MEWDS) include all of the following EXCEPT:

    A) early hypofluorescence of white dots
    B) late staining of white dots
    C) late disc staining
    D) early hyperfluorescence of white dots

76. The most common complication of multifocal choroiditis is:

    A) retinal detachment
    B) CME
    C) choroidal neovascularization
    D) epiretinal membrane

77. The electro-oculogram (EOG) is valuable in the detection and confirmation of the diagnosis of all of the following EXCEPT:

    A) carriers of Best's disease
    B) Best's disease in the pre-vitelliform stage
    C) adult onset foveomacular vitelliform dystrophy
    D) Best's disease in the vitelliform stage

78. ERG is diagnostic in cases of:

    A) Leber's congenital amaurosis
    B) Stargardt's disease
    C) both A and B
    D) neither A nor B

Questions 79–81 Match the following retinoschisis entities with the level of schisis.

79. Juvenile X-linked retinoschisis

    A) Nerve fiber layer
    B) Inner plexiform layer
    C) Outer plexiform layer
    D) Outer nuclear layer

80. Reticular retinoschisis

    A) Nerve fiber layer
    B) Inner plexiform layer
    C) Outer plexiform layer
    D) Outer nuclear layer

81. Involutional or senile retinoschisis

   A) Nerve fiber layer
   B) Inner plexiform layer
   C) Outer plexiform layer
   D) Outer nuclear layer

82. "Bull's eye" maculopathy can occur with all of the following EXCEPT:

   A) cone dystrophy
   B) thioridazine-induced retinopathy
   C) ceroid lipofuscinosis
   D) chloroquine-induced retinopathy

83. Sight-threatening complications of juvenile X-linked retinoschisis include:

   A) CME
   B) vitreous hemorrhage
   C) CNVM
   D) exudative retinal detachment

84. Oguchi's disease is characterized by:

   A) Mizuo-Nakamura phenomenon
   B) autosomal recessive inheritance
   C) golden brown fundus in the dark-adapted state and normal fundus in the light-adapted state
   D) progressive night blindness

85. Gyrate atrophy is characterized by all of the following EXCEPT:

   A) ornithine transcarbamylase deficiency
   B) peripheral RPE affected initially
   C) high serum ornithine levels
   D) abnormalities of chromosome 10

86. Which one of the following statements is FALSE?

   A) ERG amplitudes are reduced in carriers of juvenile X-linked retinitis pigmentosa.
   B) ERG amplitudes are reduced in the carriers of choroideremia.
   C) EOG light peak to dark trough ratio is normal in adult-onset foveomacular vitelliform dystrophy.
   D) EOG light peak to dark trough ratio is reduced in carriers of Best's disease.

87. A cherry red spot is seen in:

   A) Niemann-Pick disease
   B) Tay-Sachs disease
   C) both A and B
   D) neither A nor B

88. All of the following statements regarding albinism are true EXCEPT:

    A) oculocutaneous albinism usually has autosomal dominant inheritance
    B) ocular albinism is inherited X-linked or autosomal recessively
    C) retinal manifestations of albinism include foveal hypoplasia and peripheral mosaic pattern of pigmentation.
    D) decussation at optic chiasm is abnormal

89. Hermansky-Pudlak syndrome is characterized by all of the following EXCEPT:

    A) platelet dysfunction
    B) reticuloendothelial dysfunction
    C) albinism
    D) Puerto Rican heritage

90. Chediak-Higashi syndrome is characterized by all of the following EXCEPT:

    A) platelet dysfunction
    B) white forelock and silvery hair
    C) albinism
    D) recurrent pyogenic infections

91. What is the incidence of retinal tear in an eye with posterior vitreous detachment and vitreous hemorrhage?

    A) 90%
    B) 66%
    C) 50%
    D) 25%

92. Which one of the following poses the highest risk for retinal detachment?

    A) Myopia
    B) Retinal detachment in the fellow eye
    C) Lattice degeneration
    D) Family history of retinal detachment

93. What is the incidence of retinal detachment in fellow eyes of patients with giant retinal tears?

    A) 50%
    B) 25%
    C) 100%
    D) <5%

94. What is the most common location for retinal tears?

    A) 10- to 2-o'clock meridians
    B) 3 and 9 o'clock meridians
    C) 4- to 8-o'clock meridians
    D) 6 and 12 o'clock meridians

95. What is the most important factor for determining visual outcome in retinal detachment?

    A) Presence of vitreous hemorrhage
    B) Duration of detachment
    C) Number of retinal breaks
    D) Attachment of the macula

96. What is the most common cause of recurrent retinal detachment or failure of scleral buckling procedure?

    A) Scleral buckle too large causing retinal folds and fish-mouthed tears
    B) Scleral buckle too small resulting in inadequate support of tears
    C) No circumferential band to support vitreous base
    D) Proliferative vitreoretinopathy

Questions 97–100

Where is the most likely location for the primary retinal break in each of the following retinal detachments?

    A) 12 o'clock
    B) 9 o'clock
    C) 3 o'clock
    D) 6 o'clock

97. Figure 12-17

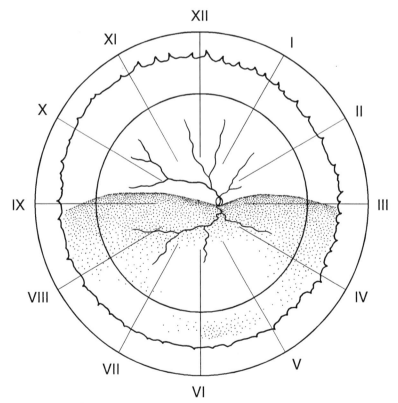

FIGURE 12-17. From Wright K. Textbook of ophthalmology. Baltimore: Williams & Wilkins, 1997.

98. Figure 12-18

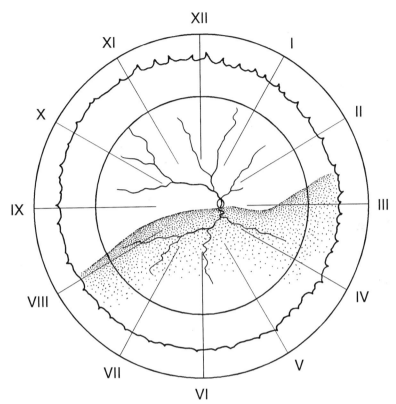

FIGURE 12-18. From Wright K. Textbook of ophthalmology. Baltimore: Williams & Wilkins, 1997.

99.   Figure 12-19

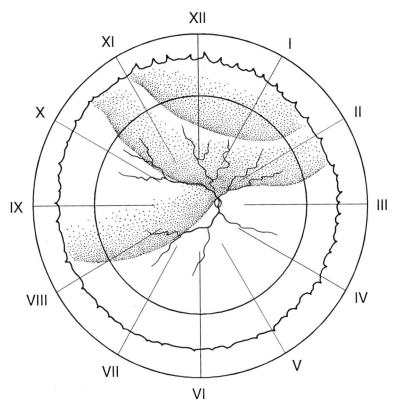

FIGURE 12-19. From Wright K. Textbook of ophthalmology. Baltimore: Williams & Wilkins, 1997.

100. Figure 12-20

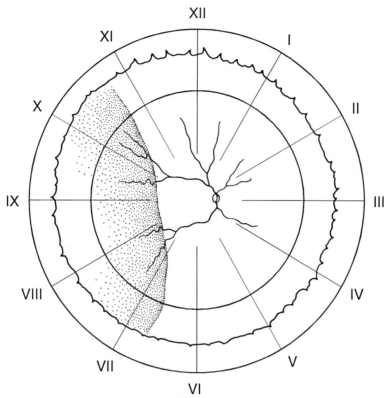

FIGURE 12-20. From Wright K. Textbook of ophthalmology. Baltimore: Williams & Wilkins, 1997.

101. Which one of the following regarding exudative retinal detachments is FALSE?

A) May occur with choroidal hemangiomas
B) May occur with choroidal melanomas
C) Should be treated with scleral buckle and vitrectomy with internal drainage of the subretinal fluid
D) Are characterized by shifting subretinal fluid

102. Tractional retinal detachments occur in all of the following EXCEPT:

A) Diabetes mellitus
B) Familial exudative vitreoretinopathy
C) Retinopathy of prematurity
D) Juvenile X-linked retinoschisis

103. Which one of the following regarding asteroid hyalosis is FALSE?

A) Represents precipitation of calcium soaps
B) Unilateral phenomenon predominantly
C) Patients asymptomatic
D) Systemic hypercalcemia

104. A patient has synchysis scintillans. Which historical feature is most probable?

A)   Previous blunt trauma with hyphema
B)   Dense arcus senilis
C)   Carotid atherosclerosis with a history of amaurosis
D)   Cushingoid appearance from long-term steroid use

105. An intraocular bubble of which one of the following gases would last the longest?

A)   Air
B)   Perfluoropropane (C_3F_8)
C)   Sulfur hexafluoride (SF_6)
D)   Perfluoroethane (C_2F_6)

106. Rate of intraocular gas expansion is fastest for:

A)   air
B)   100% C_3F_8
C)   100% SF_6
D)   14% C_3F_8

107. The surface tension of silicone oil against the retina is:

A)   greater than C_3F_8 against the retina
B)   greater than air against retina
C)   less than SF_6 against retina
D)   equal to water against the retina

108. The specific gravity of silicone oil is:

A)   greater than balanced salt solution
B)   less than water
C)   less than perfluoro-octane
D)   equal to vitreous

Questions 109–111

A patient had sudden loss of vision to the level of light perception in the left eye. The fluorescein angiogram is shown in Figure 12-21.

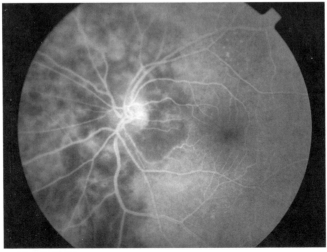

FIGURE 12-21

109. What is the MOST appropriate next step in evaluation?

    A)   Carotid Doppler ultrasound
    B)   CT scan of chest and abdomen
    C)   Erythrocyte sedimentation rate
    D)   MRI of head and orbits

110. Which one of the following ERG changes would be present in this eye?

    A)   Decreased b-wave amplitude
    B)   Increased implicit time
    C)   Absent scotopic response
    D)   Flat response to a flickering stimulus

111. What is the MOST appropriate therapy?

    A)   Systemic corticosteroids and temporal artery biopsy
    B)   Optic nerve sheath decompression
    C)   Carotid endarterectomy
    D)   Aspirin daily

Questions 112–114 (Fig. 12-22)

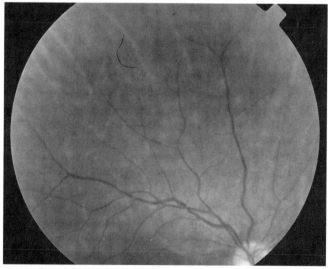

FIGURE 12-22

112. What would this patient most likely report?

    A)   Painful photophobia
    B)   Unilateral shimmering photopsias
    C)   Viral illness 2 weeks before presentation
    D)   Recurrent fevers

113. Which one of the following is a characteristic feature of this disorder?

  A) More common in women
  B) Myopic patients
  C) Usually recurrent causing progressive visual loss
  D) Often requires corticosteroids to hasten resolution

114. What is the most consistent finding on adjunct testing?

  A) Pinpoint hyperfluorescent spots that leak on fluorescein angiography
  B) Enlarged blind spot on visual field testing
  C) Multiple bright objects on T2 weighted MRI images
  D) Profoundly reduced color vision

Questions 115–117 (Fig. 12-23)

On routine examination of a 37-year-old man, you find multiple midperipheral yellowish flecks in both eyes. His fluorescein angiogram is shown in Figure 12-23.

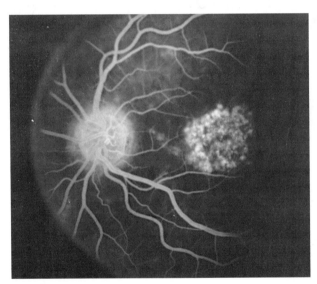

FIGURE 12-23

115. Which one of the following is a clinical characteristic of this disorder?

  A) Profoundly reduced vision in one eye
  B) Profoundly reduced vision in both eyes
  C) Autosomal dominant inheritance
  D) Autosomal recessive inheritance

116. What is the histopathologic cause of the characteristic fluorescein appearance?

  A) Choroidal nonperfusion
  B) Accumulation of gangliosides in retinal ganglion cells
  C) Accumulation of lipofuscin granules in the RPE
  D) Diffuse thickening of Bruch's membrane

117. Which one of the following electrophysiologic findings is characteristic for this condition?

    A) EOG light peak to dark trough ratio is profoundly reduced.
    B) Photopic ERG amplitudes are extinguished.
    C) Scotopic ERG amplitudes are extinguished.
    D) ERG amplitudes are often normal.

Questions 118–120 (Fig. 12-24)

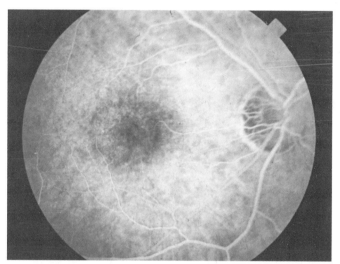

FIGURE 12-24

118. What is the most likely cause of this angiographic appearance?

    A) Thioridazine toxicity
    B) Retinitis pigmentosa
    C) Cone dystrophy
    D) Tay-Sachs disease

119. Toxicity from which one of the following medications may produce this angiographic appearance?

    A) Chlorpromazine
    B) Isoniazid
    C) Chloroquine
    D) Digoxin

120. What is the possible electrophysiologic finding?

    A) Abnormal photopic ERG
    B) Abnormal scotopic ERG
    C) Supranormal a-wave on scotopic ERG
    D) Subnormal b-wave on scotopic ERG

Questions 121–124

During which phase of the fluorescein angiogram do the following lesions initially fill? Choices may be used more than once, or not at all.

    A)   Choroidal
    B)   Early arterial
    C)   Arteriovenous
    D)   Late

121. Capillary hemangioma

122. Malignant melanoma

123. Neovascularization of the disc

124. Cilioretinal artery

125. The a-, b-, and c-waves of the ERG originate from the following retinal structures, sequentially:

    A)   RPE, ganglion cells, Müller cells
    B)   ganglion cells, bipolar cells, RPE
    C)   photoreceptors, bipolar cells, RPE
    D)   Müller cells, ganglion cells, photoreceptors

126. The following statements about Best's disease (vitelliform macular dystrophy) are correct EXCEPT:

    A)   the EOG is pathologic in affected patients and carriers
    B)   peripheral visual fields, ERG, and dark adaptation testing are normal
    C)   it is autosomal dominant
    D)   it has a poor visual prognosis

127. Select the INCORRECT statement regarding sodium fluorescein dye:

    A)   40% is bound to plasma protein
    B)   it has a molecular weight of 376 Daltons
    C)   it is excited by 465–490 nm light and emits 520–530 nm light
    D)   it stains collagen

128. Which statement concerning the events occurring in the fundus after fluorescein is injected into the antecubital vein is CORRECT?

    A)   The dye enters the choroidal circulation by way of the short posterior ciliary arteries 10 to 15 seconds after injection.
    B)   Choroidal flow is sluggish.
    C)   Arteriovenous phase occurs 10 to 15 seconds after the arterial phase.
    D)   Choriocapillaris filling is usually completed by the late recirculation phase.

129. Angiographic features of a classic or well-defined CNVM do NOT include:

A) a lacy pattern or cartwheel shape
B) speckled late hyperfluorescence
C) a well-defined net of hyperfluorescence early in the transit phase
D) staining of exudate, but not blood, in the sub-RPE space

Questions 130–131

A 50-year-old diabetic woman presents with progressive blurring of vision in her right eye. A similar episode occurred in her left eye 2 months ago. She has not had previous laser photocoagulation.

130. What angiographic features are NOT seen in the angiogram in Figure 12-25?

A) Profuse leakage from neovascularization of the optic disc (NVD) and multiple neovascularization elsewhere (NVE)
B) Hypofluorescence caused by a blocking defect
C) Diffuse punctate hyperfluorescence in the macula
D) Dilated and leaking retinal capillary bed

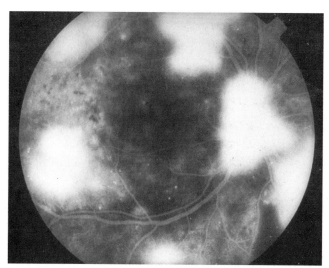

FIGURE 12-25

131. Which initial therapy would be MOST appropriate for this patient?

A) Pars plana vitrectomy
B) PRP
C) Combined PRP and focal/grid macular treatment
D) Follow-up visit in 1 month

Questions 132–140 (Fig. 12-26 to 12-33)

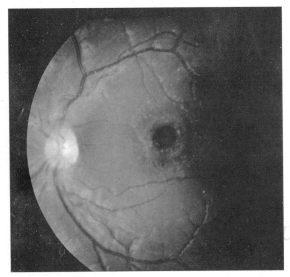

FIGURE 12-26

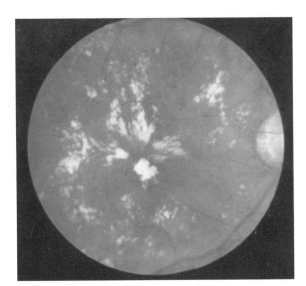

FIGURE 12-27

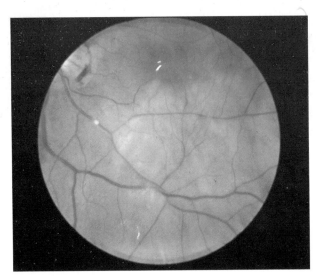

FIGURE 12-28

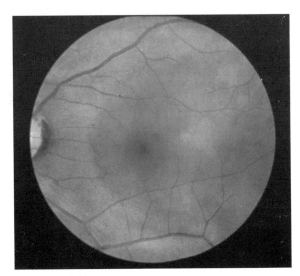

FIGURE 12-29

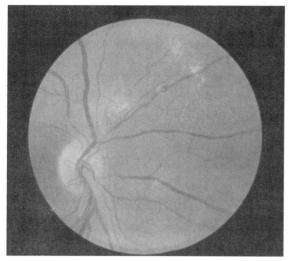

FIGURE 12-30

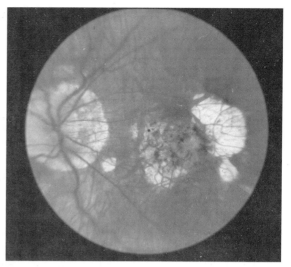

FIGURE 12-31

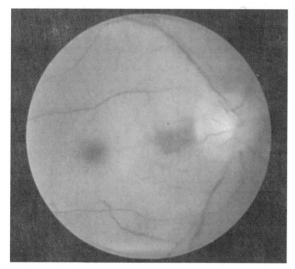

FIGURE 12-32

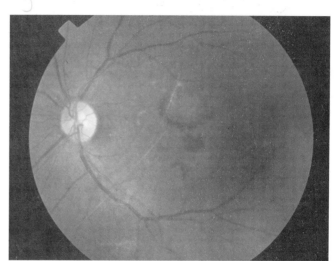

FIGURE 12-33

132. Which one of the following is NOT associated with CNVMs?

- A) Figure 12-31
- B) Figure 12-33
- C) Figure 12-30
- D) Figure 12-29

133. In Figure 12-28, which investigations would be most appropriate to perform?

- A) Fluorescein angiography
- B) CT scan
- C) Carotid Doppler and cardiac echocardiography
- D) CBC and erythrocyte sedimentation rate (ESR)

134. In which condition is laser photocoagulation inappropriate?

   A)   Figure 12-26
   B)   Figure 12-27
   C)   Figure 12-29
   D)   Figure 12-33

135. In Figure 12-30, the systemic condition most commonly associated with this disorder is:

   A)   diabetes mellitus
   B)   systemic hypertension
   C)   sickle cell anemia
   D)   thromboembolic disease

136. In reference to Figure 12-26, indications for vitrectomy could include all of the following stages of the condition EXCEPT:

   A)   Stage I
   B)   Stage II
   C)   Stage III
   D)   Stage IV

137. If a posterior vitreous detachment was present in the patient seen in Figure 12-26, in what stage would this condition be?

   A)   Stage I
   B)   Stage II
   C)   Stage III
   D)   Stage IV

138. In which of the following conditions is laser treatment contraindicated?

   A)   Figure 12-27
   B)   Figure 12-28
   C)   Figure 12-30
   D)   Figure 12-33

139. In which of the following conditions may an indocyanine green (ICG) angiogram be helpful in the management of the patient?

   A)   Figure 12-27
   B)   Figure 12-28
   C)   Figure 12-30
   D)   Figure 12-33

140. All of these conditions may give rise to the fundus appearance seen in Figure 12-27 EXCEPT:

   A)   diabetic retinopathy
   B)   radiation retinopathy
   C)   proliferative vitreoretinopathy
   D)   hypertensive retinopathy

141. Indications for vitrectomy in patients with diabetic retinopathy include all of the following EXCEPT:

    A)   nonclearing vitreous hemorrhage
    B)   extramacular tractional retinal detachment
    C)   combined rhegmatogenous tractional retinal detachment
    D)   anterior hyaloidal fibrovascular proliferation

142. Indications for vitrectomy and membrane peeling in patients with macular epiretinal membrane (Fig. 12-34) include all of the following EXCEPT:

    A)   decrease in visual acuity below 20/70
    B)   marked retinal distortion
    C)   CNVM
    D)   metamorphopsia

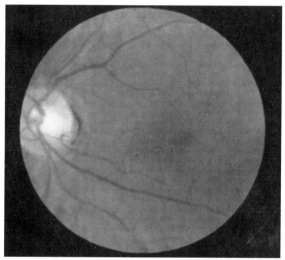

FIGURE 12-34

143. Which one of the following does not have vitreous liquefication and a vitreous that appears optically empty?

    A)   Stickler's syndrome
    B)   Jansen's syndrome
    C)   Kearns-Sayre syndrome
    D)   Wagner's syndrome

144. Which pattern seen on ICG angiography in a patient with exudative ARMD is MOST likely to be useful in guiding laser photocoagulation?

    A)   Stippled hyperfluorescence
    B)   Well-defined hyperfluorescent plaque
    C)   Hot spot
    D)   Area of hypofluorescence

Questions 145–147

A healthy, 36-year-old white man who resides in the Eastern United States presents with a loss of central vision and metamorphopsia in his left eye, associated with a serous detachment of the macula and multiple peripheral atrophic chorioretinal scars and peripapillary chorioretinal scars (Figs. 12-35 and. 12-36). There is no inflammatory reaction in the anterior chamber or vitreous.

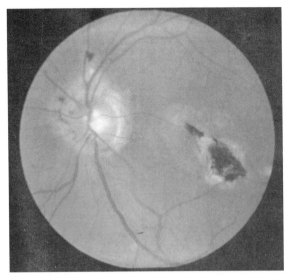

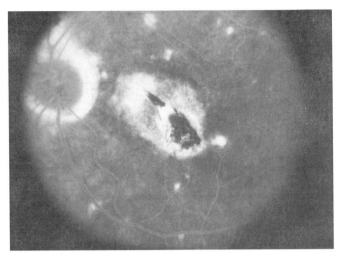

FIGURE 12-35   **FIGURE 12-36**

145. What is the most likely diagnosis?

    A)   ARMD
    B)   Toxoplasmosis
    C)   POHS
    D)   Multifocal choroiditis and panuveitis

146. Which one of the following is NOT a sign of a CNVM?

    A)   Pigment ring or mound
    B)   Subretinal hemorrhage
    C)   Chorioretinal scar
    D)   Oval or round grayish-white subretinal lesion

147. In which location has laser photocoagulation NOT been beneficial in this condition when the CNVM is well-demarcated?

    A)   Extrafoveal
    B)   Juxtafoveal
    C)   Subfoveal
    D)   Juxtapapillary

148. Which one of the following is NOT a feature of lattice degeneration of the retina?

   A)   Liquefied vitreous overlying the lesion
   B)   Sclerotic vessels traversing the lesion
   C)   Adherence of the vitreous to the edges of the lesion
   D)   Operculated holes secondary to vitreous traction

149. Which phakomatosis does NOT have characteristic retinal findings?

   A)   Louis-Bar
   B)   Wyburn-Mason
   C)   Bourneville's
   D)   von Hippel-Lindau

150. Macular complications of retinitis pigmentosa include all of the following EXCEPT:

   A)   macular atrophy
   B)   epiretinal membrane
   C)   CME
   D)   subretinal scarring

540 *Review Questions in Ophthalmology*

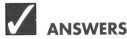 **ANSWERS**

1. D) Carotid stenosis

2. A) Hypopyon

3. A) Ophthalmodynamometry

    Pictured in Figure 1 is a patient with ocular ischemic syndrome. In this condition, there are dot and blot hemorrhages in the midperipheral retina that may extend into the posterior pole. Ocular perfusion pressure on ophthalmodynamometry is reduced substantially with collapse of the central retinal artery with minimal pressure. Anterior segment manifestations include a limbal flush, anterior chamber cell and flare, neovascularization of the iris and angle, and cataract. Hypotony from decreased aqueous production or elevated IOP from neovascularization of the angle may be present. High-grade carotid stenosis is the usual cause. Many of these patients also have systemic hypertension, atherosclerosis, and diabetes mellitus. The prognosis of this condition is usually poor, especially if neovascularization is present.

    A central retinal vein obstruction would have cotton wool spots, nerve fiber layer hemorrhages, and more dilated and tortuous vessels than would this condition. In both, fluorescein angiography would have delayed filling of the retinal vasculature.

4. C) Recurrent pneumonia, weight loss, and vascular skin lesions

    The fundus photo in Figure 12-2 depicts multiple cotton wool spots and hemorrhagic necrosis of the retina after a vascular distribution. In a young patient with recurrent infections, immune deficiency should be considered, and HIV status should always be ascertained. From 15% to 40% of patients with AIDS develop CMV retinitis. Common presenting symptoms include floaters and decreased vision. Cotton wool spots and hemorrhages may be seen in branch retinal vein occlusions; however, there would be no associated vitritis.

5. A) Retinal necrosis

    CMV retinitis is a hemorrhagic necrotizing retinitis involving all retinal layers. Intranuclear inclusion bodies may be found. Loss of pericytes and macroaneurysms can be seen with diabetes. Thickening and excrescences of Bruch's membrane correspond to the drusen seen in ARMD.

6. A) Retinal detachment

    CMV retinitis can lead to significant atrophy of the retina and subsequent retinal detachment. Oftentimes, multiple retinal defects are present, and the patients need long-term internal tamponade with silicone oil to prevent recurrent detachments. Siegrist streaks are atrophic areas of the RPE overlying areas of infarction of a choroidal lobule and may be found with hypertensive retinopathy.

7. B) Retinal thickening greater than 1 disc area in size and within 1 disc diameter of the center of the fovea

CSME is defined as one or more of the following criteria:

1. Retinal thickening within 500 μm of the fovea.
2. Hard exudates within 500 μm of the fovea with associated retinal thickening.
3. Retinal thickening 1 disc area or greater, part of which is within 1 disc diameter of the fovea.

8. D) Focal laser photocoagulation

The efficacy of focal laser photocoagulation for diabetic macular edema has been demonstrated by the Early Treatment Diabetic Retinopathy Study (ETDRS). Treated patients had half the likelihood of moderate visual loss as did untreated eyes. PRP was found to exacerbate macular edema.

9. D) A pet cat at home

The picture shown in Figure 12-4 and this history are suggestive of Leber's idiopathic stellate neuroretinitis. The exact etiology of neuroretinitis is unknown but has been linked to viral infections (mumps, influenza, varicella) and other diseases (cat-scratch fever, leptospirosis).

10. B) CBC, VDRL, toxoplasma titer, viral titer screen

Differential diagnosis may include syphilis, toxoplasmosis of the optic nerve, diffuse unilateral subacute neuroretinitis, trauma, systemic hypertension, and diabetes mellitus.

11. C) Observation

The natural course of Leber's stellate neuroretinitis is spontaneous resolution over several months. The prognosis is excellent, and over 80% of patients have visual acuity better than 20/40.

12. C) Bimodal age distribution

Coats' disease (congenital retinal telangiectasias) tends to occur unilaterally in otherwise healthy boys. The majority of boys have the juvenile form, with a peak incidence within the end of the first decade. An adult form occurs after age 16 and may be associated with hypercholesterolemia.

13. B) When there is development of neovascularization of any type

The Central Retinal Vein Occlusion Study investigated the role of PRP in preventing the development of neovascularization of the iris or angle. The study found no significant benefit of PRP as a prophylaxis for anterior segment neovascularization. Patients with PRP at the onset of rubeosis had a higher rate of regression than those with prior treatment. Photocoagulation for macular edema in a CRVO was not found to be effective.

14. D) Prosthetic cardiac valves

Histopathologically, CRVO occurs as a result of thrombosis at the lamina cribrosa. Risk factors for CRVO include hypertension, glaucoma, diabetes, hyperopia, hypercoagulable states, and older age. Emboli are associated with arterial occlusion rather than venous obstruction.

15. B) Aniridia

Foveal hypoplasia has been associated with aniridia and albinism. Choroideremia shows a generalized choroidal dystrophy. Patients with juvenile X-linked retinoschisis may have foveal schisis, and Tay-Sachs disease may have a cherry red spot.

16. C) Diffuse unilateral subacute neuroretinopathy

Although the exact etiologies of AMPPE, MEWDS, and Leber's stellate neuroretinitis have not been determined, all have been linked with viral illnesses. DUSN is thought to be caused by migration of a nematode under the retina.

17. C) Outer plexiform layer

The radiating fibers of Henle in the outer plexiform layer lead to the cystic spaces in CME.

18. B) Macular hole

This patient has a Stage IV macular hole. The borders of the macular hole may develop a cuff of subretinal fluid. Punctate yellow deposits may exist within the defect. Idiopathic macular holes are thought to arise from tangential traction on the foveal region by the posterior cortical vitreous.

19. C) Central window defect

The RPE beneath the hole may undergo atrophy, leading to hyperfluorescence during choroidal filling on fluorescein angiography.

20. A) Vitrectomy with intraocular gas injection

Vitrectomy with peeling of the posterior hyaloid may help to relieve the tangential traction on the retina and allow the hole to close. Tissue adhesives, such as autologous serum, TGF-β, or plasmin/fibrinogen, have had varied success in increasing the rate of hole closure.

21. C) renal cell carcinoma

Figure 12-6 demonstrates a retinal arterial macroaneurysm. Macroaneurysms tend to occur in the elderly population and have been associated with systemic hypertension and atherosclerosis. Complications that may result include vitreous hemorrhage, macular edema, and exudates. Renal cell carcinomas may be found in up to 25% of patients with von Hippel-Lindau disease. These patients present with retinal hemangioblastomas rather than with macroaneurysms. Other systemic manifestations of this phakomatosis include pheochromocytomas, pancreatic and renal cysts, and hemangioblastomas of the CNS and visceral organs.

22. A) 1 DA isolated NVE

Presence of three or more of the following characteristics indicates high risk for PDR as outlined by the Diabetic Retinopathy Study:
1. any NV
2. NV on or within 1 DD of the optic disc

3. NVD greater than 1/3 disc area
4. NVE greater than 1/2 disc area
5. vitreous or preretinal hemorrhage

23. B) Macular edema

Idiopathic juxtafoveal telangiectasis may present in two forms. A congenital form may be a subtype of Coats' disease. Acquired forms may be found in middle-aged patients. The telangiectasias may be unilateral or bilateral. They are often located temporal to the fovea. Complications that may develop include macular edema, exudates, and choroidal neovascularization.

24. B) Focal leaking hot spot

Figure 12-37 shows a case of idiopathic central serous choroidopathy (ICSC) demonstrating the classic serous elevation of the neurosensory retina over the fovea. Notice the multiple hypopigmented patches of RPE indicative of previous episodes.

Fluorescein angiography of ICSC characteristically shows a focal site of leakage from the choroid into the subsensory retinal space. The "smokestack" of dye collecting under the retina (Fig. 12-37) is the classic description (actually seen in <20% of cases).

Other possible causes of serous elevation of the retina include optic pits (serous detachment would be adjacent to the optic nerve), choroidal neovascular membranes (gray–green subretinal lesions, lipid, and hemorrhage), and serous detachments over nevi or melanoma (choroidal nevus/tumor would be visible on ophthalmoscopy).

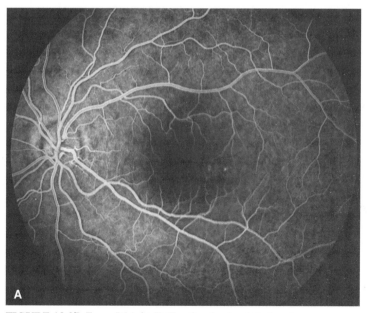

FIGURE 12-37. From Wright K. Textbook of ophthalmology. Baltimore: Williams & Wilkins, 1997.

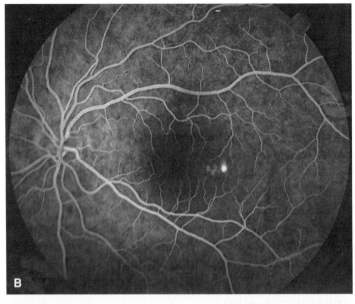

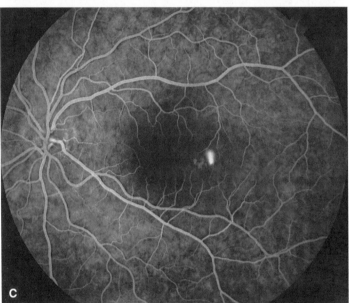

FIGURE 12-37. *Continued*

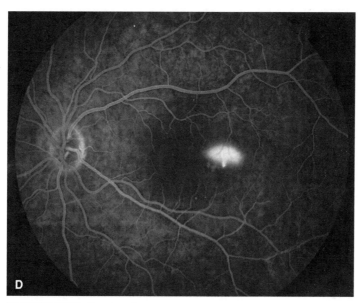

FIGURE 12-37. *Continued*

25. A) Observation

For many cases of ICSC, the serous detachment will spontaneously resolve over 3 to 4 months. Laser photocoagulation hastens reabsorption; however, there is no difference in ultimate visual acuity compared with observation. Elevation of the retina causes a hyperopic shift, and a new refraction may temporarily help until the fluid resorbs. Periocular steroids are not beneficial. Panretinal laser photocoagulation or scleral buckling is not indicated.

26. D) Punched-out chorioretinal scars

This patient has a juxtapapillary choroidal neovascular membrane secondary to POHS. Clinical findings of POHS may include a peripapillary ring of pigmentation and RPE atrophy, punched-out chorioretinal scars in the periphery and posterior pole, and linear chorioretinal scars. Bone spicules may be seen with retinitis pigmentosa, sea-fan neovascularization may be seen with sickle cell retinopathy, and snow-banking may be seen with pars planitis.

27. B) Ohio-Mississippi river valley

POHS is thought to be more prevalent in the Ohio-Mississippi river valley than in the rest of the United States. The San Joaquin valley has been linked to coccidiomycosis, and the Rocky Mountains have been linked with Lyme disease or Rocky Mountain spotted fever.

28. B) Laser photocoagulation

The Macular Photocoagulation Study demonstrated a benefit of laser treatment for juxtafoveal and extrafoveal CNVM in patients with POHS. Submacular surgery for this condition is promising but still investigational. Steroids and triple sulfa are treatments for toxoplasmosis.

29. C) Amaurosis

Temporary blockage of a retinal arteriole may cause obscuration of vision for seconds to minutes, known as *amaurosis*. In Figure 12-12, a cholesterol embolus (Hollenhorst plaque) is present at the bifurcation of a retinal arteriole. Floaters and flashing lights may indicate vitreous traction or formation of a retinal break. Metamorphopsia is more typical of conditions that cause distortion of the fovea.

30. D) Geographic atrophy (age-related macular degeneration [ARMD])

In dry ARMD, as in this case, there is atrophy and loss of the RPE. The areas may become confluent, producing geographic regions of atrophy.

31. B) Counsel and monitor with an Amsler grid

No effective treatment for dry ARMD has been found. Antioxidant vitamins and nutritional supplements may play a role in the prevention of ARMD, but once the loss of the RPE and photoreceptors has occurred, they are of no benefit. Eyes with the dry form of ARMD may rarely develop exudative changes, and monitoring with an Amsler grid is appropriate. Laser and subretinal surgery may be indicated if a choroidal neovascular membrane is present; however, they are not appropriate for the nonexudative form of ARMD.

32. A) Subretinal blood

Subretinal hemorrhage, along with a gray–green crescent, subretinal exudates, and a localized serous retinal detachment, may be indicative of an active choroidal neovascular membrane. Photocoagulation scars may indicate previous treatment for exudative ARMD, placing this eye at a higher risk of recurrence of a CNVM. Approximately 10% of patients with dry ARMD will progress onto the wet form.

33. C) Vitreous biopsy and injection of intravitreal antibiotics in patients with better than hand-motions vision did equally well as patients with immediate vitrectomy and injection of intravitreal antibiotics in final visual outcome.

The Endophthalmitis Vitrectomy Study specifically investigated the treatment of patients with endophthalmitis occurring within 6 weeks of cataract surgery. Patients were randomized to receive or not receive IV antibiotics and to undergo a vitrectomy/injection of intravitreal antibiotics or vitreous tap/injection of intravitreal antibiotics. The results of the study indicated the following:
1. There was no difference in final visual acuity/media clarity whether or not patients received systemic antibiotics.
2. Hand motions or better visual acuity on presentation did equally well with immediate vitreous biopsy or vitrectomy.
3. Eyes with light perception-only vision had much better visual outcome with immediate vitrectomy rather than vitreous biopsy.

34. A) Incontinentia pigmenti

Incontinentia pigmenti presents with vascular abnormalities in the peripheral retina; these abnormalities include capillary nonperfusion, arteriovenous shunts, and fibrovascular proliferation and neovascularization. Pathologic myopia and chorioretinitis sclopetaria have breaks in Bruch's membrane, predisposing these eyes to formation of choroidal neovascular membranes. Juxtafoveal telangiectasis, pathologic myopia, and chorioretinitis sclopetaria are associated with neovascularization in the posterior pole.

35. D)   Atherosclerosis

The causes of CRAO in children and young adults differ from those of the older population. In one study, one third of the patients had a history of migraine. Other factors include trauma (especially in males), hypercoagulable states (oral contraceptives, pregnancy), cardiac emboli, collagen-vascular disorders, and IV drug abuse. In the elderly population, atherosclerotic disease is much more common.

36. A)   Dalen-Fuchs nodules

Sickle cell retinopathy may have the following retinal findings: sunbursts (black chorioretinal scars from RPE hypertrophy and hyperplasia), salmon patch hemorrhages (subretinal blood), peripheral sea fan neovascularization, vitreous hemorrhage, and tractional retinal detachment. Angioid streaks may be associated with sickle cell disease. Dalen-Fuchs' nodules are excrescences found at the level of Bruch's membrane seen in sympathetic ophthalmia.

37. B)   Rods

Retinitis pigmentosa represents a collection of retinal degenerations with rod degeneration as the hallmark finding. A cone degeneration may occur secondarily.

38. D)   The only effective treatment is enucleation of the traumatized eye.

After penetrating ocular trauma to one eye, bilateral granulomatous inflammation and panuveitis, known as *sympathetic ophthalmia,* may occur. The injured eye is known as the *exciting eye* and the fellow eye is the *sympathizing eye.* Sympathetic ophthalmia may occur from weeks to many years after the injury, although it most often occurs within the first year. Treatment with steroids or immunosuppressive agents can be effective in suppressing the inflammation. In contrast to Vogt-Koyanagi-Harada disease, the choriocapillaris is uninvolved with the inflammation in sympathetic ophthalmia.

39. D)   nanophthalmos

POHS, angioid streaks, and pathologic myopia may lead to development of choroidal neovascular membranes. Nanophthalmos is associated with uveal effusions and serous retinal detachments.

40. B)   Retinal hole

In all patients who develop a macular pucker, the peripheral retina needs to be examined carefully to ensure that no retinal tears or holes exist. The lesions may allow migration of RPE cells, which are thought to be able to transform into fibroblast-like cells, leading to epiretinal membrane formation.

41. D)   25%

In 15% to 25% of patients, a cilioretinal artery may be present to perfuse the macula. Pulsatile flow of blood with each heartbeat may be seen in these arteries. In the case of a CRAO, the cilioretinal artery may allow preservation of central acuity. Fluorescein angiography (Fig. 12-38) shows the extensive retinal arterial nonperfusion, except in the distribution of the cilioretinal artery in a patient with a CRAO.

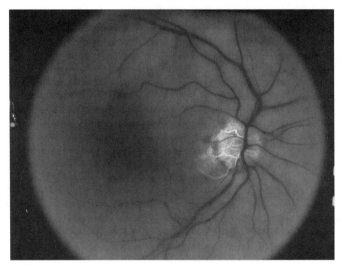

FIGURE 12-38

42. C)   Rubeosis iridis

The incidence of rubeosis may be as high as 15% to 20% after CRAO. These patients may also develop neovascularization of the disc and retina.

43. D)   Epiretinal membrane

Conditions that may have CME without leakage of fluorescein include Goldmann-Favre, retinitis pigmentosa, and nicotinic acid maculopathy. Epiretinal membranes may cause a CME that leaks from traction and distortion of paramacular capillaries.

44. A)   choroidal neovascularization

A choroidal neovascular membrane will cause subretinal hemorrhage or intraretinal hemorrhage. Preretinal hemorrhage would be very unusual. Sickle cell retinopathy, trauma (e.g., shaken baby syndrome), and macroaneurysms may cause hemorrhages at all levels of the retina.

45. C)   Anterior chamber washout

Figure 12-14 presents a patient with a hyphema after blunt trauma to the globe. The RBCs of patients with sickle cell disease are often stiff and irregular in shape and do not pass through the trabecular meshwork easily. Increased IOP may be treated initially with aqueous suppressants; however, carbonic anhydrase inhibitors may exacerbate the sickling by causing a metabolic acidosis. An anterior chamber washout removes the inflexible RBCs and will help return the IOP to normal. Vasoconstriction with phenylephrine may also increase possible thrombosis and vascular compromise. Cryopexy should be used with caution with the tenuous vasculature. Cryopexy is not used to treat the hyphema per se, but it may be indicated for retinal ischemia and neovascularization.

46. D)   headaches and nausea

47. A)   Optic nerve drusen

48. B)   Gastrointestinal bleeding

49. A)   Choroidal neovascularization

Pictured in Figure 12-15 are angioid streaks in a patient with pseudoxanthoma elasticum. The radiating hyperfluorescent lines are window defects from a break in Bruch's membrane. The predominant conditions associated with angioid streaks include Paget's disease of bone, pseudoxanthoma elasticum, Ehlers-Danlos, and sickle cell disease.

Paget's disease is a spectrum of findings, including osteoclastic hyperactivity, especially at the base of the skull and in long bones. These patients are prone to pathologic fractures.

Sickle cell patients may have a number of retinal findings, including salmon patches, sea fan neovascularization, black sunbursts, and angioid streaks. They have a higher incidence of thrombotic episodes and may autoinfarct their spleens.

Ehlers-Danlos is a genetic disorder caused by a defect in collagen synthesis. The patients may have hyperextensible joints and lax skin. Ocular findings include dislocated lenses, retinal detachment, and blue sclera.

Pseudoxanthoma elasticum classically has the findings of angioid streaks, optic nerve head drusen, and a "peau-d'orange" appearance to the retina. These patients have cutaneous manifestations with the "plucked-chicken" appearance shown in Figure 12-39. They are prone to widespread vascular malformations. Abnormalities in the mucosal vasculature of the stomach and bowel can lead to recurrent hemorrhage.

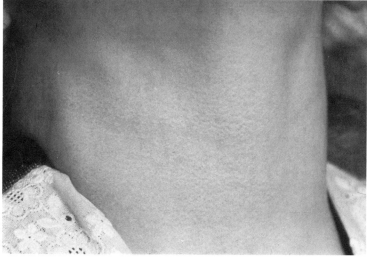

FIGURE 12-39

50. B) Krypton red

In a patient without a vitreous hemorrhage, the argon laser allows the placement of excellent laser burns. The wavelength of krypton red (647 nm) is best able to penetrate vitreous hemorrhages and deliver the energy necessary to create photocoagulation scars. This laser also penetrates nuclear sclerotic cataracts better than the argon. The xenon arc emits a large spectrum of wavelengths and has been replaced with the monochromatic lasers. The CO_2 laser is well-absorbed by water and is used for surface tissue ablation.

51. D) they occur in less than 1% of autopsy eyes

Pars plana cysts are common and occur in 16% to 18% of autopsied eyes. They contain mucopolysaccharides on histopathology and can be seen in otherwise normal eyes. Patients with multiple myeloma may have several large pars plana cysts that contain myeloma proteins.

52. C) Maroteaux-Lamy

RPE degenerations have been identified in patients with Hunter's, Hurler's, Sanfilippo's, and Scheie's mucopolysaccharidoses. Maroteaux-Lamy syndrome is not usually associated with RPE degeneration.

53. D) chloroquine

Retinal crystals may be seen in patients using tamoxifen, canthaxanthine, or methoxyflurane. Retinal crystals can also be seen in patients who have talc retinopathy. IV injection of talc crystals result in their distribution via the retinal circulation. Chloroquine or hydroxychloroquine can result in a bull's-eye maculopathy as a result of disturbance of the RPE, but crystals are not present.

54. C) Stargardt's disease

True *silent choroid* is defined as the blockage of underlying choroidal fluorescence during fluorescein angiography by material in the RPE cells. This occurs classically in patients who have Stargardt's disease. Lipofuscin accumulation within RPE cells results in the blockage of underlying choroidal fluorescence and gives the appearance of a very dark or silent choroid. Systemic argyrosis, which occurs in patients who are receiving systemic silver (e.g., from tanning agents), can also cause an angiographically dark choroid.

55. D) Vitrectomy and silicone oil tamponade

Rhegmatogenous detachments occur in up to 25% of patients with CMV retinitis. They are associated with a diffusely necrotic peripheral retina with numerous small retinal holes. These detachments cannot be repaired by conventional scleral buckling surgery, and they require pars plana vitrectomy with internal silicone oil tamponade and endolaser.

56. B) myopia

Although exudative retinal detachments may occur in CMV retinitis, it is very uncommon. Myopia is not associated with exudative retinal detachments.

57.   D)   irreversibly flat ERG

Intraocular copper foreign bodies may result in two distinct disease processes. One is a mild form called *chalcosis*. The other is a more severe suppurative form of endophthalmitis. The severity of intraocular inflammation is directly proportional to the concentration of copper within the foreign body. Chalcosis occurs in copper amalgams that contain significant amounts of nickel or other metals. Chalcosis is characterized by mild intraocular inflammation, development of a sunflower cataract, and Kayser-Fleischer rings. Characteristically, early removal of the intraocular foreign body in chalcosis can improve the amplitudes of the ERG, which have been suppressed from the presence of intraocular copper ions.

58.   D)   Coumadinization

Various treatment modalities have been advocated for CRAOs, including methods to provide more oxygen to the ischemic retina (hyperbaric oxygen, carbogen), increasing perfusion of the retina (vasodilatory drugs, lowering IOP by anterior chamber paracentesis or administration of acetazolamide or mannitol), and fibrinolytic agents (intra-arterial t-PA). Animal studies have shown that irreversible damage occurs within 90 minutes of arterial obstruction. Coumadin requires several days to reach maximal effect and would not be helpful in an acute situation.

59.   A)   It occurs in eyes with abnormally short axial length.

Uveal effusion syndrome usually occurs in eyes with abnormally short axial length. These eyes often will have thickened sclera, which are thought to impede vortex venous outflow from the eye, resulting in recurrent choroidal effusions. Treatment is often unrewarding but involves the placement of partial thickness scleral windows near the vortex vein exit sites in at least three or four quadrants of the eye. Choroidal effusions or hemorrhage can occur during or after intraocular surgery and are thought to be caused by rapid changes in IOP-shearing choroidal perforating arteries. Hypertension and atherosclerosis are risk factors for choroidal effusions.

60.   B)   Observation

Traumatic macular holes usually result from pre-existing commotio in the region of the macula. They are characterized by disruption and necrosis of retinal photoreceptors and subsequent loss of retinal tissue. Unlike idiopathic macular holes, which are caused by tangential traction on the macula where vitrectomy and gas-fluid exchange have successfully closed the hole, surgery is not, in general, the treatment for traumatic holes. There have been several reports of improvement in vision in traumatic holes with vitrectomy, gas-fluid exchange, and application of TGF-β.

61.   A)   Sand

Inert foreign bodies, such as glass, plastic, sand, stone, or ceramic, are well-tolerated in the eye. Wood incites a brisk inflammatory reaction and may harbor harmful microorganisms. Brass contains copper, which may lead to chalcosis and retinal degeneration. Iron is tolerated poorly within the eye. Intraocular iron causes siderosis, resulting in photoreceptor and RPE degeneration.

62. C)   disruption of photoreceptor elements and damage to photoreceptor cells

Commotio represents an actual disruption or destruction of retinal photoreceptor elements and photoreceptor cells in the outer layers of the retina. It does not represent retinal edema.

63. C) $3 > 4 > 2 > 5 > 1$

The most common traumatic retinal tear is an inferotemporal retinal dialysis. The vast majority of retinal dialyses occur in this quadrant. After trauma, the most common retinal tear is a superonasal dialysis, followed by giant tears, flap tears, and tears around lattice. These statistics are true only for blunt ocular injury.

64. B)   has a good visual prognosis with complete healing of retinal injuries

Shaken baby syndrome may be associated with retinal hemorrhages and cotton wool spots that have the appearance of a central retinal vein occlusion or Purtscher's retinopathy. This retinal injury often has a poor prognosis because of associated macular scarring, vitreous hemorrhage, and retinal detachment. Associated neurologic damage is common.

65. C)   both A and B

The original description by Terson consisted of both retinal and vitreous hemorrhages in patients who have subarachnoid and subdural hemorrhages. About 20% of patients with spontaneous or traumatic subarachnoid hemorrhages will present with intraocular hemorrhages.

66. D)   disseminated intravascular coagulation

Purtscher's retinopathy does not occur from disseminated intravascular coagulation. Disseminated intravascular coagulation can result in fibrinoid necrosis of the choriocapillaris, serous retinal detachments, and multiple areas of RPE changes. However, numerous cotton wool spots, subinternal limiting membrane hemorrhages, and retinal hemorrhages are uncommon in this condition.

67. D)   neither A nor B

Fluorescein leakage is not a feature of either solar maculopathy or photic injury. Both may be associated with intense staining of the damaged RPE, particularly in the acute phases of the injury. As the injured RPE heals, the fluorescein angiogram would be characterized by persistent window defects.

68. A)   is initially associated with a clear lens or minimal opacity that may later become densely cataractous

PHPV is a unilateral disorder associated with microphthalmia, and it has a variable severity of presentation. Some cases of PHPV may simply be observed or treated with lensectomy alone.

69. A)   Granulomatous keratic precipitates are found in both eyes.

Granulomatous keratic precipitates are a characteristic presentation of sympathetic ophthalmia. Sympathetic ophthalmia occurs in less than 0.1% of cases of penetrating ocular injury. It is even less common after intraocular surgery. It is thought to result from immune sensitization to melanin or melanin-associated proteins in the uveal tissues, which results in bilateral granulomatous panuveitis. Once the inflammation has started in the contralateral eye, the role of enucleation of the inciting eye in reducing inflammation is very controversial and may not be beneficial.

70. C)   Topical and systemic corticosteroids

Sympathetic ophthalmia often responds to corticosteroids with quieting of inflammation and improvement in vision. If steroids are not tolerated or are ineffective, immunosuppressive drugs may be necessary. Vitrectomy or injection of intravitreal antibiotics may be indicated for cases of endophthalmitis but not for sympathetic ophthalmia.

71. C)   Measles

White-centered hemorrhages can be found in conditions with septic emboli (endocarditis, Candida bacteremia), leukemia, and collagen-vascular diseases. Measles causes white-centered hemorrhages (Koplik's spots) on the buccal mucosa, but retinal hemorrhages are not found.

72. C)   viral prodrome

PIC is an entity that is slightly more common in myopic women in the third and fourth decades of life. It may be associated with recurrent choroidal neovascular membranes. It is not, however, associated with a viral prodrome as is acute posterior multifocal placoid pigment epitheliopathy.

73. C)   viral prodrome

APMPPE is a condition that is seen in the second to fourth decades of life. It is often preceded by a viral illness. Males and females are equally affected. Visual loss can be severe at the onset but, over the course of 4 to 6 weeks, visual acuity improves in most patients. White placoid lesions at the level of the RPE and choriocapillaris are characteristic of the acute phases of this disease. Vitritis is minimal or absent. These lesions then subsequently fade over 4 weeks and result in RPE disruption.

74. B)   late hyperfluorescence of lesions

Fluorescein angiography of APMPPE is characterized by early hypofluorescence of lesions, followed by late hyperfluorescence of the entire lesion. Rarely, perivascular staining may be seen. Because of pigmentary disturbances that occur in the healed cases, choroidal neovascular membranes can develop, although it is extremely rare.

75. A)   early hypofluorescence of white dots

Fluorescein angiography in MEWDS is characterized by early punctate hyperfluorescence, often in a wreath-like configuration, followed by late staining of the same punctate areas of hyperfluorescence. These areas of hyperfluorescence correspond to the white spots seen clinically. Late disc staining is also a common feature.

76. C)   choroidal neovascularization

Choroidal neovascularization is by far the most common macular complication of multifocal choroiditis. This is the major cause of vision loss in most patients with multifocal choroiditis.

77. C)   adult onset foveomacular vitelliform dystrophy

The EOG shows a diminished light peak to dark trough ratio, characteristically below 1.7, in patients who have Best's disease and in patients who are carriers of Best's disease. Adult onset foveomacular vitelliform dystrophy is not associated with an abnormal EOG. Patients with this particular disorder may present with a ringlike area of RPE clumping in the early phases. Over the course of many years, this area will develop into a yellowish lesion that is typically one half disc diameter in size or slightly smaller, occupying the central fovea. These lesions are much smaller than those seen in Best's disease. This disorder is associated more commonly with choroidal neovascularization than is Best's disease.

78. A)   Leber's congenital amaurosis

Leber's congenital amaurosis is a disorder of congenital blindness that often presents with an initially normal-appearing fundus in the neonatal period. However, an ERG done at this time is characteristically flat and diagnostic.

79. A)   Nerve fiber layer

80. A)   Nerve fiber layer

81. C)   Outer plexiform layer

Retinoschisis is an actual splitting of the cellular layers of the retina. Juvenile X-linked retinoschisis typically is associated with schisis at the level of the nerve fiber layer. The earliest macular changes may include parafoveal spoke wheel type appearance to these dehiscences of the nerve fiber layer. As the disorder progresses, bullous schisis cavities develop with eventual obliteration of this very thin inner layer of tissue. Retinal vessels subsequently are the only things that may remain within this inner layer of tissue. These blood vessels have a propensity for bleeding and producing vitreous hemorrhages. Once they become sclerotic, they may have the appearance of "vitreous veils." Holes in the outer layers of the retina may subsequently predispose patients with retinoschisis to the development of rhegmatogenous retinal detachment.

Reticular retinoschisis is characterized by an involutional splitting of the retina in the nerve fiber layer. This change may be seen as a spectrum of change that begins as microcystoid peripheral retinal degeneration. Reticular retinoschisis may also be seen with the more common involutional retinoschisis that is associated with splitting at the outer plexiform layer. Typical involutional retinoschisis is located most commonly in the inferotemporal quadrants of the peripheral retina. It often can be mistaken for a rhegmatogenous retinal detachment. Rhegmatogenous retinal detachments can occur in the presence of outer retinal holes.

82.   B)   thioridazine-induced retinopathy

Thioridazine may induce significant RPE atrophy alternating with areas of clumping but does not characteristically produce a bull's eye maculopathy.

83.   B)   vitreous hemorrhage

Juvenile X-linked retinoschisis may be associated with vitreous hemorrhage and rhegmatogenous retinal detachments. Although macular changes of a spoke wheel–type splitting of the nerve fiber layer can occur, it is not true CME.

84.   A)   Mizuo-Nakamura phenomenon

Oguchi's disease is an X-linked recessive form of congenital stationary night blindness. It is associated with the *Mizuo-Nakamura phenomenon,* which is the appearance of a golden brown fundus in the light adapted state with a normalization of the color of the fundus on dark adaptation.

85.   A)   ornithine transcarbamylase deficiency

Gyrate atrophy is a metabolic disorder that is seen mainly in Scandinavian Laplanders. It is associated with a deficiency in the ornithine aminotransferase enzyme, critical in the urea cycle. This results in an accumulation of serum ornithine. The end result is that of an RPE degeneration that begins in the periphery and is characterized by scalloped areas of RPE loss with eventual loss of choriocapillaris and medium-sized choroidal vessels. Recent research has suggested that the ornithine aminotransferase gene is located on chromosome 10; therefore, abnormalities on chromosome 10 may result in gyrate atrophy.

86.   B)   ERG amplitudes are reduced in the carriers of choroideremia.

ERG amplitudes in carriers of choroideremia are typically normal, unlike carriers of juvenile X-linked retinitis pigmentosa. However, female carriers of choroideremia do show midperipheral pigmentary changes and choroidal atrophy.

87.   C)   both A and B

Gangliosidoses can be associated with a cherry red spot in the macula. They occur because the retinal ganglion cells accumulate gangliosides, which characteristically opacify the normally clear retina. This opacification is extensive, particularly in the macula, because the macula has the highest concentration of retinal ganglion cells. The underlying pigment that is present in the fovea is contrasted against the opacified retina and results in the appearance of a cherry red spot. Generalized gangliosidoses types GM_1 and GM_2 type I (Tay-Sachs) and type II (Sandhoff) all cause cherry red spots. Niemann-Pick disease is a sphingomyelin lipidosis, and its infantile forms (Type A) and childhood forms (Type B) are both associated with cherry red spots.

88.   A)   oculocutaneous albinism has autosomal dominant inheritance

Oculocutaneous albinism is inherited typically in an autosomal recessive manner. Other ocular manifestations include iris transillumination defects and nystagmus secondary to poor vision from foveal hypoplasia.

89.   B)   reticuloendothelial dysfunction

90.   A)   platelet dysfunction

Hermansky-Pudlak syndrome and Chediak-Higashi syndrome are both potentially lethal autosomal recessive diseases that present with albinism. Hermansky-Pudlak syndrome has abnormal platelets that may lead to a bleeding diathesis. In Chediak-Higashi syndrome, a disorder in microtubule formation results in leukocytes that cannot release enzymes from lysosomes. This disorder increases the risk of recurrent pyogenic infections.

91.   A)   90%

The presence of vitreous hemorrhage in association with a posterior vitreous detachment is highly suggestive of the presence of a retinal tear. Repeat examination is advised in the first 2 weeks after onset of posterior vitreous detachment and vitreous hemorrhage if a retinal tear is not found initially. Ultrasound evaluation may also be useful.

92.   B)   Retinal detachment in the fellow eye

Although myopia, lattice degeneration, and a family history of retinal detachments are important factors and are associated with higher-than-normal risk of retinal detachment, retinal detachment in the fellow eye increases the chance of retinal detachment to approximately 10% to 15%. Myopia, especially moderate myopia, is the next highest risk factor (7% to 8%), followed by family history and lattice degeneration.

93.   A)   50%

Patients with a giant retinal tear in one eye are at very high risk of retinal detachment in the fellow eye. However, this risk is not 100%.

94.   A)   10- to 2-o'clock meridians

Retinal tears are much more frequently located between the 10- and 2-o'clock meridians when associated with a posterior vitreous detachment. Nearly 70% of tears occur within these meridians.

95.   D)   Attachment of the macula

The most important factor that determines visual outcome in the presence of a retinal detachment is whether the macula is attached or detached at the time of presentation. The duration of macular detachment may also play a role in determining final visual outcome, especially if the macula has been detached for less than 24 hours. Vitreous hemorrhage and pigment cells in the vitreous increase the risk of proliferative vitreoretinopathy, but these are not factors in determining visual outcome.

96.   D)   Proliferative vitreoretinopathy

Proliferative vitreoretinopathy is the most common reason for failure of scleral buckling surgery. A 5% to 10% chance of failure of primary scleral buckling exists in cases of rhegmatogenous retinal detachment.

97. D) 6 o'clock

Figure 12-17 shows an inferior retinal detachment with an equal level of subretinal fluid progression nasally and temporally, suggesting that a break is probably present at approximately 6 o'clock.

98. C) 3 o'clock

Figure 12-19 shows an inferior detachment. However, the fluid level is higher on the nasal side than on the temporal side. In this situation, the most likely position for the break is on the side where the subretinal fluid level is higher.

99. A) 12 o'clock

In Figure 12-19, the break may be located anywhere between the 10- and 2-o'clock meridians, but it is most likely located between 10 and 12 o'clock.

100. D) 9 o'clock

In Figure 12-20, the fluid level is higher on the temporal aspect (9 o' clock), and the break is most likely present temporal. The fluid has not reached the 12-o'clock meridian. The area between 3 o'clock and 12 o'clock should be examined for breaks as well.

101. C) Should be treated with scleral buckle and vitrectomy with internal drainage of the subretinal fluid

Exudative retinal detachments are not treated with scleral buckle, vitrectomy, or scleral drainage of subretinal fluid. The etiology of such detachments must be determined. Exudative retinal detachments typically are characterized by shifting subretinal fluid, and they can be quite bullous. Many intraocular tumors may be associated with serous retinal detachments, including choroidal melanomas and hemangiomas.

102. D) juvenile X-linked retinoschisis

All of the conditions listed in this question cause traction retinal detachments except juvenile X-linked retinoschisis, which typically is associated with rhegmatogenous retinal detachments and vitreous hemorrhages.

103. D) Systemic hypercalcemia

Asteroid hyalosis is a common, unilateral finding that represents calcium soaps suspended in the vitreous gel. Patients are remarkably asymptomatic and do not often complain of decreased vision or floaters. No association with any systemic abnormalities exists.

104. A) Previous blunt trauma with hyphema

Synchysis scintillans can be seen in patients after resolution of a vitreous hemorrhage. Refractile, yellow, cholesterol crystals usually float freely in the liquefied vitreous and will settle inferiorly with time. A systemic hyperlipidemic state is not necessary.

105. B)   Perfluoropropane (C_3F_8)

Intraocular gases can provide tamponade of retinal breaks. The longest lasting gas is C_3F_8 in which over 50% of the gas will still be present in 3 weeks. The duration is less with C_2F_6, SF_6, and shortest with air.

106. C)   100% SF_6

SF_6 has the highest expansile rate for any intraocular gas. It can cause dramatic increases in IOP in the early postoperative period.

107. C)   less than SF_6 against retina

Surface tension of silicone oil is significantly less than the surface tension of all gases, including air.

108. B)   less than water

Silicone oil is buoyant when placed in a fluid-filled eye. The specific gravity of gases, such as perfluoro-octane, is much less than that of water or any liquid.

109. C)   Erythrocyte sedimentation rate

110. A)   Decreased b-wave amplitude

111. A)   Systemic corticosteroids and temporal artery biopsy

Figure 12-21 is an arteriovenous phase of fluorescein angiogram that reveals nasal choroidal nonperfusion. This is most consistent with an ischemic event that involves the nasal short posterior ciliary arteries. This has resulted in not only an anterior but also a posterior ischemic optic neuropathy in the left eye. This is a characteristic presentation of patients with temporal arteritis. Erythrocyte sedimentation rate often is elevated dramatically. Immediate treatment with systemic corticosteroids and temporal artery biopsy are indicated to confirm the diagnosis.

The ERG measures the mass response of the retina to a light stimulus. The a-wave measures the depolarization of the photoreceptors. The b-wave records the function of the inner retinal elements (Müller and bipolar cells). This wave would be affected most profoundly by a CRAO. The implicit time is the time between the trough of the a-wave and the peak of the b-wave. Increased implicit times may be found in various hereditary conditions. The flicker stimulus is used to selectively measure the cone response because rods are unable to cycle quickly enough.

112. B)   Unilateral shimmering photopsias

113. A)   More common in women

114. B)   Enlarged blind spot on visual field testing

The patient in Figure 12-22 has characteristic multiple evanescent white dot syndrome. This disorder typically occurs in females in the third and fourth decades of life. It is often associated with symptoms of shimmering photopsias and paracentral scotomas. Some patients may have a flu-like illness preceding their symptoms. These scotomas often correspond to an enlarged physiologic blind spot on visual field testing. The disorder is typically self-limited, with resolution occurring between 3 and 10 weeks after onset. Usually, no treatment is necessary. However, patients may have decreased vision despite resolution of the syndrome as a result of pigmentary changes in the fovea that have a characteristic granular appearance. In addition, 10% to 15% of patients may have recurrent episodes in the same eye or in the fellow eye.

Mild to moderate myopia has been found in many patients with PIC.

115. D) Autosomal recessive inheritance

116. C) Accumulation of lipofuscin granules in the RPE

117. D) ERG amplitudes are often normal

The fluorescein angiogram in Figure 12-23 reveals the characteristic silent choroid appearance of this patient with Stargardt's disease. This disorder is inherited in an autosomal recessive fashion. Patients are often asymptomatic. Vision may be good on presentation. Clinical examination may reveal yellow flecks in the posterior pole and pigmentary changes in the macula. On fluorescein angiography, these pigmentary changes show up as window defects, and there is blockage of underlying choroidal fluorescence and the appearance of the classic dark or silent choroid. Yellow flecks in the retina are not hyperfluorescent. These flecks are caused by lipofuscin granules that have accumulated in the RPE, blocking underlying choroidal fluorescence. Electrophysiologic testing in these patients often is not helpful. Examination of family members may be useful.

118. C) Cone dystrophy

119. C) Chloroquine

120. A) Abnormal photopic ERG

The fluorescein angiogram in Figure 12-24 is characteristic of a bull's eye maculopathy. It may be seen in cone dystrophy, chloroquine toxicity, Batten's disease, and rarely in retinitis pigmentosa. Other toxic retinal pigment epitheliopathies may result in an appearance similar to a bull's eye maculopathy, but true bull's eye maculopathy is rare. In cases of cone dystrophy, electrophysiologic findings suggest a diminished cone ERG response.

121. B) Early arterial

122. A) Choroidal

123. B) Early arterial

124. A) Choroidal

The timing of the filling of a lesion with fluorescein depends on its source of blood. Choroidal lesions (e.g., malignant melanomas, cavernous hemangiomas) will fill with the choroidal phase early in the angiogram. The cilioretinal artery also fills with the choroid because it is a branch of the posterior ciliary artery rather than the ophthalmic artery. The capillary hemangioma and NVD would fill with the retinal circulation.

125. C)   photoreceptors, bipolar cells, RPE

Ganglion cells do not contribute to the ERG response. The ERG may be normal in the presence of total disc cupping. The negative a-wave (late receptor potential) originates in the photoreceptors. The positive b-wave originates in the bipolar cell layer, probably in response to increased potassium concentration in the extracellular space of the bipolar cells. The positive c-wave appears to originate from the RPE.

126. D)   it has a poor visual prognosis

Visual prognosis is good. Most patients retain reading vision in at least one eye throughout life. The progression of visual loss is slow and occurs for the most part beyond the age of 40 years.

127. A)   40% is bound to plasma protein

Fluorescein is 80% bound to plasma protein. Blue light at 465 to 490 nm excites the fluorescein molecule causing it to emit green light at 520 to 530 nm. Special filters in the camera selectively block the blue light while allowing transmission of the green light onto the film.

128. A)   The dye enters the choroidal circulation by way of the short posterior ciliary arteries 10 to 15 seconds after injection.

Choroidal flow is extremely rapid. The arteriovenous phase occurs 1 to 2 seconds after the arterial phase. The choriocapillaris filling is usually completed in the arteriovenous or early venous phase.

129. B)   speckled late hyperfluorescence

Figure 12-40 depicts a well-defined choroidal neovascular membrane demonstrating the lacy pattern hyperfluoresent in the transit phase. Later frames will show leakage. Speckled late hyperfluorescence is an angiographic feature of some occult CNVMs.

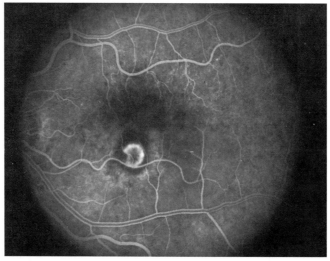

FIGURE 12-40

130. B)   Hypofluorescence caused by a blocking defect

Figure 12-25 demonstrates features of PDR, showing extensive leakage from NVD and NVEs (along the arcades and inferonasal to the disc). The capillary bed is dilated with diffuse leakage, and there is punctate hyperfluorescence and leakage (from microaneurysms in the macula). At the bottom right edge of the frame, the hypofluorescent wedge represents an area of capillary nonperfusion. There are no blocking defects as a result of pre-retinal hemorrhages seen on this frame.

131. C)   Combined PRP and focal/grid macular treatment

This patient has PDR with high-risk characteristics, and the Diabetic Retinopathy Study has shown that PRP decreases the risk of severe visual loss by 50%. Because this patient has more than three high-risk characteristics, the results of the Diabetic Retinopathy Study show that a significant risk of severe visual loss exists. However, because there is angiographic evidence of macular edema (accompanied by clinically significant macular edema) and PRP will exacerbate the macular edema, it is recommended to combine PRP with macular grid/focal treatment in cases like this.
   Note: High-risk characteristics include three or more of the following:
   1.   Any neovascularization of the fundus
   2.   Neovascularization on or within 1 disc diameter of the optic disc
   3.   Preretinal or vitreous hemorrhage
   4.   Neovascularization of moderate or severe extent

132. C)   Figure 12-30

Retinal artery macroaneurysms are NOT associated with CNVMs. They are abnormal outpouchings of the retinal vasculature, usually seen in elderly hypertensive females. The other three conditions mentioned, idiopathic central serous chorioretinopathy, myopic macular degeneration, and exudative ARMD, may all be associated with CNVMs.

133. C)   Carotid Doppler and cardiac echocardiography

Figure 12-28 shows a Hollenhorst plaque and inferotemporal branch retinal artery occlusion. A source of the emboli must be sought. The most common origin is either from the heart or from an atherosclerotic plaque in the carotid arteries, especially at the junction of the external and internal carotid arteries.

134. A)   Figure 12-26

Figure 12-26 depicts a stage IV idiopathic macular hole. The diagnosis of a full-thickness macular hole can usually be made on clinical and biomicroscopic grounds alone. Treatment (vitrectomy surgery) depends on factors such as stage of the hole, visual acuity, and length of time that the hole has been present. There is no place for laser photocoagulation in this condition.

135. B)   systemic hypertension

Retinal artery macroaneurysm is encountered most commonly in elderly hypertensive females.

136. A) Stage I

Stage I corresponds to an impending macular hole. In a randomized control trial, vitrectomy has been shown NOT to be indicated for impending macular holes because the natural history results in a better outcome than in patients undergoing vitrectomy surgery. Vitrectomy surgery results in improved visual acuity in patients with stage II, III, and IV macular holes.

137. D) Stage IV

Stage IV macular hole is defined as a full-thickness hole in the presence of posterior vitreous separation. In *stage I macular holes,* there is foveal separation but no actual retinal break. In *stage II and III macular holes,* by definition, the posterior hyaloid is still attached.

138. B) Figure 12-28

There is no role for laser therapy in managing branch retinal artery occlusions. The risk of retinal neovascularization in branch retinal artery occlusion is almost nonexistent. Diabetic macular edema, retinal artery macroaneurysms, and exudative ARMD may all be treated with laser photocoagulation.

139. D) Figure 12-33

Exudative ARMD and pigment epithelial detachment. If the fluorescein angiogram shows evidence of an occult CNVM, ICG demonstrates a treatable lesion in up to 40% of ARMD patients with a fibrovascular pigment epithelial detachment.

140. C) proliferative vitreoretinopathy

Proliferative vitreoretinopathy results in cellular proliferation on the surface of the retina and not an exudative maculopathy with edema, as can be seen in the other three conditions.

141. B) extramacular tractional retinal detachment

If a tractional retinal detachment is present without a rhegmatogenous component, and if the macula is still attached, the patient can be monitored closely. If the macula detaches, or if there is progression of the detachment and the macula is threatened, vitrectomy surgery should be considered.

142. C) CNVM

CNVM is rarely seen accompanying a macular pucker. Its presence is not, however, an indication for surgery.

143. C) Kearns-Sayre syndrome

Jansen's and Wagner's syndromes are characterized by vitreous liquefaction without associated systemic manifestations. Stickler's syndrome is related to these with the addition of a flat facies and Pierre-Robin sequence abnormalities. Kearns-Sayre syndrome is associated with retinal pigmentary changes, CPEO, and cardiac abnormalities.

144. C) Hot spot

A hot spot is a well-defined small bright area that appears within 3 to 5 minutes and lasts for 20 minutes but loses definition late. *Stippled hyperfluorescence* is a term used to describe a feature of occult CNVM seen on fluorescein angiography, NOT on ICG. *Well-defined hyperfluorescence* is an area of homogenous fluorescence with well-defined, easily determined borders that appears within 5 minutes, lasts for 15 minutes, and fades thereafter. Hypofluorescence represents areas of diminished fluorescence either caused by a blockage defect or by some insult to the integrity of the choriocapillaris in that area.

145. C) POHS

ARMD is usually seen in patients above the age of 50 years. They have drusen and RPE changes in the macula.

Toxoplasmosis is usually accompanied by anterior chamber, vitreous cell, and focal retinitis lesions often occurring at the edge of a previous scar. Multifocal choroiditis and panuveitis may present like POHS but have the following differences: (1) vitreous inflammation; (2) inactive lesions are generally smaller than those in POHS; (3) anterior uveitis occurs in 50% of cases; (4) most patients come from areas nonendemic for histoplasmosis and have a negative histoplasmin skin test; (5) about 50% demonstrate a subnormal ERG; (6) female gender predilection; and (7) more frequent in children.

146. C) Chorioretinal scar

Although a CNVM may arise from a chorioretinal scar, the scar itself is not a clinical sign of CNVM as are the other findings.

147. C) Subfoveal

According to the results of the Macular Photocoagulation Study, eyes with POHS with well-defined extrafoveal or juxtafoveal CNVMs that were untreated were at a much greater risk of a 6-line decrease in visual acuity from the 1-year through the 5-year examination than were eyes treated with laser photocoagulation.

148. D) Operculated holes secondary to vitreous traction

Patients with lattice retinal degeneration are at higher risk for retinal detachments because of the strong attachments of the vitreous to the edges of these lesions. Traction causes horseshoe tears. Holes found in lattice are more atrophic with no associated tractional component.

149. A) Louis-Bar

Wyburn-Mason has arteriovenous malformations, von Hippel-Lindau has retinal hemangioblastomas, and Bourneville's syndrome (tuberous sclerosis) may have astrocytic hamartomas. Louis-Bar, or ataxia-telangiectasia, does not have characteristic retinal changes.

150. D) subretinal scarring

Subretinal scarring is an uncommon complication of retinitis pigmentosa. Pigment disturbances, which may be perivascular and appear as bone spiculing in the midperiphery, are common. CME and epiretinal membrane formation also commonly occur. Large areas of macular atrophy have also been described. Optic disc drusen may also occur in patients with retinitis pigmentosa.

Notes